# Unreliable

# Unreliable

## *How Industry and Government Corrupt Medical Knowledge*

Brandon Novick

BLOOMSBURY ACADEMIC
NEW YORK • LONDON • OXFORD • NEW DELHI • SYDNEY

BLOOMSBURY ACADEMIC
Bloomsbury Publishing Inc, 1359 Broadway, New York, NY 10018, USA
Bloomsbury Publishing Plc, 50 Bedford Square, London, WC1B 3DP, UK
Bloomsbury Publishing Ireland, 29 Earlsfort Terrace, Dublin 2, D02 AY28, Ireland

BLOOMSBURY, BLOOMSBURY ACADEMIC and the Diana logo are trademarks of Bloomsbury Publishing Plc

First published in the United States of America 2027



ISBN: HB: 979-8-216-37364-3
PB: 979-8-216-37363-6
ePDF: 979-8-216-37365-0
eBook: 979-8-216-37366-7

Typeset by Newgen KnowledgeWorks Pvt. Ltd., Chennai, India

For product safety related questions contact productsafety@bloomsbury.com.

To find out more about our authors and books visit www.bloomsbury.com and sign up for our newsletters.

*To Mom, Dad, Zach, and Rachel, who continue to give me inspiration and purpose on all and especially the darkest of days. Your love and support will not go in vain.*

# Contents

# Figures

Acknowledgments

First and foremost, I need to thank my brother, Zach. He devoted countless hours to helping me both develop this book and go through the publishing process. Through reading chapters, leaving comments, and dealing with multi-hour-long phone calls with me to review those and my own comments, he undoubtedly made this book much better than it otherwise would have been. As a new author, much of the publishing process was foreign to me, but—even without experience himself—he spent additional countless hours aiding me to get where we are today. I am eternally grateful to Zach's love, dedication, patience, and support.

Thank you as well to Mom, Dad, my sister Rachel, and every family member and friend who supported me through this journey. Special thanks to my friend Ben McNutt, who was the first one to suggest I could turn my research into a full book. To each of you, your steadfast support and belief in me strengthened my resolve for which I am immensely grateful.

I also must thank the man whose work inspired me to write this book in the first place: Dr. John Abramson. His book *Sickening: How Big Pharma Broke American Health Care and How We Can Repair It* (2022) identifies key issues with medical knowledge that struck and drove me to conduct my research. Dr. Abramson was kind enough to not only respond to my questions, but he also repeatedly spoke with me in long conversations, offering his expertise and consequential suggestions.

Thank you to my editor, Saville Bloxham, for showing immediate interest in this project and advocating to lock in my collaboration with Bloomsbury. Thank you to the three anonymous reviewers who provided constructive feedback, improving this book.

Thank you to my colleague, Dr. Eileen Appelbaum, for green-lighting my initial outreach to Dr. Abramson and providing support to this project since. Thank you to Dean Baker who advised me as I began my research, read over an initial draft, and lent his expertise to answer my questions. Thank you to all my colleagues at the Center for Economic and Policy Research who expressed nothing but support for this book and who conduct vital work of their own.

Lastly, thank you to each of the researchers who conducted the vital research that made this book possible. I especially want to thank each of the researchers who shared with me their works, answered my questions, and took time out of their days to speak with me, such as Drs. Reshma Ramachandran, Christopher Morten, and Ximena Benavides.

# Introduction

Trust is a fragile thing. On March 8, 2023, the US House Select Subcommittee on the Coronavirus Pandemic held its first hearing.[1] This hearing heard four witnesses to investigate the origins of the COVID-19 virus. The Republican majority called three witnesses: virologist and 2018–21 director of the Centers for Disease Control and Prevention (CDC) Dr. Robert Redfield, Atlantic Council senior fellow Dr. Jamie Metzl, and former editor for the scientific journals *Science* and *Nature* along with *The New York Times* Nicholas Wade. The Democratic minority called the clinical director of the Division of Infectious Diseases at Johns Hopkins University School of Medicine, Dr. Paul Auwaerter.

While all the witnesses recognized the uncertainty of the pandemic's origins, the three Republican-selected witnesses thought it more plausible that COVID-19 leaked from the Chinese Wuhan Institute of Virology, whereas Dr. Auwaerter believed the evidence backed a natural origin hypothesis. However, a key aspect of the hearing was not the differing conclusions of the expert witnesses, it was the question of whether it was proper to question public health officials at all. Representative Debbie Dingell (D-MI) exclaimed:

> The U.S still lacks two things in the public healthcare arsenal: people and trust ... I say it's critical to rebuild trust and that continued attacks on public health officials only serves to further discredit people's confidence in our Public Health institutions ... it undermines people's trust in science.[2]

Indeed, the hearing and the existence of the committee itself focused on scrutinizing the behavior of American public health institutions and key figures within them. In the introductory remarks to the March 8 hearing, Chairman Brad Wenstrup (R-OH) outlined that National Institute of Allergy and Infectious Diseases (NIAID) director Dr. Anthony Fauci had "prompted the drafting" of a piece to disprove the lab leak hypothesis and "that the author skewed evidence to achieve that goal, and that the current chief scientist of the World Health Organization was an uncredited coauthor even though he appears to have contributed to the piece."

Representatives Dingell's and Wenstrup's comments illustrate the declining trust in scientific and medical institutions that has emerged since the pandemic began.

According to official estimates, COVID-19 has killed over 7 million people globally, including over 1.2 million deaths in just the United States.[3] The pandemic placed a significant spotlight on the role of medical and public health experts in society, including their unique grasp on medical knowledge. The Pew Research Center found that Americans' trust in medical scientists to act in the public interest declined from 89 percent in 2020 to 77 percent in 2023, remaining similar at 78 percent in 2024.[4] The share of Americans with little to no trust in medical scientists to act in the public interest rose from 11 percent in 2020 to 22 percent in 2023 and 2024.

Trust in public health institutions specifically is sharply divided based on partisan affiliation.[5] In a September 2023 Kaiser Family Foundation (KFF) survey, most Democratic respondents trusted public health institutions: 88 percent for the CDC, 86 percent for the Food and Drug Administration (FDA), and 87 percent for their local public health department. In contrast, 40 percent, 42 percent, and 51 percent of Republicans trusted the CDC, FDA, and their local public health department, respectively. Noticeably, after Republican Donald Trump won the presidency, a 2025 KFF survey noted similarly low trust by Republicans, but Democrats reported significantly lower trust in the CDC (61 percent), FDA (53 percent), and state and local public health officials (54 percent).[6]

The pandemic particularly challenged the levels of trust in the COVID-19 vaccines predominantly made by large pharmaceutical companies and supported by the federal government. A March 2023 Pew Research Center survey recorded 62 percent of Americans believing that COVID-19 vaccine benefits outweighed the harms compared to 36 percent saying the opposite, representing a much sharper divide than that of general trust in scientists.[7] The same survey showed significant levels of uncertainty with vaccine information. Fifty-seven percent of Americans believed that public health officials were not telling the public everything they knew about the vaccines and that society didn't "really know yet if there are serious health risks from COVID-19 vaccines."[8] Additionally, 54 percent of Americans found it difficult to make sense of COVID-19 vaccine information. In January 2025, 26 percent of Americans believed that the COVID-19 vaccines killed more people than the virus, including 40 percent of Republicans; both numbers increased from 20 percent and 25 percent, respectively, in 2023.[9]

In the select subcommittee hearing, trust in public health institutions among members of Congress fell sharply on partisan lines. Democratic members demanded the cessation of critiques against public health officials for the sake of trust, and Republicans accused such officials of significant misconduct. This division has not been limited to the question of the COVID-19 origins nor to just the trustworthiness of government. In November 2023, Republican attorney general of Texas Ken Paxton sued Pfizer for illegally misrepresenting the effectiveness of their COVID-19 vaccine.[10] Contrastingly, in a February 2024 House select subcommittee hearing entitled "Assessing America's Vaccine Safety System's Part I," Ranking Member Rep. Raul Ruiz (D-CA) warned against "the manufacturing of distrust in public health norms and institutions that we have held true for so long will make us less prepared to combat a future pandemic."[11]

While recent debates over trust in public health institutions have centered around the COVID-19 pandemic, their results impact the entire American health care system. Public health institutions live in an environment of medical knowledge born out of significant entanglements between government and industry. The question of whether to trust this current public-private system underlying the medical knowledge that all Americans, including doctors and patients alike, rely upon is nonpartisan. Lack of trust is indicative of a significant issue: either Americans are not capitalizing on guidance that would greatly improve their health, or the institutions themselves are worthy of distrust and fail to keep people safe. Medical experts have debated this question well before the COVID-19 pandemic, and they will likely do so long after.

Indeed, Americans have faced the harsh consequences of the opioid epidemic, showing the potential for US institutions to fail on a massive scale. From 1999 to 2023, nearly 806,000 Americans died from drug overdoses involving opioids, and the problem has been the most severe in recent years.[12] In 2010, over 21,000 Americans died from opioids, and this figure nearly quadrupled to a peak of 82,000 in 2022.[13] This crisis originated from the mass marketing of addictive medical treatments by pharmaceutical companies, which was unchecked by medical experts and public health institutions. In the 1990s, marketing for opioid medications sharply intensified, led by the pharmaceutical company Purdue Pharma for its drug OxyContin.[14] From 1999 to 2014, sales of prescription opioids almost quadrupled, and since Purdue Pharma launched OxyContin in 1996, the company earned over $35 billion by 2023.[15]

Purdue pushed OxyContin, the brand name for oxycodone, on physicians as a pain reliever that is weaker, less addictive, and lower risk than other narcotics—one that doctors should prescribe broadly to the US population. Yet, the evidence did not back this claim, as clinical trial data has not shown OxyContin to be less addictive than other narcotics, and the drug is twice as strong as morphine.[16] While opiates had typically been used to treat cancer pain, a 2003 Government Accountability Office (GAO) report found that Purdue intentionally promoted OxyContin to physicians "for noncancer pain conditions that can be caused by arthritis, injuries, and chronic diseases."[17] Their efforts especially focused on primary care doctors, who became half of OxyContin prescribers by 2003. Consequently, from 1997 to 2002, the annual number of OxyContin prescriptions for noncancer pain exploded by nearly tenfold from 670,000 in 1997 to around 6.2 million in 2002. To achieve this success, Purdue more than doubled its number of sales representatives—individuals who effectively lobby doctors to prescribe their products—from 318 in 1996 to 767 in 2002. These numbers don't count the additional 300 representatives that Abbott Laboratories provided as part of a copromotion agreement.

In 2007, Purdue Pharma pled guilty to illegally misleading federal regulators, doctors, and patients, and the company had to pay $600 million in fines, which was $400 million less than it earned in OxyContin sales that year.[18] US attorney John Brownlee stated that "Purdue ... acknowledged that it illegally marketed and promoted OxyContin by falsely claiming that OxyContin was less addictive, less subject to abuse and diversion, and less likely to cause withdrawal symptoms than other pain medications—all in an effort to maximize its profits."[19] Indeed, the company admitted in court that it pushed the drug "with the intent to defraud or mislead."[20] However, the company continued to push the drug and make even more money following 2007. In 2005, 2006, and 2007, Purdue took in over $1.3 billion, $752 million, and $1 billion, respectively, in sales from OxyContin; in 2010, the company made $2.3 billion in net sales from the drug.[21]

In 2018, CBS News interviewed former Purdue sales representative Carol Panara, who claimed that Purdue continued to misleadingly market OxyContin after the 2007 settlement.[22] For example, she alleged the company instructed her to tell doctors concerned that their patients were becoming addicted that they were only experiencing "pseudoaddiction," and that the remedy was a higher dose of OxyContin. Asked about the evidence behind such a claim, Panara responded, "we did not have any studies."

Ultimately, Purdue pled guilty again as part of an $8 billion settlement in November 2020 for defrauding the government, violating the Federal Anti-Kickback Statute, and marketing opioids to over one hundred health care providers whom it had knowledge were illegally writing prescriptions without a legitimate medical purpose.[23] Since then, Purdue Pharma has faced lawsuits over its role in the crisis, and, in March 2022, it reached a bankruptcy settlement with state attorneys general to pay $6 billion in compensation for fueling the opioid epidemic.[24] This deal would have granted immunity to the Sackler family, who owned the company, from future lawsuits. However, in a June 27, 2024, decision, the Supreme Court struck down the deal ruling that bankruptcy law does not authorize such a grant of immunity without consent from creditors.[25] State attorneys general announced a new $7.4 billion settlement in January 2025 "built on consensual releases" from liability that all fifty states agreed to in June.[26]

While Purdue Pharma ultimately filed for bankruptcy, its successful marketing campaign over twenty-five years for OxyContin fueled the opioid crisis that killed hundreds of thousands of Americans by getting them addicted to narcotics. Purdue Pharma's success in pushing a dangerous narcotic on millions of Americans did not just come from within. The company garnered aid from institutions of medical knowledge that doctors relied upon to help them treat their patients. Purdue funded nonprofit organizations such as the American Pain Society, the American Academy of Pain Management, and the American Geriatric Society that all recommended opioid use for chronic pain unrelated to cancer.[27] From 1996 to 2002, Purdue funded more than 20,000 educational programs related to pain treatment through direct sponsorship or financial grants.[28] In 2001, the Joint Commission on Accreditation of Healthcare Organizations (JCAHO) decided that pain was a "fifth vital sign," encouraging the testing for and treatment of pain. Purdue funded a series of nine programs in 2001 and 2002 to "educate" hospital doctors and staff on how to comply with the new JCAHO pain standards. An agreement between JCAHO and Purdue made Purdue the sole drug company permitted to distribute various JCAHO educational materials on pain management.

The 2017 final report of the President's Commission on Combating Drug Addiction and the Opioid Crisis found that JCAHO's fifth vital decision led doctors—under the pressure of administrators, insurers, and regulatory bodies—to compulsively seek, find, and treat pain, namely "to prescribe opioids beyond traditional boundaries of treating acute, postoperative, procedural pain and end-of-life care."[29] Yet, the report noted that while getting funded from Purdue, the JCAHO did not know that "the science behind their claims and the advice of experts in the field were erroneous." In an interview with the *New York Review*, the report's lead author, Harvard Medical School professor Dr. Bertha Madras, lambasted opioid manufacturers: "They literally bought off, and I don't use that phrase lightly, they bought off the Joint Commission (which accredits hospitals and sets medical policies), they bought off the Federation of State Medical Boards, they bought off several American pain associations."[30]

Furthermore, one of the most influential marketing materials that fueled the opioid epidemic and OxyContin's rise was a published letter in a prestigious, elite medical journal: the *New England Journal of Medicine* (*NEJM*).[31] In 1980, *NEJM* published a letter that looked at the records of nearly 40,000 monitored hospitalized medical patients, finding that there were only four cases of documented addiction in patients without a history of addiction.[32] Yet, Purdue used this very limited work, which offered no information on factors like treatment dosing, duration, and timing, to mislead the public and physicians, claiming that less than 1 percent of people prescribed opioids become addicted.[33] Subsequent articles cited the letter over 600 times by 2017. Among these citations were supposedly reputable sources like *Scientific American* and the Institute for Clinical Systems Improvement, which each respectively called the article an "extensive study" and "landmark report." In *The New York Times*, Dr. Abigail Zuger explained why most doctors wrote so many prescriptions for dangerous narcotics: "Mostly we were just well-intentioned schlubs with prescription pads, dutifully following then-current practice guidelines."[34] Accordingly, the 2017 President's Commission report found that the dramatic rise in opioid use in the decades following the 1990s was driven by how "the medical community … relapsed into liberal use of medicinal opioids."[35]

A 2003 *NEJM* review of the available evidence of using opioid therapy to treat chronic pain identified significant pain reduction without much risk of addiction.[36] According to the lead author, Dr. Jane Ballantyne, "very few studies … suggested that any more than 8 percent of people on prescription opioids exhibited addiction-type behaviors."[37] However, most of the studies included in the review were sponsored and funded by the pharmaceutical industry. Among the sixteen clinical trials the *NEJM* review used, nine (56.3 percent) were industry-sponsored or had coauthors employed by a drug company, including six (37.5 percent) where Purdue Pharma sponsored the study or employed a coauthor. Additionally, the trials employed biased designs, where researchers did not systematically check for signs of addiction or withdrawal symptoms. Rather, the examined side effects included constipation and dry mouth. By 2012, Dr. Ballantyne was a key critic of opioid overprescription, and she admitted that the true percentage of prescription-opioid users who exhibit addiction-type behaviors could be as high as 50 percent.

Additionally, the published results of the trials that the *NEJM* review relied upon did not include the full underlying data from the clinical trials, which are owned by trial sponsors. Thus, the authors could not vet if sponsors were withholding or twisting information. For example, in 2000, *Archives of Internal Medicine* published one of the

Purdue-sponsored trials included in the *NEJM* review, which concluded that around-the-clock controlled-release usage of oxycodone appeared safe and effective for patients with moderate-to-severe chronic, osteoarthritis-related pain.[38] While the researchers stopped giving doses six times during the trial, the results did not report withdrawal problems as a significant adverse event.[39] Purdue then bought 10,000 reprints of the study from the journal for its sales representatives to present to doctors so that they would use OxyContin. However, documents made publicly available from Purdue's 2007 settlement revealed that at least eleven patients reported experiencing adverse withdrawal symptoms compared to the two reported in the published journal article. According to one of the authors of the peer-reviewed published article, Purdue gave them the data and "we reported on the data which was provided to us."

Purdue's success also depended on the corruption and failures of federal regulators. In 1995, the FDA's medical review officer examining OxyContin, Curtis Wright, recommended approval for the drug, and the FDA-approved label claimed that it "delayed absorption" and was less prone to abuse even though Purdue had not conducted any studies proving this to be true.[40] Wright left the FDA and joined Purdue two years thereafter, and another key FDA reviewer also left the agency to join the drugmaker.[41] Also, the FDA in 1995 generally required that drugmakers submit two "adequate and well controlled" randomized controlled trials (RCTs) to prove efficacy in support of their application for regulatory approval.[42] However, the FDA approved Oxycontin with only one study that was adequate and well-controlled and which lasted just two weeks.[43] Ultimately, the FDA approved OxyContin for a much broader set of indications (uses) than the evidence backed, allowing the company to pursue its strategy of getting doctors to prescribe the drug for chronic pain and common conditions.

While the FDA removed the delayed absorption claim from OxyContin's label in 2001, the agency did not use its authority to require Purdue to conduct post-approval high-quality clinical trials examining safety issues with OxyContin.[44] In 2002, an FDA advisory committee met to recommend whether the approved indication of the drug should be narrowed so that Purdue could not market the drug broadly for chronic conditions.[45] The committee voted against narrowing the approved indication, and eight of the ten committee members had financial ties to pharmaceutical compánies, including five who had worked as consultants, speakers, or investigators for Purdue Pharma. Three years after Purdue pled guilty to illegally misbranding OxyContin in 2007, the FDA approved a reformulation of the drug that the agency believed to be less prone to abuse; yet, overdose deaths from prescription opioids still increased in the years that followed.[46]

The case of Purdue Pharma, OxyContin, and the opioid epidemic may be among the most extreme and well-known; however, it is not unique. Industry controls and drives the research agenda directing scientific and medical progress, and it is entrusted with conducting the very trials that test its own products. As a result, industry's massive marketing operations dramatically overstate the benefits of new products that predominantly do not provide much added clinical benefit compared to existing treatments. In search of maximizing market control and profit, drug and device companies spend large sums of money to influence doctors, journals, guidelines, and other organizations that can increase the usage of their products. Federal regulators often fail to hold these companies accountable, and they have even grown to share similar priorities. However, how far reaching are the consequences of these problems?

Several estimates show that Americans have not just fared poorly under the current system, but many are dying because of it. In 1998, the *Journal of the American Medical Association* (*JAMA*) published a meta-analysis of thirty-nine US studies, which looked at all adverse drug reactions from when patients were either in a hospital or when the reactions were the cause of their admission.[47] An estimated 106,000 Americans died annually from adverse drug reactions, representing the fourth leading cause of death at the time. These deaths were often not officially tied to drugs as doctors rarely reported them. For example, in 1994, the authors estimated around 106,000 deaths even though only 156 death certificates cited drug reactions as the cause and the FDA received just 3,500 voluntary reports of such deaths from doctors.[48] Yet, even the FDA has cited this study to recognize that adverse drug reactions in hospitalized settings could be the fourth leading cause of death.[49]

For several reasons, this estimate could significantly underestimate the number of deaths from adverse drug reactions. First, the *JAMA* study only examined deaths from correctly prescribed medications. In 2000, the Institute of Medicine (IOM)—currently the National Academy of Medicine—estimated that around 98,000 Americans die from medical mistakes each year in hospitals, including 7,000 deaths from medication errors in 1993.[50] These numbers are relatively outdated, and later estimates have found more deaths due to error. In 2010, the Office of Inspector General (OIG) of the US Department of Health & Human Services (HHS) nearly doubled the IOM estimate to 180,000 deaths annually for just Medicare patients.[51] In 2013, the *Journal of Patient Safety* published an analysis that used a weighted average of four studies conducted between 2008 and 2011, estimating that 210,000–400,000-plus Americans died annually from medical errors in hospitals.[52] A separate 2016 analysis in the *BMJ*—formerly the *British Medical Journal*—estimated around 251,000 deaths in the United States annually from such medical errors.[53] These studies do not distinguish between the causes of medical error, meaning that the proportion of deaths due to drugs specifically is unknown. However, they provide good reason to suggest that deaths from properly prescribed medications underestimate total deaths regardless of whichever estimate is the most accurate.

Second, most Americans take medications out of a hospital setting. In 2021, there were nearly 5.1 billion retail prescriptions for drugs (those filled in an outpatient setting) in the United States compared to 3.7 billion non-retail prescriptions (those dispensed in an inpatient environment like a hospital, clinic, or physician's office).[54] Therefore, thousands of Americans at a minimum die from prescribed drugs outside of the hospital. For example, the CDC reports that around 15,000 Americans died annually from overdosing on just prescription opioids from 2010 to 2023.[55] Tracking deaths outside of the hospital setting is also very difficult for researchers and government bodies, as there is no regular monitoring of medication usage and consequent outcomes. A coroner may determine that someone overdosed on an opioid; however, is it as easy to determine if fatigue or dizziness induced from a drug causes a fatal fall?

Third, the *JAMA* estimate is from 1998, and medication usage has significantly increased over the last quarter century. From just 2009 to 2022, dispensed drug prescriptions rose from around 3.9 billion to 6.7 billion.[56] Greater usage of drugs generally may also mean that more people are dying from them. Ultimately, regardless of how much the 1998 *JAMA* estimate underestimates deaths from adverse drug reactions, hundreds of thousands of Americans die from medications.

Outside of drug-induced deaths specifically, Americans do not achieve good health outcomes given that the United States is the wealthiest nation in the world.[57] While life expectancy was similar to comparable nations in 1980 (0.9 years less), the gap increased to 3.8 years before the pandemic in 2019.[58] In 2023, the gap was 4.1 years. A 2025 *JAMA Health Forum* letter noted that excess mortality in the United States was −42,109 in 1980, meaning that 42,109 fewer Americans died than they otherwise would have with the average death rate in twenty-one other wealthy nations.[59] By 2019, 631,247 more Americans died than they otherwise would have with the death rate of comparable countries, peaking at 1,098,808 excess deaths in 2021 and lowering to 705,331 in 2023. From 2007 to 2022, US children were 80 percent more likely to die than comparator nations.[60] The Commonwealth Fund conducts regular analyses of the US health care system compared to other wealthy nations, consistently finding that the United States spends far more for significantly worse outcomes.[61] Meanwhile, a 2023 KFF survey found that 61 percent of American adults reported taking prescription medicines in 2023, with 27 percent taking four or more medicines.[62]

While the United States has significantly worse health outcomes compared to other nations, Americans also spend nearly twice as much per person on health care compared to comparable wealthy nations ($13,432 vs. $7,393 in 2023).[63] The disparity is greater when looking at just prescription drugs. A 2024 RAND Corporation estimate measured that the United States spent 2.78 times more on prescription drugs than comparable countries in 2022.[64] Globally, the United States accounted for 52.7 percent of all prescription pharmaceutical sales while also only taking in 12.6 percent of the volume of drugs sold.[65] A previous 2018 Brookings Institute and Schaeffer Center analysis estimated that American consumers could account for 64–78 percent of global pharmaceutical profits.[66] The Commonwealth Fund found that utilization does not account for higher spending; the prices of drugs are simply higher.[67] Moreover, medical device spending is similarly more expensive in the United States compared to peer nations. A 2018 *Health Affairs* study found that cardiac implant devices were two to six times more expensive in the United States compared to countries like Germany and the UK.[68]

There are many problems with the American health care system and many other societal factors—such as the quality of the food we eat, our financial situations, the places we live, and so on—that play into the poor health outcomes of Americans.[69] I do not attempt to touch upon most of these topics. Additionally, it is not my place, nor is it the aim of this book, to make any medical decision for any individual. Rather, Americans hold some degree of trust that an authority is making sure that the medical products they use work and will not harm them. The COVID-19 pandemic and debates resulting from it have placed a spotlight on such trust and whether it is deserved. Knowing the extent to which our current system proves that trust to be well placed is important to every American, including myself. Regardless of whether public health institutions were or were not reliable during the pandemic specifically, the last few years have called into question the entire system. Thus, this book examines the state of the medical knowledge that Americans of all stripes rely upon.

Some people may look poorly on this attempt to conduct such a critical examination, as it could further call into question the reliability of doctors and public health institutions and decrease public trust where it is already too low. I agree that a healthy society should have trust in its public health system. Without it, individuals, families, and entire communities can be ill-equipped to protect themselves and their loved ones. If a future pandemic arises—perhaps one significantly deadlier than COVID-19—the FDA, CDC, and other public health institutions can only protect Americans insofar as people trust and listen to them. Outside of another pandemic, people should ideally be able to know that their doctors and hospitals are providing the best, evidence-based care possible that is reasonably safe and effective.

However, trust is earned, not given, and it should not be the equivalent of blind faith. A healthy society should have trust in its institutions because those institutions are trustworthy. If they are not and if there are substantial issues of reliability that call into question the safety and effectiveness of medical care, then the public has a right and duty to themselves, their families, and their communities to be skeptical. Such skepticism is not ideal, but it is made necessary when the individuals, organizations, and companies who should be acting in the interests of public health are not fulfilling their duties. Even if health institutions are not the sole contributor to mistrust, their contributions justifiably weaken faith in the system. Thus, a critical appraisal of the state of medical knowledge is not an unjustified exercise in reducing trust; it is an essential step to identify the necessary changes so that our institutions can earn the public's trust back.

Chapter 1 delves into the industry control of the clinical trials that federal regulators use to determine if a medical product is safe and effective. This control affects what questions are studied, how trials are designed, what results get published, and who has access to the underlying data necessary to truly vet study findings. Chapter 2 explains the efforts in the United States to increase transparency over the last several decades along with how these efforts still leave Americans and the world in the dark about the evidence behind our medical products.

Chapter 3 examines peer-reviewed medical journals' role as the premier source of medical knowledge for doctors and medical professionals. Yet, the journals also maintain significant ties to industry, and their peer review process largely fails to truly vet companies' claims about their products. Chapter 4 examines the similar state of clinical guidelines, which are often funded by industry and written by authors with significant conflicts of interest (COI). Guidelines, while extremely influential in directing the decision-making of clinicians, often fail to obtain and properly evaluate high-quality evidence.

Chapter 5 details the thirty years of faster approvals and weakening standards of evidence at the FDA, where the regulatory agency with actual access to underlying clinical data has increasingly approved products under a weakened standard for deeming them safe and effective. Chapter 6 buttresses these findings by examining the FDA's even more lax regulatory standards for medical devices. Chapter 7 then investigates the regulatory capture of the FDA—the agency charged with ensuring products are safe and effective—through its revolving door, reliance on conflicted advisors, sources of funding, and fundamental priorities. Chapter 8 investigates why doctors, whom patients ultimately rely upon for their care, accept the current system through exploring their education, sources of influence, and limitations.

Chapter 9 provides an overview of the patent system that creates the incentives for medical research in the United States, including both its rationale and limitations. The chapter explores two alternative systems that similarly seek to promote innovation while also tying financial rewards to health outcomes. Chapter 10 analyzes arguably the most salient test of medical knowledge in the United States in recent memory: COVID-19 vaccination policy. To what extent did the government help develop the vaccines, rein in corporate control, base its decision-making on high-quality evidence, and honestly communicate with the American people?

Given the significant challenges facing the medical knowledge that Americans rely upon, Chapter 11 provides a path forward with policy solutions that can help create a more trustworthy, transparent health care system. The afterword examines whether the second Trump administration's policies thus far have addressed these core challenges. Ultimately, this book concludes by addressing the question facing Americans and troubling lawmakers: should we trust our medical and public health institutions?

# 1

# Industry Control

For any product to get onto the market in the United States, it must meet requirements set by the FDA. Except for most medical devices (see Chapter 6), manufacturers conduct studies to prove to the government that their products are safe and effective. However, this process places control of medical research and the agenda for such research in the hands of industry. According to the chief scientist at the Center for Bioethics and Humanities at the University of Colorado Anschutz, Dr. Lisa Bero:

> [The production of research] is a cyclical process and is vulnerable to industry interference at every step, including (a) setting the research agenda and framing research questions, (b) designing the methods of the study, (c) conducting the study, and (d) publishing the study.[1]

Industry is ultimately responsible for funding the majority of the research behind pharmaceutical products and medical devices.[2] A 2015 *JAMA* analysis found that there were more than three times the number of industry-funded trials registered on the federal registry ClinicalTrials.gov compared to National Institutes of Health (NIH)-funded trials in 2006, and this increased to a roughly 6:1 ratio by 2014.[3] A 2023 *JAMA* analysis of the 600 most frequently cited clinical trials from 2018 found that 68.2 percent of trials had industry funding, and a slight majority (50.5 percent) had exclusive industry funding.[4] In comparison, only 17.3 percent of these trials were publicly funded. In 2020, industry funding comprised two-thirds of all medical research and development (R&D) spending compared to a quarter for federal spending.[5]

The US federal government does fund a significant amount of medical research that is directly responsible for new medicines and interventions, but government funding mostly targets the basic research that is theoretical and experimental in nature and provides foundational medical knowledge.[6] Examples include how the brain stores memories or how cancer cells develop. The government funds to a lesser degree applied or translational clinical research that uses the findings of basic research and directs them toward specific goals like creating new, practical medical technologies. Industry capitalizes on the foundation of government-funded research to fund development and phased clinical trial testing of its products. For example, the NIH funded the basic research and applied research behind the mRNA COVID-19 vaccines along with the actual vaccine development program for companies like Moderna.[7]

Accordingly, a 2023 investigation published in *JAMA Health Forum* examined the phased clinical trials of 387 drugs approved by the FDA between 2010 and 2019.[8] The researchers found that out of the $247.3 billion the NIH spent on research, only $8.1 billion (3.3 percent) related to phased clinical development. NIH funding represented roughly one-tenth of estimated amounts of industry spending on clinical development. The vast majority, $209.9 billion (84.9 percent), of NIH spending went to basic research while $29.3 billion (11.8 percent) went to applied research not including phased clinical trials.

The same authors in another 2023 study found that $187 billion in NIH-funded research contributed to 354 (99.4 percent) of 356 FDA-approved products from 2010 to 2019.[9] The authors concluded that the NIH's discounted investment in the decade of approved drugs "was not less" than pharmaceutical industry investment. This finding essentially means that while industry spent more money, public funding was not worth less than private spending because of the value and risk of the government's early investing.

Regardless of federal funding's importance for eventual product development, industry ultimately does most of the work for the development and testing of products themselves. The aforementioned numbers can understate the role of industry funding for research, as they reflect the proportion of industry funding for trials posted in registries and published journal articles along with general research spending. Regarding the required research to achieve FDA approval so that a company can market its product, the responsibility of funding trials falls on the company.[10]

Industry often contracts with third parties to conduct research for its products, including mostly for-profit entities rather than academic institutions. Industry sponsors significantly moved from using independent, academic investigators and academic medical centers (AMCs) to oversee and design clinical trials in the early 1990s to predominantly hiring for-profit companies—contract research organizations (CROs)—by the mid-2000s. A 2005 *NEJM* article highlighted how 80 percent of industry funding for clinical research went to AMCs in 1991.[11] By 2004, this percentage had plummeted to 24 percent, and there is no indication that companies have returned to AMCs. Companies shifted toward CROs due to their greater efficiency, principally in bypassing academic red tape and increasing the speed of clinical trials, allowing for millions of dollars in higher earnings.[12] Contracts with these for-profit actors also grant industry sponsors control over study design, making clinical trials and their results tools of industry marketing.[13]

In a 2001 letter, editors from major medical journals—such as *Annals of Internal Medicine*, *JAMA*, *NEJM*, and *The Lancet*—explained that competition between CROs and AMCs for industry funding granted undue influence to industry through industry-favorable terms in clinical trial agreements (CTA).[14] They wrote:

> Corporate sponsors have been able to dictate the terms of participation in the trial, terms that are not always in the best interests of academic investigators, the study participants or the advancement of science generally. Investigators may have little or no input into trial design, no access to the raw data, and limited participation

in data interpretation. These terms are draconian for self-respecting scientists, but many have accepted them because they know that if they do not, the sponsor will find someone else who will.

Academic researchers increasingly turned to industry for funding, especially with higher industry investment and harder-to-secure NIH grants in the 1970s and early 1980s.[15] Explaining the situation, *Science* news editor Barbara Culliton wrote in a 1982 article, "scientists who 10 years ago would have snubbed their academic noses at industrial money now eagerly seek it out."[16]

The emergence of CROs spread industry influence over study design to trials managed by academics as well. The power imbalance between industry sponsors and academic researchers—where the latter relies on the former and not vice versa—has made academic institutions set up clinical trial offices to court industry rather than uphold academic and medical integrity.[17] This industry control over study design is a phenomenon created over the last thirty years that scientists, researchers, and academics previously rejected. However, as researchers have increasingly relied on industry financing for their work, the ethical guidelines have changed.

Courting industry to finance research has produced extreme bias, as the case of the 2018 Moderate Alcohol and Cardiovascular Health (MACH) trial reveals.[18] Beginning in 2013, National Institute on Alcohol Abuse and Alcoholism (NIAAA) officials and alcohol researchers sought funding from top alcohol companies for a randomized trial with the predetermined intention of showing that moderate alcohol consumption provided health benefits. The researchers allowed industry to choose the trial investigators and approve its design. An NIH advisory committee report documented how NIAAA-industry interactions "appear[ed] to intentionally bias the framing of the scientific premise in the direction of demonstrating a beneficial health effect of moderate alcohol consumption."[19] Design flaws like small participant sizing, insufficient follow-up, and inadequate outcome measures meant "the trial could show benefits while missing harms." After public reporting, congressional hearings, and internal reviews, the NIH ended the trial in June 2018.[20]

## Industry Sponsorship Bias

Pervasive industry sponsorship bias results in industry-sponsored trials being significantly more likely to produce results favorable to manufacturers because of factors like directing the research agenda, the manipulation of study designs, and selective reporting. Analyses of industry-sponsored studies in comparison to others in the field of biomedical research have consistently shown a significant association with industry-favorable results. A 2003 *JAMA* paper examined thirty-seven quantitative biomedical studies between 1980 and 2002, finding that industry-sponsored research was 3.6 times more likely to have pro-industry conclusions compared to non-industry-sponsored research.[21] A 2017 Cochrane review examined seventy-five papers between 1986 and 2015 that themselves investigated the effect of industry sponsorship on the results of drug and device research.[22] The review found that the body of literature examining research across various diseases and treatments showed that results and conclusions of industry-sponsored studies were significantly more likely to support the sponsors' products. According to *JAMA* in 2023, the most frequently cited clinical trials in 2018 were also more likely to produce industry-favorable conclusions when sponsored by industry.[23]

## Biasing the Research Agenda

Given industry domination, companies bias research by deciding what topics are on the research agenda. In 2015, researchers in *JAMA* found that out of $121 billion in US medical and health services research in 2011, around $116 billion (95.9 percent) went toward new drugs and devices compared to just around $5 billion (4.1 percent) for better delivery of health services and the health and wellbeing of individuals and communities.[24] Looking at industry medical R&D spending specifically in 2020, only 1.4 percent of spending went toward health care services while the remaining 98.6 percent went toward biopharmaceuticals (75.5 percent), medical technologies (13.0 percent), and other sectors (10.1 percent) like contracting with computer firms.[25]

At the same time, according to the social determinants of health, medical care only determines up to 20 percent of population health. The other 80 percent is determined by health behaviors (30 percent) like diet and exercise, social and economic factors (40 percent), and one's physical environment (10 percent).[26] However, conducting studies on ways to improve people's health only makes sense from the perspective of for-profit industry if it serves their bottom line. For example, testing the efficacy of an obesity drug may lead to a profitable product, but assessing the best lifestyle modifications like particular diets and exercise regimes would not. There is no profit motive to conduct research on the 80 percent of factors that determine population health that would not sell more medical products.

In 2018, researchers in the *American Journal of Public Health* (*AJPH*) conducted a scoping review of how industry sponsorship influences the research agenda.[27] Identifying thirty-six relevant systematic reviews involving both quantitative and qualitative analyses published from 1986 to 2017, they found that industry-sponsored research was more likely to focus on areas that can be commercialized rather than those that were best suited to benefit public health. Most of the studies focused on medical research, and these revealed a focus on funding research into drugs and devices—namely in markets that could yield higher sales—rather than public health or behavioral interventions. Industry also prioritized research on areas that bolstered its policy and legal positions. For example, the sugar industry funded research into other ways to limit tooth decay without having to reduce the amount of sugar people consume.

Ultimately, with most funding for medical R&D coming from industry, these companies get to decide what questions researchers will answer. Given that the purpose of for-profit entities like pharmaceutical companies is to make as much money as possible, it is inevitable that most research will investigate products that can generate the most profit. Along with developing products that the most people can use—as I will further discuss in Chapter 9—companies also look to areas where they can charge the highest prices, namely through exploiting patent monopolies.

Industry control over the research agenda does not just mean that there is a concentrated focus on drug and device research. By controlling what questions are asked, Dr. Bero notes, companies "may not ask a question or fund researchers to ask questions that they do not want answered."[28] One way this manifests is that companies are not financially incentivized to compare their products to potentially more effective means of treatment. For example, in 2002, the publicly funded Diabetes Prevention Program Research Group conducted a study where researchers tested the effect of intensive lifestyle modification—consisting of physician-directed diet and exercise—against metformin regarding the incidence of type 2 diabetes.[29] They found that lifestyle changes were significantly more effective at reducing the risk of type 2 diabetes compared to those treated with the drug metformin. Compared to placebo, lifestyle intervention reduced the incidence of diabetes by 58 percent compared to just 31 percent for metformin, and lifestyle intervention was 39 percent more effective when compared directly to metformin.

This bias not only prevents research comparing a medical product to a lifestyle change, but also examinations of competing products. In 2010, the *European Journal of Clinical Investigation* published research examining 577 randomized clinical trials published in ClinicalTrials.gov in 2006 from the fifteen companies that sponsored the most registered trials, such as Merck, Eli Lilly, Wyeth, Pfizer, and Roche.[30] They found that two-thirds of the trials only included a treatment owned by the industry sponsor and that all the companies "strongly preferred to run trials where they were the only industry sponsor or even the only owner of the assessed interventions." Manufacturers are not incentivized to spend billions on trials that run the risk of finding that their products are less effective than a competitor's, especially given that companies deal with the risk that their products do not work at all.

## Study Design Manipulation

A significant cause of industry sponsorship bias is the manipulation of study designs. Most clinical trials testing drugs' safety and effectiveness are randomized—meaning participants are randomly sorted into treatment and control groups—which is critical to ensure there is no bias from differences in the types of people in each group.[31] Yet, all study designs—even for randomized controlled trials—are not made equally, and companies have a vested interest in testing their products in whatever manner possible that generates positive results, better marketing of their products, and, thus, the most profit. For example, the stock price of pharmaceutical companies behind twenty-three oncology drugs rose by 13.7 percent on average following the public announcements of positive trial results from 2000 to 2009.[32] Yet, the stock price only declined by 0.7 percent following the announcement of negative results.

There are many methods to alter study designs to manufacture positive results and/or hide negative outcomes. Designers can test the effect of a treatment against a placebo rather than an existing, effective treatment.[33] For most conditions, new products are not the first treatment. Trial results are not important just to show that a treatment is safer and more effective than placebo, but whether it provides an added clinical benefit compared to existing treatments. Indirect comparisons between treatments relying on different treatment versus placebo trials provide weaker evidence than direct comparisons between treatments.[34] It is more informative for doctors' decisions to read trial results in published articles showing that a new treatment will provide greater benefit to their patients than existing therapies. A 2012 analysis published in *JAMA Internal Medicine* found that among ninety-one trials registered in ClinicalTrials.gov prior to October 2009 that tested the effectiveness of biologic treatments for rheumatoid arthritis, only five trials (5.5 percent) tested the respective treatment head-to-head against an existing treatment.[35] Even head-to-head trial designs can have flaws, such as using lower quality comparative treatments and improper doses of comparators.[36]

Furthermore, the participants included in a clinical trial may inaccurately represent the actual population of people who would use the treatment. For example, Vioxx (rofecoxib) represents one of the largest drug scandals in American history. The pharmaceutical company Merck hid and distorted serious cardiovascular adverse events that Vioxx caused, such as heart attacks and strokes, leading to the estimated deaths of 30,000–60,000 Americans.[37] In 1999, Merck introduced Vioxx as an alternative anti-inflammatory treatment to reduce pain from osteoarthritis; Merck advertised that Vioxx caused less gastrointestinal side effects compared to existing anti-inflammatory drugs.[38] However, in Merck's Vioxx gastrointestinal outcomes research (VIGOR) trial, it enrolled enough patients that were taking steroids like prednisone so that they represented half of the study population even though steroid usage was not representative of the target patient population.[39] The trial results for patients not taking steroids showed that Vioxx caused no reduction in gastrointestinal side effects compared to the comparative treatment naproxen. Thus, in addition to the fact that Vioxx caused deadly cardiovascular adverse events, it did not produce the gastrointestinal benefit that Merck advertised for the actual population that would use the drug.

Along with including types of participants to bias results, a clinical trial can exclude certain demographics who would likely use the treatment.[40] For example, researchers may exclude patients who are more likely to experience adverse events due to complex risk profiles, such as the elderly, women, the impoverished, and certain racial groups. Pretrial tests can reveal particular groups of people who have better/worse reactions to a treatment along with those who have strong/weak placebo responses. This information can inform the design of trials to increase the chance of industry-favorable results.

By designing clinical trials to be relatively short-lived, results can fail to record a drop-off in efficacy or emergence of adverse events that appear later.[41] Even if a trial is sufficiently long, lack of data transparency to peer reviewers can distort results.[42] In a 2000 *JAMA* article on Pfizer's Celecoxib Long-Term Arthritis Safety Study (CLASS) trial, the authors cited only six months of data even though the trial ran for twelve months.[43] While the article claimed that celecoxib (brand name Celebrex) resulted in less gastrointestinal adverse side effects than older anti-inflammatory drugs, the full twelve months of data showed that there was no statistically significant advantage.[44]

Moreover, there are many more ways to influence study design. Researchers can manipulate treatment doses depending on the desired outcome. In head-to-head trials, using a lower dose of a comparator drug can inflate the relative efficacy of a tested treatment, and using a higher dose for the comparator can deflate the relative risks of adverse events for the tested product.[45] In placebo-controlled trials, altering doses can similarly distort results, such as by using a higher-than-necessary dose to functionally unblind participants so that they know they are receiving a treatment rather than placebo.[46] Blinding is essential so participants do not alter their conscious or unconscious behavior based on getting treatment or placebo.

Unblinding the physicians and researchers administering treatments about who is getting treatment or placebo is another source of bias.[47] In two separate studies in *BMJ* and the *Canadian Medical Association Journal*, Hróbjartsson et al. examined the impact of non-blinded trial outcome assessors—those who observe and assess treatment outcomes—in twenty-one randomized clinical trials with binary outcomes and twenty-four with measurement scale outcomes.[48] They found that trials with non-blinded assessors significantly exaggerated the treatment effects by 36 percent and 68 percent, respectively. Considering that treatments often do not have a claimed effect as significant as 36 percent, failure to blind those conducting trials can bias results and make them unreliable.[49] Overall, this chapter describes only a portion of the potential avenues for trial designers to manipulate results, as trials are tools and not guaranteed arbiters of truth, and there are many innovative ways for irresponsible actors to abuse a tool.

Along with design elements affecting how a trial is conducted, researchers can take many divergent paths when statistically analyzing results. Researchers examining the exact same data set can reach entirely different conclusions based on employing different statistical methods. In a 2020 *Nature* study, the authors provided 70 different research teams with the exact same data to investigate the results of functional magnetic resonance imaging (fMRI).[50] The authors found that no research team used the exact same analytical technique, and the results varied across the teams. They also found "an overestimation of the likelihood of significant findings," meaning that researchers were more likely to have statistically significant findings than they should have been.

When determining if a drug has statistically significant effects that show efficacy or risk of adverse events, the conclusion often hinges on probability values ($p$-values). Frequently, if a $p$-value is below 0.05, observers determine the result to be statistically significant. In a drug trial finding that a medication lowers mortality, a 0.05 $p$-value means that there is just a 5 percent chance of observing the same or more extreme mortality effect assuming there was no relationship between taking the drug and lower mortality. So, lower $p$-values suggest a lower likelihood of observing the mortality decrease by chance alone. Yet, it can take very little for design biases and varying statistical methods to make a $p$-value below or above the required threshold of statistical significance. This allows sponsors and investigators to reinterpret data until they find a statistical result that aligns with their interest.[51] According to the cofounder of the Cochrane Collaboration and medical researcher Dr. Peter Gøtzsche, while RCTs are "the most reliable design we have for evaluating treatment … we have accepted much too readily that what comes out of these experiments should be believed if the trial was blinded and the main result is accompanied by a significant P value."[52]

Ultimately, there are many ways that biased actors can jeopardize the integrity of clinical trial results, highlighting the need for general guidelines, thorough peer review, and data transparency. Industry reliance on for-profit CROs exacerbates this dynamic, as sponsors control study design and CROs are incentivized to meet industry demands to receive more contracts.

## Selective Publication

Selective publication is another major form of bias. Not all research is published in journals, and incentives bias researchers to publish positive, exciting, and career-advancing findings.[53] However, industry-sponsored research is especially likely to reach publication with positive results due to the financial incentive to increase the likelihood of higher product usage and industry profits. In a 2008 *NEJM* article, researchers examined the FDA reviews of seventy-four trials of twelve antidepressant medications and found that twenty-three (31 percent) were not published in journals.[54] In twenty-two out of these twenty-three unpublished trials, the FDA reviewers determined that the efficacy results were negative or questionable. Among the published trials, 94 percent showed positive outcomes for the antidepressant medications, while the FDA analyses documented that just 51 percent of the 74 trials had such positive results. This issue is not limited to just antidepressants. In a 2017 systematic review and meta-analysis published in the *Journal of Clinical Epidemiology*, researchers identified eighty-five studies that tracked cohorts of different clinical trials from trial launch through journal publication.[55] Trials with positive results were more than twice as likely to get published compared to the other studies.

Selective publication inherently involves industry and its allies knowingly misleading doctors and patients. In May 2000, Dr. Charles Schulz presented his data analysis based on four clinical trials to compare AstraZeneca's antipsychotic drug Seroquel with an older, generic antipsychotic drug haloperidol to the American Psychiatric Association (APA).[56] His presentation claimed that Seroquel was significantly more effective in treating schizophrenia than haloperidol. An AstraZeneca press release claimed that the drug was "significantly superior" while Schulz expressed his hope that the "findings help physicians better understand the dramatic benefits of newer medications like SEROQUEL … because, if they do, we may be able to help ensure patients receive these medications first."[57] Yet, just two months prior in March 2000, internal emails from AstraZeneca showed that their analysts reached the opposite conclusion. In a March 23 email, an AstraZeneca official wrote:

> The data don't look good. In fact, I don't know how we can get a paper out of this. My guess is that we all (including Schulz) saw the good stuff … What seems to be the case is that we were highlighting the only good stuff and that our own analysis support the "view out there" that we are less effective than haloperidol and our competitors.[58]

Yet, Schulz still appeared before the APA to present his cherry-picked findings two months after AstraZeneca officials knew that Seroquel was less effective than haloperidol. While Dr. Schulz was an academic researcher at the University of Minnesota and was not an AstraZeneca employee, he had significant financial ties to the company.[59] From 2002 to 2007, Schulz received $112,000 in consulting fees and university grants from the company along with an additional $450,000 from another drug company, Eli Lilly.

This was not the first time that AstraZeneca employees internally admitted to lying to the public about Seroquel. The company sponsored a trial called COSTAR comparing Seroquel with haloperidol; however, the results were not favorable to AstraZeneca: patients taking haloperidol had better symptom ratings and fewer psychotic relapses.[60] An employee stated in December 1999 that the "disadvantages are obvious" if they chose to publish COSTAR due to "potentially damaging data."[61] An entire email thread involved various employees debating whether to hide the study results and, if they did publish them, how to "diminish the negative findings."[62] Ultimately, AstraZeneca did not publish the negative results; rather, it cherry-picked positive elements from the study and got them published in the journal *Schizophrenia Research* in January 2002.[63] The abstract stated that higher doses of Seroquel in comparison to haloperidol appear "to have a positive impact on important domains of cognitive performance that have been found to predict role function and community outcomes in patients with schizophrenia."

COSTAR was not the only suppressed trial. As an employee noted, there was "a precedent set regarding 'cherry picking' of data"; in fact, he stated, "thus far, we have buried Trials 15, 31, 56, and are now considering COSTAR."[64] He highlighted the issue of outside pressure calling for public access to industry-sponsored clinical trial data, worrying about how AstraZeneca would respond "when they begin to criticize us for suppressing data." A suggested response to such criticism was to "say that our competitors indulge in this practice." In other words, the public should not go after AstraZeneca because other pharmaceutical companies also cherry-pick findings and hide negative trial results.

Selective publication can also work in tandem with biased trial designs. GlaxoSmithKline (GSK) published around twenty-four trials by 2012 comparing its migraine-relieving drug sumatriptan against placebo, showing sizable positive results.[65] Examining GSK's trial registry, a 2009 investigation found that the company did not publish five trials comparing the drug against comparative treatments, where only one of the trials found more than half of patients to have received headache relief from the drug.[66]

Selective reporting bias has decreased since the creation of the federal register ClinicalTrials.gov, International Committee of Medical Journal Editors (ICMJE) trial registration requirements, and the subsequent passage of the Food and Drug Administration Amendments Act (FDAAA) in 2007. These shifts (discussed in the following chapters) required trial sponsors to publicly disclose that their trials took place and post limited summary data. However, selective reporting is still a significant issue within the medical literature that doctors rely upon. The creation of a national registry and requirements for most clinical trials to register and report basic results data did prevent researchers and industry sponsors from de facto hiding the existence of trials with negative outcomes. Yet, many trials still fail to register with ClinicalTrials.gov. Additionally, doctors and medical professionals rely on publications in medical journals as the premier source of medical knowledge rather than very limited data posted on public registries. While overall reporting bias has decreased, the selective publication of trials with positive results in medical journals still allows industry sponsors to misrepresent the actual efficacy of their products.

## Industry Control of Data

Predominantly, the funders/sponsors of clinical trials own the data resulting from their research. However, when the federal government funds nonprofit and academic research institutions for clinical research, the recipients control the data while also being subjected to NIH requirements, such as registering trials with ClinicalTrials.gov.[67] In 1980, Congress passed the Bayh-Dole Act, giving nonprofit research institutions the right to patent and commercialize inventions their researchers made with federal funds.[68] Congress passed the Shelby Amendment in 1998, allowing members of the public to file Freedom of Information Act (FOIA) requests for research data in relation to published findings from federally funded research.[69] Ultimately, the institutional recipients of federal funds largely control the data from their clinical trials.

In industry-sponsored clinical trials, the sponsors almost always own the study data, including the metadata, summary data, and individual participant/patient data (IPD). This reality is true regardless if the industry sponsors hire a private CRO to design and manage the study or an academic medical center. When pharmaceutical companies and device makers fund clinical trials outside of the academic arena, they own and store the data. An internal Pfizer document states that, in the companies' view, "Pfizer-sponsored studies belong to Pfizer, not to any individual" (see Figure 1).[70]

In contrast, when industry sponsors have contracted with AMCs, they have not always had exclusive access to the clinical trial data. However, the increased desire and need for industry funding among academics has yielded a greater willingness to grant industry ownership of clinical data. In a 2005 study published in *NEJM*, researchers sent out a questionnaire to medical school administrators in charge of negotiating clinical-trial agreements with industry sponsors, receiving responses from 107 medical schools.[71] They found that 80 percent of the administrators would allow the sponsor to "own the data produced by the research."

The best indication of industry ownership of clinical trial data comes from the pharmaceutical companies trade association: Pharmaceutical Research and Manufacturers of America (PhRMA). Their publicly available "Principles on Conduct of Clinical Trials and Communication of Clinical Trial Results" clearly state that industry sponsors own clinical trial data:

> As sponsors, we are responsible for receipt and verification of data from all research sites for the studies we conduct; we ensure the accuracy and integrity of the entire study database, which is owned by the sponsor.[72]

**Pfizer's Internal Recognition of Data Ownership Rights and Usage**

1. "Pfizer-sponsored studies belong to Pfizer, not to any individual"
2. "Purpose of data is to support, directly or indirectly, marketing of our product" through:
   a. "[U]se in label enhancements," supplemental new drug applications
   b. "[P]ublications for field force use"
   c. "[O]ff-label data dissemination"
3. "[C]ommercial marketing/medical need to be involved in all data dissemination efforts"

**Figure 1** Quotes from an internal Pfizer document, stating that "Pfizer-sponsored studies belong to Pfizer" and that the "purpose of data is to support ... marketing of our product." *Source*: Glen I. Spielmans and Peter I. Parry, "From Evidence-Based Medicine to Marketing-Based Medicine: Evidence from Internal Industry Documents," *Journal of Bioethical Inquiry* 7 (January 21, 2010): 13–29, https://doi.org/10.1007/s11673-010-9208-8.

PhRMA makes it clear that the investigators who sponsors hire to conduct the trials don't have complete access to the data. Rather, the sponsors provide "meaningful access," meaning the investigators can see the data for the research participants they directly oversaw along with a summary of the results that "could be the primary manuscript submitted for publication, a slide presentation, or a synopsis of the sponsor's Clinical Study Report (CSR)."[73]

Further demonstrating industry control, when independent researchers, research organizations, and even government institutions seek access to IPD or other forms of unpublished information, they have requested data from the pharmaceutical/device manufacturer directly. After the development of their COVID-19 vaccines, the coauthors of a study on the safety of the vaccines wrote an open letter in the *BMJ*, pleading for Moderna and Pfizer to give independent researchers access to IPD from their clinical trials.[74] When people request such data from the FDA, the agency alerts the industry sponsors and allows them to object to disclosure of confidential information.[75]

Industry control of clinical trial data severely limits the ability for anyone outside the FDA to understand study results. For any actor to fully understand the results of clinical trials, they require access to three key types of data: metadata, IPD, and summary data. Metadata is data that describes the data from clinical research (the data about the data).[76] Principally, metadata involves the full protocol of a clinical trial. This involves the entirety of how the study is designed: the type of study, the eligibility and exclusion criteria for participants, the different interventions and treatment groups, how researchers administer different treatments, the primary and secondary hypotheses and corresponding outcome measures, the study endpoints, and much more. Other information included in metadata involve information about the key people involved: the investigators, sponsors, funders, data management and analysis teams, committee members, and so on. Amendments to the trial protocol are also recorded along with information on participant flow: how participants are assigned to treatment groups and how they progress through the trial (including if they drop out).

Metadata includes the statistical analysis plan (SAP) created before the start of a trial and describes how researchers will handle and analyze the data they collect over the course of the study.[77] This contains which data the researchers will analyze and what statistical methods they will employ. The SAP contains critical definitions of important variables, such as adverse and serious adverse events. While amendments to trial protocol are standard, deviation from SAPs is significant, as it can bias results and represent efforts by researchers to manipulate outcomes. A *BMC Medicine* analysis of randomized trials published in medical journals from January to April 2018 found that most trials (60.7 percent) had unexplained deviations from their SAP.[78] Accompanying the SAP is a trial's analytic code that describes the choices researchers made to turn data sets into scientific results.[79] The analytic code is a critical element for reproducibility of research, meaning that it allows other researchers to reproduce the original authors' findings. Without access to the SAP and analytic code, independent investigators cannot check if the trial researchers followed their study design nor can they conduct their own reanalyses of the data.

Data sharing agreements are another form of documentation often required to register trials and publish them in medical journals. This agreement details if, to what extent, when, and for how long the owners of clinical trial data will share data with outside sources such as journals, independent researchers, and the public. Yet—as Chapter 2 discusses—these data sharing agreements are very ineffective in actually getting companies to publicly disclose trial data.

IPD provides the most complete picture of trial results. Raw data is the original source information collected over the course of a clinical trial. This information includes demographic information of participants, patients' medical history, baseline measurements like weight and blood pressure, clinical outcome measures, and anything else investigators track during a trial. Raw data is usually stored on case report forms, where different types of information are recorded in alignment with the coding outlined in the trial protocol. The researchers then computerize the information collected on case report forms, loading them onto electronic data sets. Through this process, quality control and data "cleaning" is essential to ensure the completeness and accuracy of the recorded data. On its own, it is difficult for researchers to conduct in-depth analysis of raw data. However, raw data serves as the foundation of all recorded information from a clinical trial.

Researchers transform raw data into analyzable data sets for them to conduct any form of data/statistical analysis. This process often involves mathematically transforming the raw data, creating new variables, and overall setting up the data set so that the researchers can carry out the SAP and utilize their analytic code. While the data is the resource from which researchers conduct all their analyses to derive primary and secondary outcomes, information on adverse events, and more, most of the data is never used. Therefore, analyzable data sets are the best source for identifying key findings not discovered by the original researchers under their SAP. Yet, individual data is also the data least likely to be shared to anyone outside of the sponsor. Even the FDA relies mostly on summary information; but, it also has access to IPD.[80]

While IPD provides the most information, it requires the highest level of in-depth analysis by researchers well-versed with the metadata. Summary data serves to turn the large data sets into something more manageable. There are several different types of summary data, but they all are supposed to present the key findings from the analyzable data according to the prespecified SAP. When clinical trial sponsors seek FDA approval, they submit clinical study reports (CSRs).[81] According to the FDA, a CSR is "an 'integrated' full report of an individual study of any therapeutic, prophylactic, or diagnostic agent (referred to herein as drug or treatment) conducted in patients."[82]

Encompassing thousands of pages, CSRs should provide practically all the necessary information for the FDA to gauge the safety and efficacy of a particular treatment. Along with summaries, tables, and graphs of key measurements, such as primary outcomes and adverse events, CSRs also include considerable amounts of supplemental data. As CSRs are predominantly only prepared for and read by clinical trial investigators and sponsors along with the FDA, they may include personally identifiable information of participants and/or commercially sensitive information.

Industry rarely voluntarily shares CSRs or IPD with anyone outside federal regulators. Instead, the public has access to much more limited summary information. Trial registries, such as the congressionally-created ClinicalTrials.gov, provide public audiences with basic trial information far less detailed than that included in a CSR.[83] Trial data registered on ClinicalTrials.gov largely include surface-level information on characteristics of participants and main outcomes.[84]

FDA reviewers representing various scientific disciplines, rather than clinical trialists, produce another form of summary data: they conduct discipline-specific reviews to determine whether the FDA should approve the product. These reports include data from various clinical studies conducted for a particular product. Since the reviewers have access to significantly more data than the public, their analyses can reveal information otherwise not found publicly or in medical publications.[85] While FDA review documents may reveal otherwise nonpublic information, they, in no way, approach the full documentation of IPD and CSRs.

Before 2020, the FDA posted all the officers' reports reviewing a drug/biologic through the lens of different disciplines.[86] The FDA has since adopted an "integrated review" process, where the public no longer has access to all the individual reviews. Instead, the FDA posts an integrated assessment that consolidates the findings of the various disciplines. Supporters of the new model tout the improved ability for readers to comprehend the information due to removing duplicative information and streamlining.[87] Critics argue that it reduces the amount of information available to researchers and the public, and it can both hide disagreements between reviewers and stifle dissent within the FDA.[88]

Product labels are also summary data available to the public. Labels are primarily meant to guarantee patient safety by providing summary information on how to dose and administer the treatment along with its safety and efficacy.[89] Therefore, the label contains information on topics such as dosage and administration, indications (approved reasons for usage), contraindications (harmful usage circumstances), interactions (the effect of a drug when taken alongside another drug), the most frequent adverse reactions (those reported at or above a specified rate), and a brief overview of clinical trial results. Drug companies draft labels, and the FDA approves them with the primary intended audience of medical professionals rather than the public.[90]

Perhaps the most relevant form of summary data for patients is when trial researchers seek to publish their work in medical journals. They submit a manuscript that includes limited and selective summaries of trial data. While different journals have their own requirements, these summaries come from manuscripts written by clinical trial researchers, which include selected elements of the data. Typically, manuscripts include similar data points to those submitted to trial registries. Yet, journals and their peer reviewers cannot verify the completeness and accuracy of the summary data in submitted manuscripts due to a lack of access to either IPD or CSRs. While researchers may sometimes gain access to IPD at the discretion of clinical trial sponsors, this often occurs years after initial article publication in medical journals.[91]

Overall, independent researchers, health care professionals, and the public do not have access to the underlying clinical data, instead relying upon limited summary data. As the Institute of Medicine recognized, the "primary method for sharing clinical trial data with the scientific and medical communities, as well as the public" is through publication in peer-reviewed scientific journals.[92] The peer review process involves experts in a relevant field vetting the findings and claims made by researchers. Yet, when pharmaceutical companies and researchers behind clinical trials submit manuscripts to journals, the peer reviewers do not have access to the underlying clinical trial data necessary to actually vet their claims. Consequently, the vetters of the most important means of disseminating medical knowledge take at face value the claims of manuscript authors and pharmaceutical companies seeking favorable reviews of their products.

## What about the FDA?

For medical products to reach the market, they must undergo testing through phased clinical trials.[93] Phase I clinical trials test the safety and side effects of a particular intervention in a small group of participants (typically 20–80 people), phase II trials primarily investigate effectiveness along with safety in a larger participant pool (roughly 100–300 people), and phase III trials test both safety and effectiveness in even larger scale populations (1,000–3,000+ people, depending on intended patient population). The FDA collects data from all three phases when deciding if a product is sufficiently safe and effective for regulatory approval for specific uses. Manufacturers and researchers may also conduct phase IV clinical trials after FDA approval to track effectiveness and safety as the public uses the intervention.

While the FDA regulatory approval process strives to ensure that pharmaceuticals, biologics, and medical devices on the market are reasonably effective and safe for specific uses, it has significant limitations. Regulatory agencies have limited resources and can have trouble detecting important details about efficacy and safety, such as adverse events, throughout the tens or hundreds of thousands of pages of clinical trial information.[94] For example, in 2005, an FDA advisory committee recommended approval of the drug muraglitazar.[95] However, independent researchers who managed to access underlying data from phase II and III clinical trials conducted their own analysis, finding that the drug had serious adverse side effects like major cardiovascular events including strokes and even death.[96] Luckily, the outside analyses prevented FDA approval for muraglitazar; however, preapproval access to clinical data is the exception rather than the rule. A 2017 *JAMA* analysis found that 32.0 percent of novel pharmaceutical drugs and biologics approved by the FDA from 2001 to 2010 had significant safety issues after approval.[97]

The FDA does not require clinical trials to test medical interventions against existing, comparable treatment methods; they often test against a placebo.[98] Therefore, FDA approval does not inform doctors and patients whether a particular treatment is better than existing therapies. Additionally, a drug may statistically provide a benefit on average, but it could also have a poor number needed to treat (NNT). In other words, a drug may statistically benefit a tested population of 3,000 people, but only 1 out of 300 people who receive the treatment would get the benefit. Similarly, the same drug could have a poor number needed to harm (NNH), where the likelihood of an adverse event, even if lower than the likelihood of receiving a benefit, is unreasonably high in relation to the actual chance of benefit.

Furthermore, the FDA relies on the integrity of industry-sponsored research. A pharmaceutical company tests its own product; the FDA merely reviews the data from any relevant trials. Thus, the regulating agency—which the public entrusts with guaranteeing the safety and effectiveness of medical products—itself relies upon industry to sponsor scientifically sound research. While companies used to predominantly contract with academics to conduct research, they dramatically shifted to using for-profit CROs and used their leverage to make academic institutions they still contract with more subservient to their interests.

Additionally, the FDA's role does not involve verifying whether published articles in medical journals are misleading as to the actual effect of an approved product. As long as manufacturers do not illegally market their product—such as advertising unapproved, off-label uses—the FDA leaves them alone.[99] Therefore, without appropriate vetting by peer reviewers, published articles in medical journals rely on potentially biased and limited summary data.

The FDA's regulatory capacity is especially limited given widespread off-label usage of drugs. As noted by Dr. Gail Van Norman: the FDA regulates the marketing of drugs and devices but "it does not regulate the practice of medicine, and physicians are legally free to use them for purposes other than that for which they were approved."[100] While the exact number of drug prescriptions for off-label use is unknown, estimates show that they can constitute up to a third of prescriptions for common drugs. As off-label uses inherently are not for approved purposes, they also are often based on little to no scientific evidence. This places significantly more control into the hands of industry to manipulate and/or hide whatever evidence exists because the FDA likely has either not evaluated the data to determine safety and efficacy or it has but not approved those particular uses.

In 2010, a Massachusetts jury found Pfizer guilty of illegally marketing its epilepsy drug Neurontin for off-label uses—namely treatment of neuropathic or nerve pain, bipolar disorder, and migraines—mandating that the company pay $142 million.[101] The FDA approved Neurontin initially in 1993 for treatment of epilepsy, and subsequent indication approvals did not permit marketing of the drug for general neuropathic pain. In fact, the FDA told Pfizer in a May 2001 meeting, "the general neuropathic pain indication cannot be granted for Neurontin."[102] Yet, as of September 2001, Pfizer's own data showed that 93.5 percent of Neurontin usage in the United States was for unapproved, off-label uses, and the company's operating plans for Neurontin revolved around off-label prescriptions. One internal Pfizer document explicitly stated that "Growth of Neurontin Is Outside Epilepsy."

As part of the trial, Dr. John Abramson served as an expert witness, writing a report finding that the original owner of the drug, Parke-Davis, and later Pfizer spread false and misleading information to deceive insurers and physicians. These duplicitous methods were, in part, controlling and manipulating the "research design, analysis, and publication of clinical trials" along with hiding evidence.[103] For example, Parke-Davis knew a 1997 company-sponsored study showed that Neurontin was likely no better than placebo in treating diabetic neuropathy, yet this finding was not published. Rather, opposite conclusions of the study claiming that Neurontin could be effective were presented at a conference for the American Academy of Neurology and published in the *Journal of Neurology, Neurosurgery & Psychiatry*.[104] This was done by ignoring the study design and simply showing that Neurontin-treated patients indeed experienced less pain over time without showing that the same was true for the placebo group.

While *JAMA* published a company-sponsored study in 1998 showing that Neurontin significantly reduced diabetic neuropathic pain compared to placebo, the study design was heavily biased.[105] The researchers increased the dosage of Neurontin given to participants over the length of the study to more than twice the FDA-approved limit. The drug caused so many side effects that it unblinded the study participants, biasing the results. An independent analysis done with the IPD obtained as part of the litigation found that 90 percent of the reported pain reduction came after the onset of side effects, meaning after patients were de facto alerted that they had received the treatment.[106] A larger 1999 study with a different design that didn't unblind the participants through increasing the provided dosage found that Neurontin did not reduce pain compared to placebo. After absorbing Parke-Davis as a subsidiary in 2000, Pfizer did not publish this study as an independent paper, and a Parke-Davis employee revealed in an email that a Parke-Davis medical director "made it very clear that we should take care not to publish anything that damages neurontin's marketing success."[107] Pfizer did attempt to publish positive spins of the results but was rejected by several medical journals for poor statistics and unjustified conclusions.

Another expert report from Dr. Jeffrey Barkin buttressed Dr. Abramson's findings: directly resulting from "the concealment of misrepresentation of critical Level 1 Evidence, many psychiatrists became falsely convinced that Neurontin was a safe and effective treatment for bipolar disorder."[108] Barkin lambasted Pfizer and Parke-Davis for pushing such a conclusion based on "the illusion of scientific support." The Neurontin case is one where the government took industry to trial and where trial documents have become publicly available. Yet, while off-label prescribing is common, such accountability and transparency into the internal workings of industry is not.

Moreover, the lack of clinical trial data transparency outside of the FDA leaves health care professionals unequipped to provide the best care to American patients. The FDA only approves medical products, it does not examine the relative clinical and cost-effectiveness between treatments. In the United States, public and private payers individually conduct these types of analyses; however, they do so without access to the underlying clinical trial data. Therefore, the ability for public and private health insurers to cover the most clinically- and cost-effective treatments is significantly limited. Similarly, physicians who rely upon the published literature in peer-reviewed medical journals are not properly equipped to prescribe the optimal treatments for their patients.

## Tamiflu

Industry sponsorship bias and control of trial data not only can misinform doctors but it can lead to governments spending billions on products that do not work as advertised. This was the case with Roche's drug oseltamivir, more commonly known as the brand name Tamiflu. In 1999, the FDA approved Tamiflu as a treatment for influenza within adult populations.[109] The FDA approved Tamiflu for the prophylaxis or prevention of influenza in everyone aged thirteen years and older in November 2000 and then everyone aged one year and older when presenting symptoms for a maximum of two days in December 2000. Other countries followed in approving the drug with Japan doing so in December 2000, the European Medicines Agency (EMA) in June 2002, and India in October 2005.

In 2003, a *JAMA Internal Medicine* meta-analysis assessed the effect of using Tamiflu to treat patients aged thirteen through ninety-seven with influenza-like illness.[110] The meta-analysis included ten Roche-sponsored, placebo-controlled, and double-blinded RCTs. The study examined influenza-like illnesses because often when people discuss getting the flu, that refers to not just influenza but similar illnesses like rhinovirus and coronavirus, and doctors usually don't test to distinguish between them when treating patients.[111] The meta-analysis reported that Tamiflu significantly reduced lower respiratory tract complications (LRTCs), antibiotic use, and hospitalization for both healthy adults and those in higher risk groups. Yet the FDA, which had access to the same clinical trials, had concluded that Tamiflu did not reduce complications, and it even sent a letter to Roche in 2000 for marketing misleading claims like that Tamiflu "reduces the incidence of secondary complications (i.e., bacterial infections) by 45%."[112]

The global nonprofit organization known as the Cochrane Collaboration or Cochrane conducts systematic reviews of the medical literature to provide conclusions on what the evidence shows regarding specific questions for various health interventions.[113] The organization has been a widely respected source of medical knowledge for health care professionals and policymakers. In April 2005, Cochrane reviewed neuraminidase inhibitors (NIs)—the class of drug that Tamiflu belongs to—for preventing and treating influenza in adults.[114] The review relied on the 2003 meta-analysis and concluded that NIs should not be used seasonally to control influenza due to low effectiveness, but "in a serious epidemic or pandemic, NIs should be used with other public health measures."

In the following years, governments across the globe spent billions stockpiling Tamiflu: the only NI available in oral form.[115] In 2006, HHS sent a letter of intent to Roche stating that the United States sought to purchase enough of the drug to treat 46 million people.[116] As of 2014, the United States spent $1.5 billion on stockpiling Tamiflu while the UK spent £424 million or $710 million.[117] Globally, Roche earned $18 billion from Tamiflu from its launch in 1999 to 2014.[118] The World Health Organization (WHO) designated Tamiflu as a "core" medication, defined as those needed for a basic health care system that are "the most efficacious, safe and cost-effective medicines for priority conditions."[119]

In April 2009, the UK government commissioned an update of Cochrane's systematic review of NIs to add a safety assessment component to their 2008 review following the outbreak of H1N1, otherwise known as the swine flu.[120] However, a Japanese pediatrician, Dr. Keiji Hayashi, sent a comment to the Cochrane authors pointing out that they had not made their previous conclusions on NIs based on their own calculations. Only two of the ten Roche-sponsored RCTs from the 2003 meta-analysis had been published in peer-reviewed medical journals. Thus, eight of the studies had never been examined by peer reviewers in addition to the fact that the Cochrane authors generally lacked access to the underlying trial data.

Due to Hayashi's comment, the Cochrane authors lead by Dr. Tom Jefferson requested the full CSRs for all ten RCTs from Roche. Jefferson and two of his fellow authors Drs. Peter Doshi and Chris Del Mar wrote a *PLOS Medicine* article titled "The Imperative to Share Clinical Study Reports: Recommendations from the Tamiflu Experience."[121] They sought access to CSRs rather than published articles from peer-reviewed biomedical journals due to the fact that they are far larger, have much more detail, "and represent the most complete synthesis of the planning, execution, and results of a clinical trial." However, it took four years of persistent requests and efforts from the Cochrane team from 2009 to 2013 until Roche provided the full CSRs in 2013.[122]

Armed with most of the underlying clinical trial data, the authors updated the Cochrane review in 2014. They found that NIs like Tamiflu had very minimal impacts on treating and preventing influenza, reducing the time to first alleviation of symptoms from 7 to 6.3 days for adults, with similar effects in healthy children and no effect in asthmatic children.[123] Tamiflu reduced the risk of symptomatic but not asymptomatic influenza, and it had no impact on serious complications, hospitalizations, and death. No data suggested the drug stopped viral transmission. At the same time, the review found harms of Tamiflu treatment, such as for every twenty-eight and twenty-two people treated with the drug, one would have nausea and vomiting, respectively. Additionally, for every thirty-two and ninety-four people treated with Tamiflu, one person would have headaches and psychiatric adverse events, respectively. The Cochrane authors also noted significant "evidence of selective reporting" bias from studies of Tamiflu along with other issues like performance bias from "non-identical presentation of placebo" and attrition biases stemming from participants leaving during the studies.

Even though the FDA had access to Roche's clinical trials and had even sent a letter to stop Roche's misleading marketing practices in 2000, industry control of the clinical trials led to widespread, global purchases of Tamiflu worth billions of dollars. Selective reporting and concealment of underlying clinical trial data allowed for Roche to get a positive meta-analysis published in one of the worlds' leading peer-reviewed medical journals without the ability for outside actors to vet its claims. Only years after the Cochrane authors got access to the full CSRs, the WHO downgraded Tamiflu in 2017 from a core to a complementary drug, meaning it is part of a group still deemed to include "essential medicines for priority diseases."[124] However, such drugs are also less cost effective and/or are used in specialized settings. This action came after roughly a decade of global health leaders believing that Tamiflu was a necessary and significantly effective drug.

While Tom Jefferson and his coauthors eventually got ahold of the full CSRs for the ten Roche-sponsored trials, this is an exception to the current rule with clinical trial data. Pharmaceutical companies and other industry sponsors control and conduct impactful research for the many medical products Americans use, doctors prescribe, and governments even purchase even though these actors don't have access to the underlying data. Just as access to the CSRs for Tamiflu revealed significant biases within the conduct of the studies and their selective reporting, how many studies underlying the treatments that Americans rely upon are similarly biased and not as effective or safe as industry claims?

# 2

# Less Opaque Is Still Opaque

Over the past several decades, Congress has passed multiple pieces of legislation, and agencies have consequently promulgated regulations to increase clinical trial transparency. While these efforts have significantly increased the amount of information readily available to the public, this outcome is largely due to the severe lack of any transparency that existed beforehand. Thus, these improvements have contributed toward an illusion of progress while industry still protectively guards against public disclosure of the underlying data behind their clinical trials.

Before the twenty-first century, the United States lacked any federal, centralized database for clinical trial information. Registries and databases were highly fragmented and usually specific to certain diseases.[1] According to a 2003 estimate in *JAMA* by Drs. Kay Dickersin and Drummond Rennie, only about half of clinical trials were publicly reported from the 1950s through 2003.[2] The number of trials with meaningful amounts of data available to the public was certainly far lower.

Advocates of trial registration argued that it would reduce the publication bias that existed with just published clinical trial results. In a 1986 article, researcher R. J. Simes called for an international registry of clinical trials.[3] Simes reasoned that published clinical trials are likely biased with positive or promising results for treatments, while a registry of clinical trials would require trial registration before participant enrollment, reducing the chance of bias.

The first federally funded registry for clinical trials was the AIDS Clinical Trials Information Service (ACTIS) that the FDA and NIH established in 1989.[4] The first reported cases of HIV/AIDS in the United States came in 1981, and the disease progressively became an epidemic through the 1980s.[5] As the disease represented a relatively new area for clinical research, critical information about potential treatments came from clinical trials occurring around the time.[6] In 1988, the National Institute of Allergy and Infectious Diseases found that a centralized telephone service would ideally provide information about clinical trial results to health professionals and the public. Patient advocates also lobbied Congress to increase their access to innovative treatments from clinical trials.[7]

Consequently, Congress passed the Health Omnibus Programs Extension (HOPE) Act in 1988.[8] The legislation tasked the HHS secretary in consultation with the FDA commissioner, the Clinical Research Review Committee, and the director of the Office of AIDS Research to create a data bank of information on clinical trials and AIDS treatments. The data bank would include both NIH-funded and privately funded clinical trials. Additionally, HHS had to disseminate such information to the public, affected AIDS patients, health care professionals, and researchers.

By 1989, the NIH, FDA, and CDC enforced the HOPE Act through the creation of ACTIS. In May 1989, the ACTIS phone service—where trained professionals could educate callers on clinical trial information—became operational.[9] By August 1989, the NIH's National Library of Medicine (NLM) made the information in the ACTIS database searchable online. However, the online database only became available on the World Wide Web in 1996, as the Web became available to the public in 1993.[10]

The ACTIS database's purpose was primarily to promote trial participation and interest in the treatments tested in clinical trials. As the CDC described, ACTIS information pertained to the purpose of study protocols, locations, eligibility requirements, exclusion criteria, and the names and telephone numbers of contact people.[11] The database was not created to provide detailed levels of results data; it just included "bibliographic references to published results."[12]

## The Creation of ClinicalTrials.gov

Patient advocacy led to the creation of the first version of ClinicalTrials.gov: the contemporary national registry of clinical trial data in the United States. In the mid-1990s, lobbying and advocacy by breast cancer community members pushed for federal funding of a publicly available clinical trial data resource.[13] In 1997, Congress passed the Food and Drug Administration Modernization Act (FDAMA).[14] The legislation required the FDA through the director of the National Institutes of Health to "establish, maintain, and operate a data bank of information on clinical trials for drugs for serious or life-threatening diseases and conditions." Thus, this data bank was limited, being restricted to investigational new drug (IND) applications—which all new drugs without FDA approval must complete—and only for those drugs targeted to treat diseases and conditions that the FDA deemed to be serious or life-threatening.[15] Simultaneously, Congress intended for the data bank's audience to include the public, especially those with a vested interest in trial results like cancer patients.

The bank contained a registry of federally funded and privately funded clinical trials, including eligibility criteria for participation in the trial, descriptions of trial site locations, and a point of contact for people seeking to enroll in the trial. FDA guidance in March 2002 would further specify that the data bank would also include information on study design.[16] The FDAMA allowed the data bank to include information on the results of the clinical trials; however, this was not a requirement and was conditional on "the consent of the sponsor." Thus, the pharmaceutical company sponsoring a particular drug trial would have to give consent for the data bank to include data showing whether their treatment was safe and effective.

FDAMA Section 113 required that clinical trial sponsors submit the required information within twenty-one days after the trial became open for participant enrollment. Within two to five days of submission, the NIH would then publish the information on the data bank.[17] However, the legislation did not include any penalties for noncompliance.

On February 29, 2000, the NLM launched ClinicalTrials.gov as part of what it called "the first phase of a consumer-friendly database."[18] In this first phase, most of the information registered on the online database pertained to NIH-funded clinical trials. Information for over 4,000 trials were available upon launch. However, the limited and often voluntary nature of trial registrations on ClinicalTrials.gov allowed drug and device companies to avoid disclosure.[19] Members of Congress and the Senate introduced two similar versions of the Fair Access to Clinical Trials Act of 2004 to create mandatory trial registration; however, neither became law.

In 2007, Congress passed the Food and Drug Administration Amendments Act, significantly increasing the number of trials that responsible parties—trial sponsors or principal investigators designated by the sponsor—had to submit to ClinicalTrials.gov.[20] Section 801 of the FDAAA expanded the types of clinical trials contained in the database to include any "controlled clinical investigation" of any drug or biologic for any disease or condition that is regulated by the FDA except for phase I clinical investigations.[21] Phase I investigations have small patient populations and test for safety rather than effectiveness. The legislation also required clinical trials that prospectively test an intervention with a medical device against a human control group to register with the database. It additionally required sponsors to submit postmarket surveillance of marketed devices for pediatric care. Thus, the FDAAA represented a significant increase in the scope of the ClinicalTrials.gov database from the FDAMA.

The FDAAA similarly increased the amount of information responsible parties submitted to ClinicalTrials.gov, including limited results data. Along with descriptive information about the study itself—participants and participant eligibility, trial location and contact information, and administrative data—the legislation requires the submission of results data for applicable drug and device clinical trials. This results information includes a summary of prespecified primary and secondary outcome measures for each treatment/comparison group including statistical analyses of such measures.[22] Additionally, the sponsor or principal investigator must submit a summary of both anticipated and unanticipated adverse event data that exceed a 5 percent frequency threshold within each treatment group.[23] Lastly, ClinicalTrials.gov submissions must include data on participant flow (how individuals progress through the trial) and demographic and baseline characteristics.

To bolster transparency, the legislation required responsible parties to submit summary information in both "non-technical, understandable language for patients" and a technical manner.[24] Although regulators could limit this requirement based on determining whether parties can submit summaries without being misleading or promotional. Along with making language more accessible, the FDAAA required submission of each applicable trial's full protocol and statistical analysis plan so that observers could determine to what extent the trial results mirror what researchers intended to investigate.

The FDAAA mandated responsible parties to register clinical trials on ClinicalTrials.gov no later than twenty-one days after the enrollment of the first participant. The NIH would then publicly post the submitted information online within thirty days of submission. For results data, the legislation and subsequent rulemaking mandated that responsible parties submit data within one year of the trial's primary completion date, meaning the date of the final data collection for the trial's prespecified primary outcome measures.[25] However, the legislation allowed for delaying of the results submission deadline if the drug/device had not received FDA marketing approval, if the manufacturer had filed or would file an application for a new approved use, or if a responsible party's extension request "demonstrates good cause for the extension and provides an estimate of the date on which the information will be submitted."[26] Congress prescribed civil monetary penalties and the withholding of grant funds as penalties for failure to comply with the FDAAA.

As a result of the FDAAA, results data became publicly available on ClinicalTrials.gov by September 2008.[27] However, submission of adverse event data did not become mandatory until September 2009. At the same time, HHS did not finish rulemaking to better implement Section 801 of the FDAAA until September 2016, nearly a decade after the legislation's passage (see Figure 2).[28] Various elements required for submission under the legislation were optional until the 2016 final rule. These included but were not limited to the primary purpose of the trial, the interventional study model, and the number of arms (e.g., placebo and treatment groups) in the study along with information about each arm.[29]

Moreover, the final rule also took advantage of rulemaking discretion granted from the FDAAA to expand the applicability of clinical trial transparency requirements. For example, the rule required all applicable clinical trials, even those for unapproved products, to submit results data.[30] It enhanced the levels of specification for outcome measures, making sure that data included the name of a specific measure, a description of the used metric, and the points in time when the assessment for the measurement occurred. The rule required submission of the timeline of adverse events along with the inclusion of all-cause mortality. Additionally, the rule mandated that the responsible party must submit a trial's statistical analysis plan at the same time as its results data to ensure that viewers could contextualize the information.

On the same day as the final rule, the NIH issued a final policy to expand transparency for NIH-funded clinical trials.[31] The policy mandated that all clinical trials receiving funding from the NIH register with and submit information to ClinicalTrials.gov. This requirement applied to all trials including those otherwise not covered by the FDAAA.

In *Seife v. U.S. Department of Health & Human Services* (2020), the US District Court for the Southern District of New York further solidified the final rule's expanded result reporting requirements for unapproved products.[32] Prior to the case, HHS interpreted the final rule to not require submission of results data for clinical trials where the trial was completed between the effective dates of the FDAAA (September 27, 2007) and the final rule (January 18, 2017) and the relevant drug/device had not received FDA approval before trial completion. Investigative reporter Charles Seife and Center for Science in the Public Interest president Peter Lurie sued HHS for depriving them of access to data that the FDAAA required to be publicly available on ClinicalTrials.gov. Ultimately, the court rejected HHS' interpretation, ruling that the results data for the previously exempted clinical trials completed between 2007 and 2017 had to be submitted to ClinicalTrials.gov.

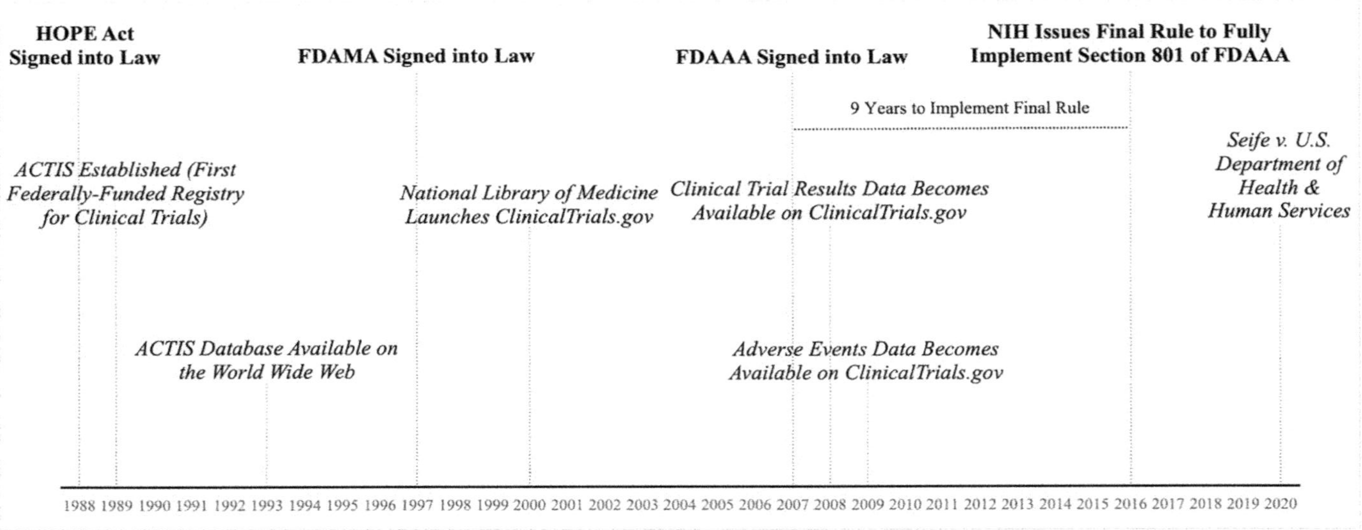


**Figure 2** A timeline of major legislative and regulatory actions surrounding the creation of a national registry of clinical trials in the United States.

## Limitations of ClinicalTrials.gov

While registrations on ClinicalTrials.gov have increased over time, the FDA and NIH have failed to enforce statutory requirements for registration and data submission. An *NEJM* analysis of clinical trial registrations from 2012 to 2014 found that nearly a third (32.8 percent) were registered late; a majority of late registrations (57.0 percent) were late by over a year.[33] A *PLOS One* study of 400 randomly selected clinical trials completed in 2008 found that 29.5 percent did not publish their primary outcomes in a medical journal and/or post results data to ClinicalTrials.gov within four years of completion.[34] Another analysis in *BMJ* examined trials registered on ClinicalTrials.gov that were completed in 2009, fell under the FDAAA, and investigated a drug that already had approval from the FDA.[35] The researchers found that only 163 (22.1 percent) of the 738 trials within their criteria had reported results within the one-year deadline.

Although the NIH designed its 2016 final rule to better implement the FDAAA, many clinical trials still fail to register with ClinicalTrials.gov. An analysis in *The Lancet* tracked all applicable trials due to report results under the FDAAA from March 2018 through September 2019.[36] The authors found that only 1,722 (40.9 percent) of the 4,209 trials reported results within the one-year deadline, and just 63.8 percent of the trials had results submitted at all. A 2020 investigation by *Science* examined 4,700 clinical trials from 184 sponsor organizations that should have registered with ClinicalTrials.gov under the 2016 rule.[37] *Science* found that twenty-nine of the sponsor organizations (15.7 percent) never met a deadline as of September 25, 2019 and had at least five trials due.[38] The twenty-nine sponsors did not report any results for two-thirds of their trials and were 268 days late on average for all trials that missed a deadline.

While there is evidence that the number of trials registered on ClinicalTrials.gov is improving over time, there has been an increasing discrepancy between the number of trials registered and those that posted results. According to the FDAAA Trials Tracker run by the University of Oxford, the percentage of trials reported on ClinicalTrials.gov has increased from 66 percent in May 2019 to 78.3 percent in July 2025.[39] However, an *NEJM* article tracked the cumulative number of trials registered on ClinicalTrials.gov between 2007 and 2018 as of May 8, 2019.[40] The authors found that while the cumulative number of registered trials naturally rose over the period, the gap between trials registered and trials that posted results data widened. In 2010, the difference was around 15,000 articles, and the discrepancy grew to over 40,000 by 2018.

Even though there has been significant noncompliance with the FDAAA over its lifespan and that of ClinicalTrials.gov, the government has failed to use its enforcement authorities to penalize unlawful behavior. After the investigation by *Science*, Lyric Jorgenson—then deputy director of the NIH—said the NIH had been "trying to change the culture of how clinical trial results are reported and disseminated; not so much on the 'aha, we caught you,' as much as getting people to understand the value, and making it as easy as possible to share and disseminate results."[41] Another FDA official, Patrick McNeilly, remarked, the "FDA has limited resources, and we encourage voluntary compliance." Since the enactment of the FDAAA in 2007, it took fourteen years for the

FDA to issue its first notice of noncompliance in 2021.[42] The agency has now issued seven notices of noncompliance.[43] According to the FDAAA Trials Tracker, the federal government could have levied nearly $95.2 billion in fines for noncompliance as of July 2025, but it has claimed $0.[44]

Even if the widespread failure of trial reporting required by the FDAAA did not exist, ClinicalTrials.gov is severely limited as a source of clinical trial data. Responsible parties are not required to submit complete metadata, detailed summary data (e.g., CSRs), or any form of individual participant data. Therefore, the registry does not provide peer reviewers of medical journals, doctors, other health care professionals, or members of the public sufficient information to vet and investigate safety and efficacy from clinical trials. Dr. John Abramson, an expert witness in multiple drug trials, wrote, "drug companies' posting of unaudited summary results on internet registries is hardly a substitute for genuine transparency and independent analysis of clinical trial data."[45] A 2016 comparison of results data found on ClinicalTrials.gov with the FDA reviews found on the FDA's website found that 98 percent of the primary outcome data on ClinicalTrials.gov had corresponding data on the FDA's website.[46] More specifically, 95 percent of primary outcomes had concordant definitions and 78 percent had concordant results. Thus, much of the key results data on ClinicalTrials.gov is not unique on the publicly accessible landscape.

In 2012, Senator Bernie Sanders (I-VT) introduced an amendment to the Food and Drug Administration Safety and Innovation Act (FDASIA) that would have required numerous transparency measures.[47] Importantly, the amendment would have bolstered the data publicly available on ClinicalTrials.gov, including requiring drug sponsors to submit de-identified IPD that included the number of people participating in a trial at each phase, a description of the dosage given to each participant, and a description of the results for every individual. The pharmaceutical industry opposed Sanders's proposal. Andrew Emmett, managing director of science and regulatory affairs at the Biotechnology Industry Organization—a lobbying group representing biotechnology companies—sent out a memo laying out the industry's opposition.[48] Regarding de-identified participant data, Emmett argued that such a requirement would be redundant as the sponsors already report that information to the FDA even though the Sanders amendment sought to make it publicly available. Additionally, he asserted, "it would be inappropriate to publicly disclose this information" during a trial, as it "could lead to bias and weaken" the data. However, the amendment did not require disclosure prior to trial completion, and making results public would inherently not retroactively bias trial outcomes. The amendment died, as the Senate never voted on it.

## The Freedom of Information Act

Given limited data disclosure from registries like ClinicalTrials.gov, the primary means for independent researchers, interest groups, members of the public, and any other outside actor to access clinical trial data for approved drugs is to file a Freedom of Information Act (FOIA) request.[49] While individuals can make FOIA requests for any agency record, one cannot simply ask for all the safety and efficacy data for a particular drug, biologic, or medical device that the FDA has. According to the Code of Federal Regulations, FOIA requests must be in writing and "reasonably describe the agency record sought."[50] This involves describing the records' subject matter, date of creation, and the person/office that created it. For clinical trial data specifically, a requester must ask for the specific metadata, summary data, or IPD that they are looking for.

Moreover, the FDA has avenues to avoid providing requested clinical trial data, and it has a history of deference to pharmaceutical industry interests. There are currently nine exemptions to FOIA requests, such as protecting information an agency deems "classified to protect national security."[51] The exemption most relevant to FOIA requests for clinical trial data is Exemption 4, which protects information that is "trade secrets and commercial or financial information obtained from a person [that is] privileged or confidential."[52] A review of FOIA requests made to HHS from 2008 to 2017 found that the most common exemption applied to FOIA requests at the FDA was Exemption 4.[53]

FDA prescribed definitions and policy written in regulations are essential to the level of disclosure afforded by FOIA, as the Supreme Court ruled in *Chrysler Corp. v. Brown* (1979) that FOIA exemptions do not prevent agencies from disclosing information.[54] Rather, the "exemptions were only meant to permit the agency to withhold certain information, and were not meant to mandate nondisclosure."[55] Whether Exemption 4 protects clinical trial data rests squarely in the lap of the FDA, which can choose to be either very transparent or restrictive. The FDA has chosen to be very restrictive through regulation, voluntarily opting to prevent itself from making data and information that it receives "within the definitions of a trade secret or confidential commercial or financial information" available for public disclosure.[56]

The FDA defines trade secrets and commercially confidential information (CCI) in federal regulations.[57] Trade secrets involve "any commercially valuable plan, formula, process, or device" that can be used to produce a trade commodity. Thus, trade secrets apply more to information on how to make a novel drug rather than clinical trials testing the safety and efficacy of a drug. The FDA defines CCI broadly as "valuable data or information which is used in one's business and is of a type customarily held in strict confidence or regarded as privileged and not disclosed to any member of the public by the person to whom it belongs." This definition gives wide latitude to the FDA to determine what may or may not constitute CCI.

Additionally, the FDA grants clinical trial sponsors and, thus, pharmaceutical companies control over what information is CCI. Federal regulations state that anyone who submits information to the government "may designate part or all of the information in such records as exempt from disclosure under exemption 4" either at the time of submission or "within a reasonable time thereafter."[58] President Ronald Reagan issued Executive Order 12600 in 1987, requiring federal agencies to notify submitters of information containing CCI of disclosure requests.[59] As a result, the FDA notifies companies that submitted their clinical trial data of FOIA requests and provides them ten working days "to object to disclosure of any part of the records and to state all bases for its objections."[60] Ultimately, the FDA has discretion to accept or deny the objections.

Yet, the FDA has a history of not verifying submitters requests to object to disclosure and/or redact information.[61] In *Seife v. Food and Drug Administration* (2019), the District Court judge Jesse Furman wrote that the FDA redactions pertaining to requested clinical trial information for Sarepta Therapeutics' drug Exondys 51 were overbroad, the agency made mistakes in all disputed categories of redaction, and he mandated the agency to rereview the entirety of the FOIA request.[62] In a 2006 article, the nonprofit consumer advocacy group Public Citizen's Peter Lurie and Allison Zieve document several cases where Public Citizen had to sue the FDA to get access to clinical data that the FDA improperly withheld under Exemption 4, such as data showing the drug Bextra's failure to treat acute pain.[63]

Companies' ability to block clinical trial data disclosure under Exemption 4 has become easier since the Supreme Court's decision in *Food Marketing Institute v. Argus Leader Media* (2019).[64] Prior to the decision, the government considered commercial information to be confidential if disclosure would either damage the government's ability to get necessary information in the future or cause substantial competitive harm to the submitter.[65] The Supreme Court struck down this standard, creating the new relevant definition for CCI: commercial or financial information that is "customarily and actually treated as private by its owner and provided to the government under an assurance of privacy."[66] This new definition greatly expands the ability for submitters to object to FOIA requests and for the FDA to voluntarily restrict disclosure. Dissenting to the Court's new interpretation of Exemption 4, Justice Stephen Breyer wrote:

> The fact that private actors have "customarily and actually treated" commercial information as secret ... cannot be enough to justify nondisclosure. After all, where information is already publicly available, people do not submit FOIA requests—they use Google ... [G]iven the temptation, common across the private and public sectors, to regard as secret all information that need not be disclosed, I fear the majority's reading will deprive the public of information for reasons no better than convenience, skittishness, or bureaucratic inertia.[67]

Breyer's warning that the new definition will limit FOIA requests due to "bureaucratic inertia" is not without merit, as FOIA requests can both take years to fulfill and are extremely costly. From fiscal years 2019–24, the FDA received an average of roughly 10,257 FOIA requests each year (11,702 for fiscal year [FY] 2024).[68] The average number of requests still pending by the end of the fiscal year were approximately 4,017 over the same period (4,242 for FY 2024). The FOIA requests to the FDA are also more complex than other agencies, such as the Centers for Medicare & Medicaid Services (CMS), and often take more than sixty days to process.[69] However, requests can take far longer to process, especially attempts to receive detailed clinical trial data, and they do not guarantee approval.[70] In an extreme example, when scientists and medical researchers filed a FOIA request to get access to 455,000 pages of clinical information for the Pfizer-BioNTech COVID-19 vaccine, the FDA claimed it would take seventy-five years to complete the request.[71] Ultimately, the requesters sued, and the US District

Court for the Northern District of Texas ruled in 2022 that the FDA had to begin with releasing 12,000 pages before the end of January 2022 and continue releasing documents at a rate of 55,000 pages a month.[72]

Filing FOIA requests can also be very expensive, placing independent researchers at a significant disadvantage in comparison to pharmaceutical companies that want to block disclosure. Requesters must pay FOIA fees to the FDA when requesting information.[73] While the average cost in fees is not significant—as the FDA charges $0.10 per page for noncommercial requesters—requests for large amounts of data can cost tens of thousands of dollars.[74] Additionally, FOIA requesters can rack up significant costs through legal fees for preparing a request and going through litigation to successfully get access to information.

The FDA also restricts access to information by barring disclosure of clinical trial data prior to its approval decision. However, if a New Drug Application (NDA) becomes publicly known, the FDA gives itself the option to release a summary of chosen parts of the safety and effectiveness data that the agency deems "appropriate for public consideration of a specific pending issue."[75]

While FOIA requests are currently the primary mechanism for acquiring detailed clinical trial data like CSRs, requests made to the FDA are likely dominated by commercial interests. Using data acquired from responses to her own FOIA request, Margaret Kwoka found that commercial requesters made 7,615 (74.9 percent) of 10,167 FOIA requests to the FDA in 2013.[76] But rather than being pharmaceutical companies, information resellers were the dominant type of commercial requester.

Ultimately, the FOIA is not close to resembling a comprehensive, accessible means for researchers, medical professionals, and the public to get access to clinical trial data. The process is inherently reactive, so requesters must already know about the specific information they want to access. While people have, at times, gotten access to detailed trial data like CSRs through FOIA requests, the FDA has opted to restrict its own ability to release information, and the agency has given significant leeway to clinical trial sponsors to block disclosure. The Supreme Court's decision in *Food Marketing Institute v. Argus Leader Media* (2019) has amplified this reality. FOIA requests can both take significant amounts of time and cost large sums of money. Importantly, the process of requesting data through FOIA has little impact on the decision-making of doctors who predominantly rely upon medical knowledge disseminated in peer-reviewed medical journals.

## The European Model

Regarding clinical trials of pharmaceutical products and medical devices, all countries in the European Union (EU) follow the rules and regulations of the European Medicines Agency (EMA). Like the FDAAA's requirements, the EMA mandates registration for all clinical trials. While the EMA's policy is like the FDAAA in terms of clinical trial registration, the EMA provides far greater access to detailed clinical trial data, including CSRs, when compared to the FDA.

All clinical trials in the EU must register with the publicly accessible database Clinical Trials Information System (CTIS).[77] After trial completion, sponsors must report result data to CTIS within twelve months.[78] Like ClinicalTrials.gov, CTIS provides limited summary data that are searchable and publicly available online. These data include baseline characteristics of participants, primary and secondary endpoint descriptions and results, and adverse events.

In November 2010, the EMA issued Policy 0043, allowing widespread access to any documents about medicinal products for humans and animals upon freedom-of-information requests.[79] The EMA conducts redactions to protect personal information of participants and commercially confidential information. Requesters of information are limited to citizens of the EU along with natural and legal persons that reside within an EU member state. Requesters must reveal their identity and affiliation; however, they need not describe the purpose of their data inquiry. Consequently, on a case-by-case basis, the EMA's Policy 0043 has allowed release of detailed clinical trial data such as CSRs. However, as the freedom-of-information requests are reactive rather than proactive, the amount of data released has been limited. From 2010 to 2016, the EMA fulfilled 823 requests representing 380,911 released pages that, considering the great size of CSRs and other documents, is limited.[80]

In January 2015, the EMA launched phase I of a proactive data transparency program through Policy 0070.[81] For noncommercial purposes, this policy allows anyone to access metadata and clinical reports that are narrowly redacted to prevent identification of any trial participants along with revelation of commercially sensitive information. Data were only available for clinical trial data submitted to the EMA on or after January 1, 2015. Clinical reports include CSRs, clinical overviews, and clinical summaries. The CSRs also have appendices relating to trial protocol and protocol amendments, sample case report forms, and documentation of statistical methods. Additionally, Policy 0070 makes data available predominantly for clinical trials relevant to "marketing authorisation applications" (MAAs)—applications to be able to market a product within the EU.[82] Under 0070, the EMA publishes clinical reports sixty days after the European Commission makes a decision to approve an MAA.[83]

To access the data, individuals must simply register with the EMA website; afterward, they can view clinical reports but not download them. However, people can gain the ability to download clinical reports by providing more identifying information that includes their passport or ID card number.[84] Downloaded reports have a watermark to prevent commercial use. Policy 0070 was meant to include disclosure of IPD starting in May 2025, but the EMA dropped this update.[85]

While the EMA suspended the policy in 2018 due to the agency's relocation from London to Amsterdam following the UK's withdrawal from the EU, the EMA did reinstate it in September 2023.[86] During the COVID-19 pandemic, 0070 remained suspended except for data regarding COVID-19 vaccines and treatments. For the program restart, the EMA began publishing clinical data 120 days rather than 60 days after the European Commission's decision on the respective MAA.[87] By mid-2025, the EMA resumed disclosing data with the 120-day timeline for all new authorization applications excluding biosimilars, hybrids, and generics.[88]

## Canada Follows the European Model

The EMA transparency model transcends the EU, as Canada developed its data publishing program through Health Canada based on the EMA.[89] In 2019, Canada launched the Public Release of Clinical Information (PRCI) initiative to proactively make clinical data available 120 days after Health Canada provides or rejects regulatory approval for drugs and medical devices over a four-year phase-in period.[90] While the timeline for publishing data is longer, the EMA's Policy 0070 only applies to human drugs and biologics and not some medical device applications as in the PRCI initiative.[91] People can also get access to clinical data by requesting data rather than waiting for the prospective publishing. Through requests, the PRCI initiative allows access to clinical data prior to 2019. Health Canada makes the same type of data available as the EMA: clinical reports including clinical overviews, clinical summaries, CSRs, SAPs, trial protocols and protocol amendments, and sample case report forms.

Health Canada's PRCI initiative is more transparent than the EMA's policies in several key ways.[92] Unlike Policy 0043, clinical data obtained via request then becomes available on Health Canada's online database. Additionally, people outside of Canada are allowed to request data, and there is no registration requirement. However, the PRCI initiative never announced intentions to make IPD publicly available.

### The FDA's Brief Experiment

In 2018, the FDA launched the voluntary Clinical Data Summary Pilot Program. The agency planned to contact clinical trial sponsors and recruit volunteers to allow the FDA to proactively publish parts of CSRs online.[93] The pilot program aimed to include "up to" nine NDAs across different disease areas, and the FDA would publish "the parts of the CSRs that were most important to the FDA's assessment of the safety and efficacy of the drug." However, the pilot program concluded in 2020 after it had only made one CSR available for Janssen Pharmaceuticals' (subsidiary of Johnson & Johnson) drug Erleada (apalutamide).[94] While the FDA ended the pilot program, it also admitted that the pilot "identified a potential approach that could facilitate a harmonized system for disclosing study reports."[95]

### Health Technology Assessments

Along with more proactive disclosure policies, European and other wealthy nations have agencies that conduct health technology assessments (HTAs). Government bodies conduct HTAs on particular medicines and health interventions to best inform coverage decisions, as most countries either have some form of public health insurance or heavily regulated private insurance.[96] HTAs specifically examine clinical effectiveness of medicines and health interventions, especially in relation to already existing methods of care. Some countries additionally consider cost effectiveness.

In the UK, the National Institute for Health and Care Excellence (NICE) conducts HTAs to assess both the clinical- and cost-effectiveness of new medicines and health interventions in relation to comparators.[97] In a four- to twelve-week process, NICE identifies health care topics that it deems a national priority and its topic selection oversight panel decides whether to conduct an HTA.[98] Additionally, NICE is required to appraise "all medicines that are new to the U.K. market or have a significant new therapeutic indication."[99] The National Health Service (NHS)—the UK's socialized health care system—must cover all NICE recommended medicines and interventions. The primary drawback of NICE's HTAs is that the government body does not have access to underlying clinical trial data, such as CSRs and IPD, that are not publicly accessible.[100]

Canada has a very similar system as the UK.[101] The Canadian Agency for Drugs and Technologies in Health (CADTH) conducts HTAs for all new drugs, evaluating both clinical- and cost-effectiveness. As Canada has a single-payer health insurance system, the government directly uses CADTH evaluations and recommendations when determining what to cover. Furthermore, Australia similarly includes clinical- and cost-effectiveness in its HTAs that help determine coverage decisions in its universal public health insurance system. However, the government also considers the budget impact of covering a medical intervention for its recommendations, which is something that neither the UK nor Canada does. Additionally, Australia has two separate HTA-conducting bodies for pharmaceuticals and medical devices/procedures: the Pharmaceutical Benefits Advisory Committee (PBAC) and the Medical Services Advisory Committee (MSAC), respectively.

Unlike the UK, Canada, and Australia, France and Germany only evaluate clinical effectiveness; they do not conduct cost-effectiveness analyses as part of their HTAs.[102] In France, the National Committee for the Evaluation of Medical Devices and Health Technologies (CNEDiMTS) analyzes the medical benefit of interventions absolutely and in relation to existing methods of care.[103] While CNEDiMTS does not conduct cost-effectiveness analyses, it does an economic evaluation to determine recommended reimbursement rates that the government then uses in its direct negotiation of prices with manufacturers.[104] The German body that conducts HTAs—the Institute for Quality and Efficiency in Healthcare (IQWiG)—is similar to CNEDiMTS. IQWiG conducts an absolute and relative analysis of clinical benefit; however, it only does an economic evaluation if the government's price negotiations and arbitration fail.

None of the government bodies conducting HTAs have inherent, immediate, and direct access to CSRs or IPD that are not publicly available. However, the EMA's Policy 0070 should allow EU countries and other nations to have such access. In Canada, CADTH should have access to information from Health Canada. However, neither the EMA, Health Canada, or agencies in any other country have the same level of collected data as the FDA, which has the largest known collection of clinical trial data in the world.[105]

The United States was the first nation to conduct HTAs; however, Congress ended the practice in the 1990s. In 1972, Congress passed the Office of Technology Assessment Act, creating the Office of Technology Assessment (OTA).[106] The OTA's statutory purpose was "to provide early indications of the probable beneficial and adverse impacts of the applications of technology and to develop other coordinate information which may assist the Congress."[107] With health care, the OTA conducted assessments of health technologies—including pharmaceuticals, medical devices, and more—and evaluations of insurance benefits design, pharmaceutical R&D, and medical malpractice.[108] However, congressional Republicans successfully led the charge to effectively eliminate the OTA in 1995 by completely defunding it as part of the party's "Contract with America" agenda.[109]

Along with the OTA, the United States also had an Office of Health Technology Assessment (OHTA). In 1981, the OHTA replaced the National Center for Health Care Technology (NCHCT) in advising Medicare on whether to pay for certain services.[110] However, the OHTA was absorbed into the Agency for Healthcare Research and Quality (AHRQ) in 1989. The AHRQ currently conducts HTAs in a very narrow capacity; for example, the agency published four and one HTA in 2020 and 2022, respectively.[111] In the Patient Protection and Affordable Care Act of 2010, Congress created the private, nonprofit Patient-Centered Outcomes Research Institute (PCORI) with the goal of conducting comparative clinical-effectiveness research, and the AHRQ is tasked with disseminating its research.[112] By law, both AHRQ and PCORI are banned from including cost-effectiveness analyses or factoring in cost as a criterion for medical coverage in their assessments. Neither the AHRQ or PCORI has access to the same level of clinical trial data as the FDA. To conduct assessments, they rely upon publicly available sources: namely registries like ClinicalTrials.gov, systemic reviews such as Cochrane reviews, and the published literature in medical journals.[113]

While the United States lacks a national HTA program like other wealthy countries, there are nonprofit organizations that conduct HTAs. The most significant nonprofit conducting HTAs in the United States is the independent Institute for Clinical and Economic Review (ICER).[114] ICER analyses consider clinical- and cost-effectiveness along with economic and budget impacts. However, unlike national HTA programs in other nations, ICER's recommendations are not directly tied to health coverage. Public and private insurers ultimately utilize their own internal processes to decide what to cover. A 2020 comparison of ICER and NICE published in the *Journal of Managed Care & Specialty Pharmacy* found that while ICER had a comparable budget to NICE due to grants ($13.9 million vs. £12.6 million or around $16 million), it published far fewer assessments (under ten vs. fifty annually).[115] ICER also lacks access to the underlying clinical trial information available in CSRs and IPD. Relying on inadequate and/or unvetted publicly available information, its recommendations are inherently limited.

Even if the United States had a national HTA program like other nations, it would still suffer from a lack of data transparency. Without access to the underlying information from clinical trials, insurers, doctors, and patients cannot make fully informed decisions about the products they cover, prescribe, and use. The "progress" that the United States has made in terms of trial registration has been wholly insufficient in remedying this core feature of contemporary American health care. Outside of the FDA, no actors have access to the data necessary to truly vet trial results. As I discuss in the following chapter, even the source that doctors rely upon most that has historically represented the pinnacle of medical knowledge—peer-reviewed medical journals—suffer from lack of access to full clinical trial data.

3

# False Prophets and the Role of Medical Journals

Medical journals played an integral role in disseminating clinical trial results to physicians and other health professionals well before the creation of government trial registries. In 1665, the Royal Society of London created *Philosophical Transactions*, the first scientific journal.[1] A critical role of the journal was to disseminate published knowledge to the rest of the scientific community. The first journal dedicated to medical research came in 1679 through the French *Nouvelles Découvertes sur toutes les parties de la médecine*, although it would only be in 1731 when the Royal Society of Edinburgh published the first peer-reviewed collection of medical articles.[2] *The Lancet* and the *British Medical Journal* (*BMJ*)—two of the most prestigious English-language medical journals today—were created in 1823 and 1857, respectively.[3]

In the United States, the first medical journal, *The Medical Repository*, began in 1797; however, it ended in 1824.[4] Yet, one of the most prestigious medical journals, *NEJM*, came into being in 1812 as the *New England Journal of Medicine and Surgery and the Collateral Branches of Science*.[5] Another top US journal, *JAMA*, launched in 1883.

The key role of medical journals has been to collect, review, and disseminate medical knowledge. According to Leartus Connor—the president of the American Association of Medical Editors—in 1884, medical journals are "the great unifier of the past and present, the diffuser of all new facts, new thoughts, all new and better appliances for the study of the human body and for the relief of its derangements."[6] The predominant role of medical journals as disseminators of medical knowledge has not changed in contemporary times with the existence of government databases. According to *JAMA* editor-in-chief Kirsten Bibbins-Domingo in a 2022 interview, "scientific and medical journals are the way in which our scientific discoveries really reach the broadest audience."[7]

Critically, the primary audience of the published research in medical journals are doctors and medical professionals who rely upon such research as a source of ongoing education to inform how they treat patients. Chicago physician J. H. Salisbury espoused this reality in a 1906 *JAMA* piece:

> The medical school is attended, as a rule, but once in a lifetime; the meetings of the medical society are usually infrequent, but the medical journal, like the newspaper, is an ever-present friend whose influence and advice are potent for good or evil. Whoever gains control of the medical press goes a long way toward securing a paramount influence on the entire medical profession.[8]

Again, Bibbins-Domingo demonstrated the continued reliance upon medical journals, describing how the primary audience of journals are clinicians.[9] To be effective, journals must maintain those doctors' trust that they will properly vet the information in the articles they publish.

The emergence of the evidence-based medicine (EBM) movement further entrenched journals' critical role in educating clinicians. EBM directs medical professionals to combine clinical expertise with the best available evidence, principally from top-grade clinical research.[10] Exact dates differ, but the contemporary EBM movement started formalizing in the second half of the twentieth century, really taking off by the 1990s.[11] In 1992, *JAMA* published "Evidence-Based Medicine: A New Approach to Teaching the Practice of Medicine," where the authors argued that a new medical paradigm was emerging.[12] Rather than using "intuition, unsystematic clinical experience, and pathophysiologic rationale" as the backing for clinical decisions, doctors should focus on the results of clinical research. This shift would require physicians to learn academic research skills associated with sifting through the published literature in peer-reviewed medical journals (see Chapter 8).[13]

Since the 1990s, the EBM movement has changed; however, alterations have not de-anchored the medical knowledge of clinicians from medical journals. For example, in 2017, physician proponents of EBM described the difficulty individual doctors had with having enough time to sufficiently go through the medical literature.[14] Thus, many physicians relied upon "trustworthy clinical practice guidelines" (CPGs). According to the Institute of Medicine (IOM) in 2011, CPGs are "statements that include recommendations intended to optimize patient care that are informed by a systematic review of evidence and an assessment of the benefits and harms of alternative care options."[15] Rather than individual doctors reading through the medical literature, CPGs shift responsibility of research onto institutions and organizations of experts for which physicians then rely upon.[16]

While CPGs add an additional required layer of trust between CPG authors and doctors, they do not remove the root reliance on published articles in peer-reviewed medical journals. This reliance reflects the self-regulating nature of the scientific community. While the FDA approves products to let them on the market, the evidence base and clinical guidance guiding doctors' decision-making comes from the community itself outside of government. Thus, the integrity of this self-regulating, private structure is essential for the health care system overall to serve the public good.

## Industry Domination of Journal Publications

While doctors hold medical journal publications as the gold standard of medical knowledge, most published research is tied to industry. Published trial results are funded by industry, predominantly come from industry-crafted study designs, are written by employees of industry, and even the editors of journals have significant financial ties to industry. Per a 2009 IOM report, financial ties to companies—through gifts, research support, and so on—risk compromising the integrity of people's professional judgment and can bias them toward their benefactor and away from objective science.[17] Thus, rather than being repositories of advancements in medical knowledge, journals often serve as marketing arms of pharmaceutical and device manufacturers, publishing their trials to increase usage of their products and boost profits.

In 2018, a *BMJ* study examined the latest 200 publications of industry-funded trials between July 2014 and April 2017 among seven leading journals, including *NEJM*, *The Lancet*, *JAMA*, *Annals of Internal Medicine*, *JAMA Internal Medicine*, and the *BMJ*.[18] The vast majority of trials pertained to drugs (82.5 percent) compared to medical devices (13.0 percent) and vaccines (4.5 percent). In 173 (86.5 percent) of the trials, the journal publication had at least one coauthor who was an employee of the industry sponsor (see Figure 3). Yet, the corresponding author—the individual responsible for signing the publishing agreement and handling all correspondence about the article—was almost always (96.0 percent) an academic. At the same time, the lead academic author had a financial conflict of interest with the industry sponsor in 82.5 percent of trials; only 11.5 percent of trials had a lead academic author with no COIs with industry.

Along with significant influence among journal publication authors, the study found significant industry involvement in the design, reporting, and data analysis of the published trials themselves. Only 4.0 percent of trials were independent—meaning that the design, conduct, data analysis, and reporting of the trial only involved academics. However, half of these independent trials had lead authors with disclosed COIs with the industry funder for separate work. The remaining 96.0 percent of trials had significant industry involvement, such as industry sponsor involvement in the design and data analysis of 86.5 percent and 73.0 percent of trials, respectively. In fact, the industry funder and/or CRO conducted the data analysis in around half of trials without any involvement of academic authors. In just 38.5 percent of trials, all authors declared access to trial data, with some authors doing so in 72.0 percent of trials. However, just 4.5 percent of trials specified the type of data authors had access to with just 2.5 percent reporting access to raw or analyzed data. The *BMJ* study authors further believed that data access descriptions in publications may have been inaccurate. For example, 97.1 percent of study protocols for trials published in *The Lancet* did not describe academic authors' access to data while 92.8 percent of publications claimed some academic access.

The study also sent out a survey to the lead academic authors of the 200 trials with just eighty (40.0 percent) responding at least partially. Just twenty-nine (36.3 percent) out of the eighty responding authors reported that academics had final say on the trial design. Additionally, more authors reported industry control over trial outcomes rather than academic control. One academic author responded, "I drafted the introduction and discussion sections, while the company scientific writers drafted the methodology and results sections."

Industry similarly dominates highly impactful clinical trials. Among the 600 most-cited clinical trials published from 2019 to 2022, not only were a majority exclusively funded by industry, but 354 trials (59.0 percent) had industry authors.[19] A plurality of the trials (46.6 percent) used industry analysts and one-fifth exclusively used industry analysts. Ultimately, 89.0 percent of the trials reached conclusions favorable to the

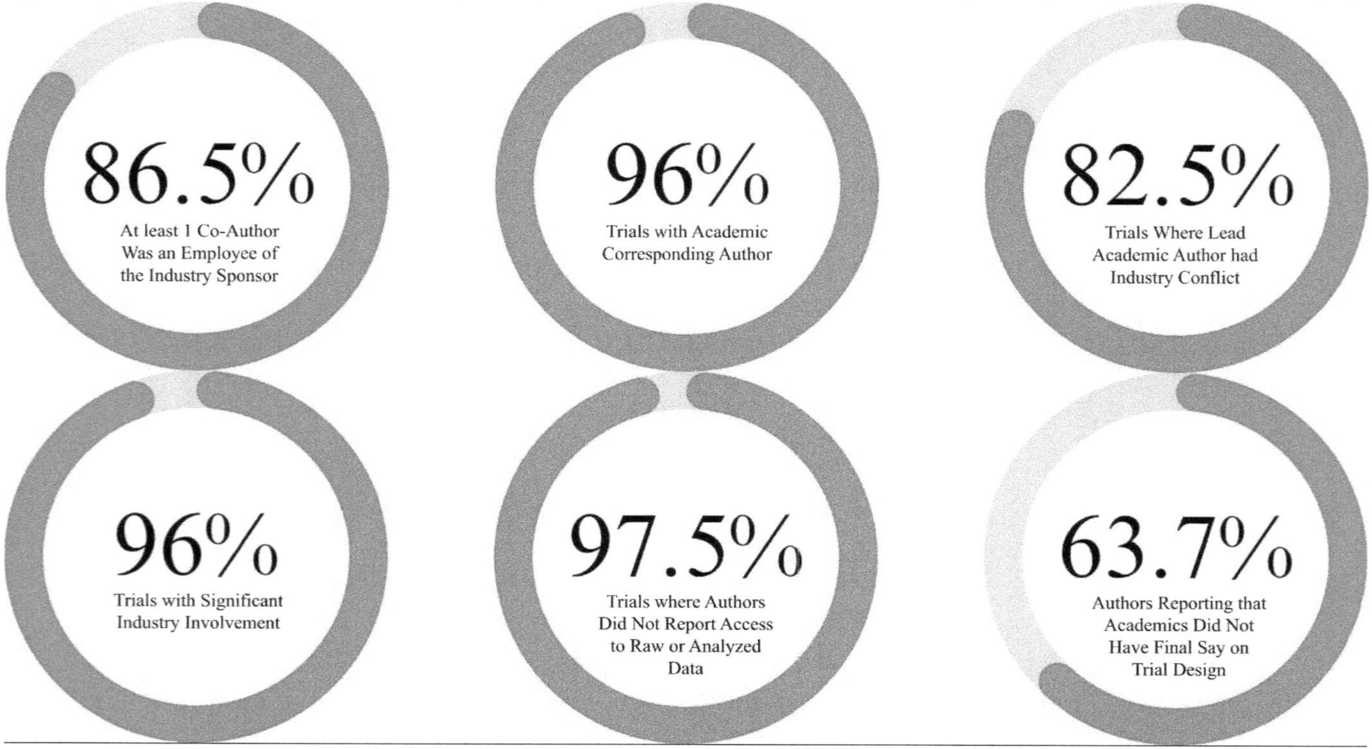


**Figure 3** Study results showing major drug and device industry control over the trials they fund, such as trial design, data access, and publication. *Source*: Kristine Rasmussen et al., "Collaboration Between Academics and Industry in Clinical Trials: Cross Sectional Study of Publications and Survey of Lead Academic Authors," *BMJ* 363, no. 8170 (October 3, 2018): k3654, https://doi.org/10.1136/bmj.k3654.

industry sponsor, and such pro-industry findings were nearly three times more likely among trials exclusively funded by industry and which had industry authors. While over three quarters of trials published an intention to share data, just 2.7 percent had data already available to others as of 2023 while most required filing requests to authors, data repositories, or the sponsor itself.

While the ICMJE requires disclosure of COIs for both authors and editors, many journals fail to disclose editors' ties to industry.[20] A 2019 *BMJ* investigation examined 130 high-impact medical journals, representing the top five journals in 2017 among each of twenty-six different medical specialties, such as immunology and cardiology, to find how often they provided COI disclosure for authors and editors.[21] While 129 journals (99.2 percent) required disclosure for authors, just 16 (12.3 percent) reported COIs for their individual editors. Simultaneously, 58 journals were on the ICMJE Recommendations subscription list and 93 were members of another professional committee, the Committee on Publication Ethics (COPE), which recommended the public declaration of COIs, ideally publicly. In a previous 2018 analysis, a random sample of 350 journals found that just 2 declared individual editors' COIs on their website while 82 percent required author disclosure.[22]

The lack of financial disclosure is significant, considering that the US government's Open Payments Program (OPP) reveals substantial financial ties to industry among journal editors. In a 2017 *BMJ* study, researchers examined reported payments to 713 physician journal editors from fifty-two journals in 2014, finding that a majority (50.6 percent) received general payments—such as consulting fees and meal/travel reimbursements—and 19.5 percent received research payments.[23] While the level of payments varied greatly—as the median general and research payments, respectively, were $11 and $0—eleven journal specialties had at least around 20 percent of their editors receiving more than $10,000 in general payments. Endocrinology and cardiology had over 20 percent and 15 percent of their editors receiving more than $100,000 in general payments, respectively. The five largest individual general payments in the one year to physicians ranged from over $325,000 to nearly $11 million. Overall, just 32.7 percent of the journals had editor COI policies accessible on their websites.

Similarly, 2018 *PLOS One* research examined industry payments in 2015 to 703 physician editors from sixty influential US medical journals.[24] Nearly half (45.5 percent) received more than 8,600 general payments, totaling over $8.1 million. The vast majority of the dollar amount of these payments (78.4 percent) came from consulting fees. While the median amount per payment was just $91, the median total amount received by each editor in one year was $4,364, and more than one-fifth (21.6 percent) of all 703 physicians and around half (47.5 percent) of those receiving payments got over $5,000. The NIH considers this $5,000 threshold a significant financial interest.[25] Only seven (11.7 percent) of the journals reported that editors received payments, and just two (3.3 percent) specified the dollar amount.[26]

Another *PLOS One* study in 2019 examined industry payments from August 2013 through 2016 to "top-tier" US-based physician editors—meaning those the researchers determined to be most directly "responsible for making manuscript decisions"—from the thirty-five journals in 2015 with the highest number of citations within seven medical specialties.[27] Of the 333 top-tier, US-based physician editors, 212 (63.7 percent) received industry payments over the period, and 42.3 percent received a direct general or research payment within the average year. Three in ten of the editors received direct payments of over $5,000 within a single year, and roughly a fifth (19.8 percent) of these editors received over $5,000 in a year on average over the period. Overall, while the results of these studies show significant levels of industry payments to editors of medical journals, the numbers are conservative in their ability to show all financial ties, as they do not include payments to editors who sit on corporate boards or payments from companies that have not yet marketed their products.[28]

The premier source of medical knowledge that doctors rely upon to inform their practices is not just entangled with industry; it is dominated by it. Industry funds most of the trials pushed for publication, has significant control on the design and conduct of trials, employs and/or has financial ties to the authors of published articles, makes direct payments to significant numbers of journal editors, and ultimately benefits from highly cited published trials providing conclusions favorable to their bottom line.

## Journals Do Not Have Access to Sufficient Clinical Data

Even though clinicians rely upon the validity of published articles in peer-reviewed medical journals, the peer reviewers and journal editors themselves almost never have access to the underlying data from clinical trials. This reality places significant control of medical knowledge into the hands of those who own the data from clinical trials: largely pharmaceutical company sponsors.

Traditionally, clinical trial researchers submit interim findings during an ongoing trial and/or final results afterward to well-respected, peer-reviewed medical journals. These journals play a crucial gatekeeping role by reviewing the submitted information, determining its validity, and accepting it for publication. Unlike the FDA approval process, clinical trial sponsors do not have to submit their underlying data—including individual participant data and clinical study reports—to journals. Researchers need only share selected summaries of their trial data within their submitted manuscripts (see Figure 4). For example, the current policy of *JAMA Network Open* is that clinical trial researchers need to submit the primary and secondary outcome measures as described in their original trial protocol along with "the main results of the study."[29] Thus, peer reviewers are dependent on the integrity and honesty of those submitting the data, as they lack the means to run their own analyses of the CSRs and IPD.

The weak foundation of the existing medical literature in medical journals is no secret. In 2015, *The Lancet* editor-in-chief Richard Horton wrote, "the case against science is straightforward: much of the scientific literature, perhaps half, may simply be untrue."[30] In the same year and in relation to the widespread prescription of statins, the

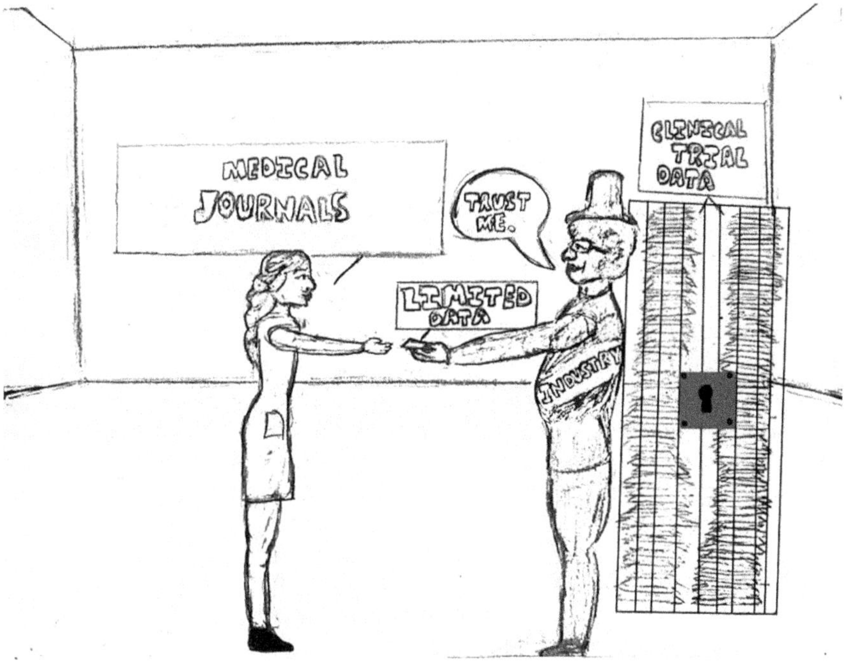


**Figure 4** An illustration showing how industry sponsors of clinical trials do not share much of the full trial data with editors and peer reviewers when seeking publication in medical journals.

editor-in-chief of the *BMJ* asked, "how can it be right to recommend mass treatment of healthy people without independent review of the patient level data, especially the data on adverse effects?"[31]

While medical journals follow their own sets of rules, most major medical journals follow the recommendations of the International Committee of Medical Journal Editors.[32] The journals that are actually members of the ICMJE are fewer and currently include *JAMA*, *NEJM*, *The Lancet*, the *BMJ*, *Nature Medicine*, *Annals of Internal Medicine*, *PLOS Medicine*, and more.[33] In 2004, the ICMJE issued a strict requirement that for anyone to have their clinical trial results published in member journals, they must register in a public trials registry, such as ClinicalTrials.gov, for trials beginning enrollment after July 1, 2005.[34] The ICMJE defined a clinical trial as "any research project that prospectively assigns human subjects to intervention or comparison groups to study the cause-and-effect relationship between a medical intervention and a health outcome."

The ICMJE justified its requirement on the primary basis of combatting the selective reporting of clinical trials that "show either a large effect of a new treatment (positive trials) or equivalence of two approaches to treatment (non-inferiority trials)."[35] Trial registrations on ClinicalTrials.gov grew from 13,153 when the ICMJE issued its policy to 22,714 after one month.[36] In 2007, the ICMJE expanded its previous definition of clinical trial by adopting the World Health Organization's definition: "Any research study that prospectively assigns human participants or groups of humans to one or more health-related interventions to evaluate the effects on health outcomes." This expanded clinical trials to include any intervention that has a health-related or biomedical impact, such as drugs, surgery, dietary changes, process-of-care changes, and more.

In 2017, the ICMJE issued another policy, requiring clinical trials to include a data sharing statement in their registrations.[37] Manuscripts submitted to ICMJE journals also had to include the data sharing statement. Data sharing statements had to indicate whether the owners of the trial data will share de-identified IPD, what data they will share at all, whether they will share related documents like the study protocol and statistical analysis plan, when they would share data and for how long, and how they would share the data (i.e., who has access, for what reasons, and by what mechanism). Critically, the ICMJE did not mandate the sharing of clinical trial data; they only required that those submitting manuscripts to journals disclose their intentions to share. This policy went into effect for manuscripts submitted to ICMJE journals as of July 1, 2018 along with clinical trials registered on or after January 1, 2019.[38]

The 2017 policy represented a diminished version of their proposed policy in 2016.[39] For submission to an ICMJE journal, the proposed policy would have required authors to share de-identified IPD behind the outcomes described in the potentially published article. However, the required sharing of the individual data would have only needed to occur within six months of publication. Thus, sharing of the data would not have necessarily involved the original peer reviewers or had an impact on the initial published article for a product's trial. Additionally, the data sharing requirement only applied to IPD of the outcomes described in the submitted manuscript; it would not have allowed access to other data with potentially important revelations. Nonetheless, the ICMJE withdrew the sharing requirement, going against its own assessment in the 2016 proposal that "sharing data will increase confidence and trust in the conclusions drawn from clinical trials. It will enable the independent confirmation of results, an essential tenet of the scientific process."

The exact reasons for the highlighted difference between the 2016 proposal and 2017 actual policy are unknown. However, the 2017 policy did cite concerns about the general proposal like feasibility, risks to trial participants, and protecting "the interests of patients and researchers."[40] Regarding the last point, the editor-in-chief of *NEJM*, Dr. Jeffrey Drazen, and Dr. Dan Longo coauthored an *NEJM* editorial arguing against the limited IPD sharing proposal.[41] Their two principal concerns were (1) that those not involved in creating and collecting the trial data may be too ignorant of the choices behind its construction and (2) that a "new class" of researcher would emerge who used the data for their own ends or "even use[d] the data to try to disprove what the original investigators had posited." Thus, among their concerns was that researchers would be able to scrutinize and potentially invalidate the published results of clinical trials.

## The Failures of Data Sharing Agreements

Inherently, ICMJE-mandated data sharing agreements do not guarantee access to clinical trial data for researchers or the public because they only reveal whether the data owners will share data and, if so, how. The existence of data sharing agreements could theoretically incentivize voluntary sharing of data. However, available evidence suggests this does not occur in either a timely or sufficiently detailed manner.

A 2018 analysis of pharmaceutical-industry-sponsored clinical trials published in medical journals between July and December 2015 found that only nine (14.8 percent) of sixty-one identified trials made IPD available to researchers two years after publishing the results data in a medical journal.[42] While only thirty-two (52.5 percent) of trials had public data sharing policies, 93.3 percent of the sponsors within the top twenty-five pharmaceutical companies by global sales had such policies. Within two years of publishing, 22.9 percent of top-pharmaceutical-company-sponsored trials provided some access to IPD compared to 3.8 percent of other drugmaker trials. Similarly, a 2019 study of the top twenty pharmaceutical companies according to 2015 market capitalizations found that a quarter made IPD available upon request for phase II and III clinical trials for novel drugs approved by the FDA in 2015 in accordance with IOM guidelines.[43] More specifically, companies had to share data six months after FDA approval or eighteen months following trial completion, whichever deadline was later.

Analyses of data availability for clinical trials relating to specific diseases similarly show a lack of access to IPD for researchers. A 2022 *JAMA* study examining sharing of clinical trial data for FDA-approved anticancer medicines from January 2011 through June 2021 found that only 136 trials (44.7 percent) were eligible for data sharing in 2021.[44] For the nearly half (44.7 percent) of trials that posted summary results on product labels within three years before the *JAMA* study, 70.6 percent were not eligible for data sharing. The trials that had summary data available on product labels for three to seven years (41.4 percent) and more than seven years (13.8 percent) had lower ineligibility rates (48.4 percent and 26.2 percent, respectively). As drug labels are created shortly after drug approval, the vast majority of anticancer medicine clinical trials failed to share data within several years of approval.[45]

A 2016 study examined randomized clinical trials that focused on cardiovascular diseases, had more than 5,000 patients, and were sponsored by a top twenty pharmaceutical company by 2014 global sales.[46] Looking at all such trials registered on ClinicalTrials.gov as of January 9, 2015, only fifteen trials (25 percent) had IPD available for data sharing to researchers as of 2015. Another fifteen trials did not share such data and the study authors could determine availability for the remaining half of trials.

Studies examining data sharing often examine the availability of IPD, finding low levels of sharing. They also do not identify if shared data is complete or if sponsors withhold relevant data. Inherent in these analyses is the fact that data sharing agreements largely do not guarantee access to detailed clinical data whether in analyzable data sets or CSRs. This is especially true considering that most major medical journals follow the ICMJE policy that mandates the posting of data sharing statements rather than actual sharing. Voluntary clinical data sharing may be less likely with the most consequential pharmaceuticals and devices, where companies want to protect their effective data monopoly the most.[47] A critical example of this phenomenon is both Pfizer's and Moderna's unwillingness to voluntarily share the IPD from their COVID-19 vaccine trials.[48] According to the CDC, 81.4 percent of the US population received at least one shot of a COVID-19 vaccine by May 2023.[49] The public has a legitimate interest in accessing the clinical trial data for such a widely taken treatment.

Among pharmaceutical companies, Johnson & Johnson (J&J) commonly ranks among the best in terms of clinical trial data sharing.[50] According to the Yale University Open Data Access (YODA) Project, J&J allows researchers to request access to full CSRs and de-identified IPD for phase II, III, and IV pharmaceutical clinical trials if three criteria are met.[51] J&J must have government authorization to market the treatment, the product must have been approved by the FDA and EMA for the relevant indication, and the trial was completed at least eighteen months prior. J&J similarly allows data sharing for medical device trials. Overall, J&J data sharing policy is positive news for proponents of detailed data sharing that allows vetting of trial results via access to CSRs and de-identified IPD.

However, the primary limitations of J&J's policy are that it is voluntary—data sharing is not guaranteed; it is contingent on the willingness of the company—and it does not apply across the pharmaceutical industry.[52] Trial sponsors ultimately decide to what extent IPD is collected from a trial along with when they share and publish the data. The YODA Project asserts that J&J typically shares data eighteen months after trial completion. While the YODA Project requires researchers writing manuscripts to disseminate their research findings with a preference for peer-reviewed journals, they generally do not share trial data before the results are submitted to such journals. This limits the benefits as journal articles have a disproportionate impact on doctors' opinions, and sponsors also determine whether sharing occurs.[53] Ultimately, usage of sufficiently complete clinical trial data in peer-reviewed medical journals in a timely manner is paramount to improve the medical knowledge that doctors rely upon.

Another caveat to the case of J&J is how its data sharing arrangement with the YODA Project beginning in 2014 closely followed a $2.2 billion settlement with the Department of Justice (DOJ) in 2013 over illegal behavior.[54] J&J pled guilty to illegally marketing off-label uses for the antipsychotic drug Risperdal, and it settled over allegations that it did the same for the drugs Invega and Natrecor. J&J also settled allegations about false claims and paying kickbacks to physicians and pharmacies. Allegedly, the company was aware of serious adverse events for Risperdal—like strokes—but it manipulated trial results by combining data between different studies to show a lower risk of adverse side effects. J&J also signed a Corporate Integrity Agreement (CIA) requiring the company to change its practices in a variety of areas.[55] Among the provisions, the CIA mandated that J&J register clinical trials and report results in accordance with federal law, "make good faith efforts" to publish results in peer-reviewed journals in a timely manner with a specified timeframe for submitting manuscripts, and implement "data dissemination plans that establish prospective publication strategies."

The J&J case study is not unique, as another large pharmaceutical company, GSK, followed a similar path toward data sharing after a CIA.[56] In 2012, GSK pled guilty for illegally promoting the drugs Paxil and Wellbutrin as well as failing to report safety data about the diabetes drug Avandia to the FDA.[57] Along with paying $3 billion, GSK signed a CIA with HHS.[58] GSK agreed to publish summaries of its trial protocols and metadata on its own Clinical Study Register and register summary results for all applicable GSK-sponsored clinical trials on ClinicalTrials.gov in compliance with federal law. GSK also agreed to seek to publish trial results in "peer-reviewed, searchable journals" and implement "data dissemination plans that establish prospective publication strategies."

Soon thereafter, while GSK did not enter into an agreement with the likes of the YODA Project, the company made de-identified IPD available to researchers upon request in May 2013 for a subset of GSK trials.[59] This subset included all clinical trials (phases I–IV) starting in and after 2013, and the company gradually made trials available all the way back to the year 2000.[60] For up to twelve months with a potential six-month extension, GSK provides researchers access to the anonymized raw data, analyzable data set, metadata (protocol and SAP), annotated case report forms, and the CSR.[61] GSK makes data available for request within six months of product approval by both the FDA and EMA or either agency when "regulatory submissions are not planned in both regions; or where development is terminated across all indications." To access the data, researchers must submit research proposals that then get reviewed by a panel of outside experts appointed by GSK. In addition, researchers must sign a data sharing agreement, promising to publish results of their analyses to a scientific journal or preprint server. While the GSK data sharing initiative falls short of public transparency and guaranteeing data access to peer reviewers prior to initial publication in a medical journal, it is much more transparent than most of the pharmaceutical industry.

The cases of J&J and GSK show that while certain drugmakers have voluntarily made more clinical trial data available than otherwise required, their actions likely reflect the successes of federal litigation and law enforcement. In this vein, data transparency shields these companies from further prosecution and federal fines.[62] Additionally, the programs of J&J and GSK are still limited, and doctors and the public do not have easily accessible means to view CSRs and IPD.

## Drug Makers' Financing of Journals

Another potentially significant concern that underlies the lack of journal requirements for authors to submit enough data is the financial relationship between drugmakers and the medical journals themselves. While the ICMJE does not require data sharing among its member journals, individual journals can require authors to share data to get their work published. Yet, without collective action, individual journals may place themselves in financially bad situations by imposing data sharing requirements.

In 2005, *JAMA* uniquely created a requirement that clinical trials funded by industry cannot submit research to the journal if only their own statisticians conducted data analyses.[63] For *JAMA* to accept submissions from these industry-funded clinical trials, they must have had an independent statistical analysis done "by statisticians at an academic institution, such as a medical school, academic medical center, or government research institute." These independent statisticians must have had access to "the entire raw data set" along with the study protocol and statistical analysis plan. The final published article had to include the details of this independent statistical analysis along with information on whether the statistician received compensation or funding.

A *PLOS One* analysis investigated the impact of *JAMA*'s policy on the number of industry-funded trials published in the journal.[64] The number of RCTs overall and the number of industry-funded RCTs decreased significantly from the three-year period before the policy compared to the three-year period afterward. Over the same periods, the number of industry-funded RCTs published in *NEJM* and *The Lancet* increased significantly. While the authors cautioned that they could not absolutely prove causality, they reasoned that "the most plausible explanation" is that, in a zero-sum environment, industry shifted the publishing of their trials to other high-impact medical journals that lacked the requirement for independent statistical analysis. Supporting this conclusion, *JAMA* dropped the requirement in 2013.[65]

## Reprints

A significant source of revenue for medical journals comes from drug reprints. A key mechanism for pharmaceutical companies to market their products is to purchase reprints of favorable articles published in well-respected, peer-reviewed medical journals and give them to doctors whom their drug representatives reach out to. In a 2005 piece entitled "Medical Journals Are an Extension of the Marketing Arm of Pharmaceutical Companies," former editor-in-chief of the *BMJ*, Richard Smith, reflected:

> For a drug company, a favourable trial is worth thousands of pages of advertising, which is why a company will sometimes spend upwards of a million dollars on reprints of the trial for worldwide distribution. The doctors receiving the reprints may not read them, but they will be impressed by the name of the journal from which they come. The quality of the journal will bless the quality of the drug.[66]

The strategy of drugmakers using reprints to persuade doctors to prescribe their products is no secret. In 2007, *PLOS Medicine* published an article derived from conversations between a former drug representative and a physician researching drug marketing.[67] The relevant finding was simple: drug representatives approach doctors tied to the doctrine of evidence-based medicine with reprints from medical journals, appealing to their faith in high-quality evidence.

Contemporary data on the significance of reprints as sources of revenue for medical journals is lacking, as there is no public access to such information and journals are reluctant to share their finances. Lundh and colleagues found that reprints constituted 41 percent and 3 percent of income for *The Lancet* and the *BMJ* in 2005–06, respectively.[68] The *BMJ*'s lower percentage of revenue coming from reprints may remain accurate, as the journal and the entire BMJ group (the publishing company that owns multiple journals) voluntarily revealed that they earned only 0.5 percent (£116,000) and 2.6 percent (£1.98 million) of their 2016 income from reprints, respectively.[69]

Handel and colleagues examined data for the most highly ordered reprint papers between 2002 and 2009.[70] Published articles with high numbers of reprint orders were nearly nine times more likely to be funded by the pharmaceutical industry, including over twelve and fifteen times more likely in *The Lancet* and the *BMJ*, respectively. Additionally, they noted that reprint orders represented "a large source of income for the *Lancet* and *BMJ*." The median reprint order costs for *The Lancet* and the *BMJ* were £287,353 and £12,458, and the highest order costs were £1,551,794 and £132,805, respectively. Both Lundh and Handel were denied access to income data from prominent US medical journals like *JAMA*, *NEJM*, and *Annals of Internal Medicine*. Commenting on Handel et al.'s analysis, Dr. Richard Smith highlighted that the study didn't reveal something that he knew from his experience previously being editor-in-chief of the *BMJ*: the profit margin on drug reprints is around 80 percent.[71] If true, *The Lancet's* reprint sale of £1,551,794 returned around £1.24 million in profit.

While US medical journals have not revealed their revenue from reprints, and data overall is very limited, the unavailability of Creative Commons Attribution (CC BY) licenses for commercially funded studies serves as an indication of reprint profitability. Most major medical journals allow academic study authors to purchase CC BY licenses so that their published articles are free to read and open-access. Additionally, the license allows anyone to copy, distribute, and make commercial use of the published material if they attribute the original publication. As of the mid-2010s, these licenses for medical journals cost between $3,000 and $5,000.[72] The cost of accessing articles is often higher due to the additional cost of subscriptions that many medical journals require, which can vary. However, most journals do not offer CC BY licenses to commercially funded research. As Dr. Smith pinpoints, the profitability of reprints far exceeds the cost of a CC BY license.[73] Thus, allowing research funded by commercial interests—primarily the pharmaceutical industry—to obtain open access via CC BY licenses would produce a significant loss in revenue.

Journals are also more likely to accept reprint fees when publication authors have COIs with industry sponsors. A 2020 *PLOS One* study examined the relationship between various commercial practices of biomedical journals and author COIs.[74] They examined 128,781 articles published in 159 journals, finding that journals that accepted reprint fees were almost three times more likely to have authors that receive payments from the pharmaceutical industry.

One journal that recently announced enhanced data sharing requirements is the *BMJ*. In March 2024, the journal announced that from the beginning of May 2024, it would "require authors of all submitted trials to post relevant trial data in an enduring, publicly accessible repository such as Vivli before publication" with the purpose of making data available for other researchers.[75] According to Vivli's website, this repository focuses on sharing IPD from completed clinical trials.[76] It is unclear to what extent the *BMJ* policy will be successful, as the journal also noted that its previous requirements for trial authors to share data "upon reasonable request" did not actually succeed, causing the sharing of data to remain "disappointingly low."[77] *BMJ*'s policy followed PLOS journals, which require data sharing for "all data necessary to replicate their study's findings" for submission, meaning only the "minimal data set" for all reported findings in a journal article rather than the entire data set.[78] Nonetheless, *BMJ* and PLOS policies go further than other journals. Notably, the *BMJ* has received far less revenue from reprints than competing journals like *The Lancet*.

### Advertising Revenues

Given that physicians rely on medical journals as the premier source of medical knowledge, pharmaceutical companies have capitalized on this reliance through purchasing advertisements in these journals.[79] Aside from promoting potentially misleading claims to increase physician prescription of advertised treatments, a consequence of advertisements is that they can create a COI for medical journals by constituting a source of revenue.

However, the significance of medical journal advertising has declined over time. A 2019 *JAMA* analysis of medical marketing from 1997 to 2016 found that medical journal advertising significantly fell from $744 million to $119 million over the two decades.[80] Yet, advertising to health care professionals grew from $15.6 billion to $20.3 billion over the same period largely due to spending on free samples, prescriber detailing, and direct payments to physicians.

Identifying how important advertising revenues are for individual journals is difficult as the information is not publicly available. A 2014 *PLOS One* analysis estimated that while *JAMA* and *NEJM* collected £3.8 million (around $5.9 million) and £3.3 million (around $5.1 million) in print advertising revenues in 2013, *The Lancet* and *BMJ* collected significantly less: £0.025 million (around $37,000) and £0.96 million (around $1.5 million).[81] Therefore, leading American journals may be more impacted by the allure of pharmaceutical advertisements than their British counterparts. Overall, individual medical journals' reluctance to impose stringent data sharing requirements may rest—at least partially—on their self-interest to receive more research for publication, especially from industry, and subsequently earn more profit via reprints.

## Consequences of Weak Peer Review

Without access to the protocols, CSRs, and de-identified IPD behind clinical trials, peer reviewers cannot vet the accuracy and completeness of submitted manuscripts. This reality in conjunction with the profit motive of pharmaceutical companies has significant consequences for the dissemination and marketing of medical knowledge published in peer-reviewed medical journals.

A 2023 *JAMA* investigation explored what drug characteristics were most associated with higher levels of direct-to-consumer (DTC) advertising.[82] Examining the 150 prescription drugs with the highest US sales in 2020, the researchers found that drug manufacturers spent more money marketing less clinically beneficial drugs compared to drugs providing more clinical benefits to patients. A 2021 cross-sectional study in *Research Integrity and Peer Review* corroborates this finding.[83] Researchers examined all 158 medical advertisements in the *Journal of the Danish Medical Association* for the thirty-five most frequently advertised prescription drugs (six or more advertisements), finding that not one of these drugs had a substantial added benefit over older treatments even though they were significantly more expensive.

Therefore, the pharmaceutical industry's spending on marketing is not based on the actual effectiveness of a drug. DTC advertising specifically works by getting consumers to ask their doctors for prescriptions for marketed products. Pharmaceutical companies are further incentivized to spend large sums of money on DTC advertising, as it is tax deductible.[84] Without access to sufficient clinical trial data, peer-reviewed journal articles do not adequately educate doctors so that they are properly equipped to know whether a drug marketed to their patients provides enough real clinical benefits.

Due to First Amendment protections, American courts may strike down a DTC advertising prohibition.[85] The United States and New Zealand are the only nations that allow direct-to-consumer advertising for prescription drugs.[86] From 1997 to 2016, pharmaceutical companies spent around $10 billion annually on DTC advertising. From January to May 2025, 24.4 percent of advertising minutes on evening news programs on ABC, CBS, CNN, Fox News, MSNBC, and NBC came from prescription drug brands.[87]

While the FDA monitors the practice, the agency only ensures information is accurate and in line with FDA-approved product labels. It does not mandate further transparency for truthful advertising that is necessary to know a drug's true added clinical benefit, such as the numbers needed to treat (NNT) and harm (NNH).[88] For example, a clinical study with a large population may find a statistically significant result for a drug, but the NNT could reveal that 300 people must receive the drug for one person to receive the benefit. If the NNH shows that 200 people must receive the drug for one to have an adverse outcome, there is additional incentive to not use the treatment. Advertisers also use emotional imagery and messaging to manipulate audiences. In addition, the FDA's regulatory oversight is significantly weaker for online and social media advertisements, allowing more promotional materials that mislead patients and hide risks.[89]

Not only do drug manufacturers spend more on marketing drugs with less added clinical benefits, but high numbers of new drugs entering the market provide little to no added clinical benefit. The German health technology assessment agency, IQWiG, conducts early benefit assessments of newly approved drugs to ascertain whether the respective drug provides an added benefit compared to currently available standard care.[90] In a 2019 *BMJ* study, researchers examined the 216 drugs IQWiG conducted early benefit assessments for from 2011 to 2017.[91] They found that 125 (57.9 percent) of the new drugs did not provide any added clinical benefit over standard care, while 2 drugs (0.9 percent) provided less clinical benefit. Only 54 (25.0 percent) of new drugs provided a considerable or major added benefit, 20 (9.3 percent) provided just a minor added benefit, and IQWiG could not quantify benefits for the remaining 15 drugs (6.9 percent).

A 2023 *JAMA Internal Medicine* analysis examined the added clinical benefit of new drugs compared to standard care entering the French market between 2008 and 2018.[92] The authors found that between 71.3 percent and 77.6 percent of new medicines originating from industry provided no added benefit, 21.1–26.1 percent provided some added benefit, and just 1.3–2.6 percent provided substantial added benefit. New drugs originating from academia provided more added benefits in comparison, but still produced little added benefit overall. Between 61.9 percent and 64.3 percent of new medicines provided no added benefit, 30.4–33.9 percent provided some added benefit, and just 1.8–7.7 percent provided substantial added benefit.

Evidence from patents within the United States further show the lack of novelty in new drug development and marketing. In a 2018 comprehensive analysis of all drugs on the US market between 2005 and 2015, Robin Feldman found that 78 percent of the drugs tied to new patents were not actually novel.[93] Rather, they were existing drugs that had inconsequential changes sufficient enough only to get extensions of government patent protections. With protection against competition, pharmaceutical companies have monopoly control over the pricing of protected drugs; thus, it is in their financial interest to forsake novelty to charge and earn more money.

Without proper peer review where the reviewers have access to the underlying clinical trial data, published articles relying on biased submitted manuscripts are less able to detect when the benefits of a medical intervention are inflated and the harms downplayed. Currently, published articles on new products are less likely to include data on all outcomes relevant to patients. This empowers manufacturers to deprioritize innovation based on added clinical benefit and prioritize innovation based on marketing and getting patent protection.

A 2013 *PLOS Medicine* article took advantage of clinical trials for which the German IQWiG had successfully requested and obtained full CSRs from pharmaceutical companies to compare results data in CSRs with those reported in publicly available journal articles and registries.[94] Among 101 clinical trials, 86 had at least one publicly available source, 65 had at least one published journal article, and 50 had results posted in a registry. While the full CSRs had data on 86.1 percent of patient-relevant outcomes, publicly available sources for trials only had data on 39.4 percent of such outcomes. The full CSRs provided more information on both benefit (84.4 percent vs. 34.6 percent) and harm outcomes (87.3 percent vs. 42.8 percent). However, given that doctors primarily rely upon published articles in medical journals, the findings about trials with publications in just journals demonstrates an even greater lack of transparency. Only 23.1 percent of trial results published in just journals had complete information on all outcomes. More specifically, 19.3 percent and 26.0 percent of trials had complete benefit and harm outcome information, respectively. On top of doctor's reliance on medical journals, the importance of the lack of complete data in journal publications is greater considering the authors failed to obtain CSRs from 62.3 percent of the trials they requested from. Of the excluded trials, a greater proportion were reported in journals (over three quarters) than registries (almost two-thirds).

Along with misleading reported results, an additional problem resulting from weak peer review is outright fraudulent data. In 2020, anesthetist Dr. John Carlisle analyzed the manuscripts of 526 clinical trials submitted between February 2017 and March 2020 to the journal *Anaesthesia* for which he was an editor.[95] Carlisle managed to successfully request access to IPD for 153 (29.1 percent) of the 526 trials. He found that 67 (43.8 percent) of the 153 studies contained false data—meaning that the underlying data included impossible values, incorrect calculations, and the duplication of tables, figures, and other data from published works. Consequently, he labeled 40 (26.1 percent) of these trials as zombies, meaning trials that—from his experience as a journal editor—he believed would have been retracted given discovery of the flaws. Out of the 74 total trials with false data, *Anaesthesia* published 24 trials (32.4 percent) and 15 zombie trials (20.3 percent). However, he could only identify 6 trials (1.6 percent) with false data and 3 zombie trials (0.8 percent) for the 373 trials that he could not get access to IPD. Without IPD, Carlisle lacked the resources to adequately check for false data.[96] He concluded that peer reviewers must have access to IPD for proper vetting, as "all scientific journals should assume that submitted papers contain false data."[97]

The issue of fake data in published medical journal articles is not limited to *Anaesthesia*.[98] In 2023, researchers applied the Cochrane Pregnancy and Childbirth Trustworthiness Screening Tool (CPC-TST) to remove potentially fraudulent RCTs and examine the effect on conclusions made in Cochrane reviews.[99] The tool removed 93 (24.9 percent) out of 374 included RCTs, reducing the total number of included RCTs in fourteen out of eighteen Cochrane reviews. Ultimately, the authors found that six (33.3 percent) out of the eighteen Cochrane reviews required updates due to significant changes in the findings, conclusions, implications for practice, and/or significance for research.

Furthermore, one 2023 analysis estimated that fake publications may have represented 28.8 percent (of around 380,000 publications) of the published biomedical literature in 2020, up from around 16 percent in 2010.[100] Even if the real proportion of fraudulent publications is much lower—such as just 14 percent—there would be a significant problem in the medical literature.[101] An unpublished *Nature* analysis found that medicine and biology have the highest proportion (3.0 percent) of articles produced by companies—predominantly in China—known as paper mills that produce fake research.[102]

Whether it's fake data, misleading results, or serving as a marketing arm for industry, lack of effective peer review in medical journals prevents these institutions from serving as successful gatekeepers of medical knowledge. Industry influence over journals corrupts the scientific community's ability to self-regulate by affecting what they publish, what data they have access to, and how they make money. Currently, no other system of private oversight and distribution of medical research has filled the hole left by the failure of journals to regulate the information that physicians rely upon. In fact, the next chapter discusses how clinical guidelines—the sources meant to aggregate the knowledge from thousands of journal articles and pieces of published research—suffer from very similar issues.

# 4

# Poor Instructors and Clinical Practice Guidelines

With adoption of evidence-based medicine principles, clinical practice guidelines arose as significant sources of medical knowledge for physicians and health care professionals alongside medical journal publications. The process of developing guidelines generally involves systematically reviewing the available evidence to produce recommendations based on the highest quality evidence.[1] Ideally, guideline authors look through thousands of pages of research to synthesize the evidence, assess the benefits and harms of health interventions, and produce recommendations to best help patients.[2] Thus, guidelines are critical to the medical profession's self-regulation by providing physicians with evidence-based direction for the diagnosis of particular patients and treatment of varying conditions and diseases. However, CPGs suffer from the same lack of transparency as medical journals. Additionally, the quality of guidelines are highly variable and lacking at the same time, as key individuals involved in their development have financial conflicts of interest with industry.

## Clinical Guidelines

Before the 1970s, the gatekeeping of who became a medical professional largely regulated the strength of medical practice.[3] In other words, the education and training for physicians and other health care workers were the primary means of ensuring that those providing care were properly equipped to aid their patients. However, this approach led to a significant degree of variety in how different doctors treated their patients and what different physicians viewed as the best avenues for treatment. Through the final quarter of the twentieth century, organizations created CPGs to standardize treatment through a systematic review of the available evidence. For example, in 1981, the American College of Physicians (ACP) began developing clinical guidelines, and it had previously contributed to the development of other guidelines in the late 1970s.[4] A conservative estimate of guideline production—mostly located in the United States—showed that 55 guidelines emerged from 1945 to 1974.[5] By 2011, there were more than 3,700 guidelines from thirty-nine countries published in the Guidelines International Network database.[6]

There are various explanations behind the rise of guidelines.[7] The proliferation of medical knowledge, procedures, and products throughout the twentieth century made it increasingly difficult for physicians to keep up with all new information relevant to their practices. While medical journals and meetings allowed health care professionals to learn, they were not realistic strategies for synthesizing large swaths of information into methods of best practice. Thus, guidelines represented a form of medical knowledge regulation and quality control. Moreover, the production of clinical guidelines also intensified during a period of quickly rising health care costs. Guidelines appeared as a method to control costs through directing physicians toward effective treatments and limiting wasteful practices. Additionally, some researchers have posited that physicians created guidelines as a method of preserving their autonomy by creating standards of diagnosis and treatment detached from administrative pressures.

While many guidelines emerged as a method of standardization and quality control, there is significant variation in the quality of different guidelines. By passing the Omnibus Budget Reconciliation Act of 1989, Congress created the Agency for Healthcare Research and Quality (AHRQ).[8] Congress charged the agency with a mandate to "enhance the quality, appropriateness, and effectiveness of health care services."[9] The AHRQ also had to form a joint public-private partnership regarding the development, dissemination, and evaluation of CPGs. Thus, the agency's Office of the Forum for Quality and Effectiveness in Health Care was tasked with arranging for the development, periodic review, and updating of CPGs.

To assist the AHRQ, the Committee to Advise the Public Health Service on Clinical Practice Guidelines within the IOM published a report in 1990 on the state of CPGs. The report found that the state of CPGs at the time was deficient "in method, scope, and substance."[10] Wide variations in terminology, technique, and the quality and quantity of evidence inhibited the effectiveness of such guidelines. The report also notes that "disproportionately more attention is paid to developing guidelines than to implementing or evaluating them." As a result, the committee proposed numerous solutions to improve the CPG landscape. Broadly, the committee recognized that "scientific and clinical evidence should take precedence over expert judgment" and that the AHRQ should focus on ensuring CPGs are valid, reliable/reproducible, clinically applicable, clinically flexible, clear in language, developed by multiple disciplines, having scheduled reviews for possible revisions, and having fully documented development procedures.[11]

Yet, a 1999 *JAMA* study revealed that the majority of CPGs failed to adhere to recognized standards for guideline development.[12] The authors developed an instrument to measure adherence to key elements for guideline development and reporting based on the views of the IOM and other major actors, such as the National Library of Medicine, the ACP, and the AHRQ. Examining 279 guidelines published by sixty-nine unique developers from 1985 through June 1997, they found that the average adherence to the standards was only 43.1 percent, meaning that CPGs failed to meet most key standards on average. Adherence was especially poor with standards for evaluating evidence, at 33.6 percent. While adherence to measures of guideline development and format improved from prior to 1990 (41.5 percent) compared to after 1995 (55.9 percent), poor evaluation of evidence did not significantly change (34.6 to 36.1 percent).

On top of failing to meet recognized elements of adequate quality, various methods CPGs used to grade the quality of evidence all suffered serious limitations. In a 2004 *BMC Health Services Research* analysis, researchers compared and contrasted six of the most prominent systems that fifty-one CPG-sponsoring organizations used to create guidelines.[13] They found that the reproducibility of judgments made using all six systems was low and that all systems at least sometimes would result in guidelines lacking necessary information.

In 2008 and 2011, the IOM published reports updating the state of CPGs.[14] In the 2008 report, the IOM concluded that "it is not yet possible to say that the development of clinical guidelines is based on a scientifically validated process."[15] This stems from how guideline developers make conclusions that go beyond what the available evidence says, and there is insufficient distinction between the state of evidence and the subsequent recommendations. Even in situations with consensus for existing scientific evidence for a particular issue, different actors produce a variety of interpretations of the same evidence for clinical practice.

Guidelines' failure to make recommendations based on high standards of evidence is reflected by a 2009 *JAMA* article examining the scientific evidence underlying recommendations in the joint cardiovascular practice guidelines of the American College of Cardiology (ACC) and the American Heart Association (AHA).[16] Among the sixteen guidelines from 1998 through 2008 including reports of the level of evidence used, only 314 (11.6 percent) of the 2,711 total recommendations were based on evidence of multiple RCTs or meta-analyses. In contrast, the guidelines made 1,246 recommendations (46.0 percent) based on the lowest tier of evidence: expert opinions, case studies, or standards of care. Thus, a plurality of recommendations were not based on even a single RCT or nonrandomized study.

Furthermore, the 2011 IOM report on CPGs did not report much progress, noting that while the quality of guidelines had improved "over the past several decades, improvement has been too slow, and the quality of many guidelines remains subpar."[17] The report noted that guidelines not only suffer from significant gaps in research and low-quality research and systematic reviews, but also from "the dominance of industry-funded research and guideline development."[18] The majority of published evidence underlying CPGs comes from industry-sponsored studies, which are biased to produce conclusions favorable to sponsors. Additionally, the studies themselves are predominantly conducted by "profit-making research companies" rather than academic medical centers. The IOM ultimately considered industry-sponsored research to be "severely limited" because these studies used for FDA approval "follow patients for relatively brief periods of time, involve comparatively small numbers of younger and healthier patients than the drug's target population, may rely on comparison with placebo only, and often use surrogate endpoints" (more on surrogate endpoints in Chapter 5).[19]

Following the IOM report, a 2012 *Archives of Internal Medicine* (now *JAMA Internal Medicine*) analysis found that CPGs failed to meet IOM standards after independently reviewing 114 unique guidelines selected at random from the website of the National Guideline Clearinghouse (NGC)—a database of guidelines that was maintained by the AHRQ.[20] The researchers measured how the guidelines adhered to eighteen out of the twenty-five recommendations from the 2011 IOM report, excluding seven recommendations pertaining to the articulation of recommendations, external reviews, and consistent monitoring of the literature after guideline publication. The median number of IOM standards satisfied by the guidelines was 8 (44.4 percent), and just 49.1 percent of guidelines met most IOM standards. Additionally, 35.1 percent of guidelines did not provide the evidence backing the individual recommendations given, and 98.2 percent did not include the unpublished data behind their conclusions. While 94.7 percent of guidelines explained the benefits of their recommendations, just 72.8 percent described potential harms, meaning that over a quarter (27.2 percent) did not.

In 2017, the AHRQ announced that it would require guidelines posted on the NGC to demonstrate "the extent to which clinical practice guidelines (CPGs) submitted adhere to the standards for trustworthiness."[21] These standards included transparency, minimizing COIs, proper evidence evaluation, and more. According to Dr. John Abramson, the NGC attracted around 200,000 visitors per month.[22] However, the AHRQ shut down the NGC in 2018 due to a lack of funding.[23] Thus, the opportunity for the NGC to provide physicians with a source of high-quality, unconflicted guidelines vanished.

The numerous issues with CPGs, such as poor evaluation of evidence, add to the reality that guideline developers—just like peer reviewers in medical journals—lack access to the underlying clinical trial data. In fact, guidelines rely on a systematic review of the available evidence that predominantly comes from the published data and results in medical journals themselves. Therefore, the developers of guidelines rely on practically unvetted information from industry sponsors. One major example of the limitations of CPGs relating to the lack of high-quality evidence is the case of statin therapy, especially for women and people undergoing treatment for primary prevention of cardiovascular disease—meaning prevention for people without a history of cardiovascular conditions like heart disease or stroke.

## Statins

In May 2001, the National Cholesterol Education Program (NCEP) released guidelines about the detection, evaluation, and treatment of high blood cholesterol in adults.[24] They recommended that healthy men over forty-five years old and healthy women over fifty-five years old use cholesterol-lowering statin drugs for primary prevention of coronary heart disease (CHD) if they had (1) a 10–20 percent risk of heart disease over ten years, (2) LDL cholesterol levels of at least 130 mg/dL even with lifestyle change efforts like dieting, and (3) at least two other major risk factors—such as high blood pressure and a family history of heart disease. Yet, the guidelines did not make this recommendation for women based on clinical trial evidence. In Table VIII.2–1, the guidelines stated, "clinical trials of LDL lowering generally are lacking for this risk category: rationale for therapy is based on extrapolation of benefit from men of similar risk."[25] This admission was not transparent to most physicians, as the information was buried in the guidelines, while a summary posted in *JAMA* suggested that clinical trials had shown statin therapy providing favorable outcomes for women without a history of heart disease.[26] Moreover, these guidelines represented a dramatic shift from the previous 1993 guidelines to the extent that nearly three times as many Americans were prescribed statins under the 2001 recommendations.[27]

The guidelines made this recommendation to middle-aged women without clinical trial evidence at the same time as there were known alternatives to lower the risk of cardiovascular disease. The guidelines themselves recognized that lifestyle modifications, namely dietary changes and exercise, are extremely beneficial for reducing the chance of heart disease. In fact, lifestyle factors like lack of exercise, poor diet, and tobacco use account for around 80 percent of cardiovascular disease.[28]

In 2004, new NCEP guidelines further lowered the aforementioned threshold for statin therapy from those with LDL cholesterol levels of at least 130 mg/dL down to 100 mg/dL.[29] Yet, only one of the five new trials incorporated into the updated guidelines included this risk group of women. Women did not experience any benefit from a statin drug, Lipitor (atorvastatin), for the study's primary endpoint of nonfatal heart attacks and fatal CHD.[30] Less than one-fifth of the trial participants were women, and the authors recognized the trial shared a flaw with most other large statin studies by mostly including white male participants.

Over time, guidelines continuously lowered the threshold for when physicians should prescribe statins for primary prevention without high-quality clinical trial evidence of widespread benefit among men or women. The aforementioned trial did not show that Lipitor reduced the incidence of death for men and women compared to placebo. Thus, even against no alternative method of treatment, such as lifestyle modification, Lipitor did not reduce mortality rates. A 2010 *JAMA Internal Medicine* meta-analysis of eleven RCTs supported this finding, recognizing a lack of "evidence for the benefit of statin therapy on all-cause mortality" for primary prevention in high-risk groups.[31]

In 2013, the ACC and AHA issued guidelines further reducing the threshold for statin usage in adult populations for primary prevention, lowering the required level of heart disease risk from 10 percent to 7.5 percent while removing the LDL level requirement entirely.[32] These new guidelines were based on a 2012 meta-analysis from the Cholesterol Treatment Trialists' (CTT) Collaboration, which has access to private, underlying clinical trial data from statin manufacturers to conduct such studies.[33] Yet, the guideline writers at the ACC and AHA did not have access to this data. Even without access to the underlying data, however, independent reanalysis of the published results showed that statins did not reduce mortality and serious illness in populations at low risk of heart disease (<10 percent over five years).[34] While the data did show a reduction in nonfatal heart attacks and strokes for low-risk people, the number needed to treat was 140 over five years, meaning that 140 people need to take a statin for five years for one person to not have a nonfatal heart attack or stroke. According to one of the authors of the reanalysis, Dr. John Abramson, 99 percent of the low-risk population recommended for statin therapy under the 2013 guidelines would not derive meaningful benefit.[35] Therefore, the 2013 guidelines recommended statin therapy for a low-risk population where the vast majority of individuals would not derive a benefit, alternative methods to reduce heart disease risk exist, and the evidence that showed minimal benefit was sponsored by industry where the underlying clinical data were not known to the guideline writers.

Responding to the independent reanalysis published in the *BMJ*, one of the authors of the CTT Collaboration meta-analysis, Dr. Rory Collins, called on the journal to retract the paper due to one error in reporting statin side effects based on an observational study that was corrected prior to the complaint.[36] The *BMJ* commissioned an independent panel to review the call for retraction and ruled against doing so, upholding the validity of its primary claims. The panel highlighted the importance of the CTT making its data publicly available due to how two different meta-analyses of statins for primary prevention reached completely different conclusions—one claiming they reduced total mortality and the opposite for the other—because of a difference of just half of a percent in their statistical conclusions.[37]

Proponents and critics of widespread statin usage largely agree that people benefit from such therapy for secondary prevention: prevention for people who have already experienced cardiovascular conditions/events. Here, the CTT Collaboration study found that the absolute risk reduction (ARR) for a recurrent episode was 3.3 percent, meaning that thirty people need to receive treatment over five years for one person to not suffer another cardiovascular event.[38] Regarding mortality, the ARR was 1.25 percent, meaning that eighty people would need to receive treatment over five years to prevent one death. Thus, twenty-nine (96.7 percent) out of thirty people and seventy-nine (98.8 percent) out of eighty people over five years would not benefit from not having a recurrent cardiovascular episode or dying. While these numbers show a higher benefit to secondary prevention patients, they can provide nuance that physicians or industry advertisers may not present to patients.

Guidelines continue to recommend statin therapy to millions of Americans, including for primary prevention and those at low risk of heart disease, while the available evidence does not suggest clinical benefits for most users. A 2022 *JAMA Internal Medicine* meta-analysis examined twenty-one RCTs investigating statin therapy's effects on total mortality, cardiovascular outcomes, and strokes in adults.[39] These trials were at least two years long, enrolled over 1,000 participants, used a placebo/usual care comparator, and reported absolute changes in LDL cholesterol levels. They found that the overall ARR for all-cause mortality, heart attack, and stroke was 0.8 percent, 1.3 percent, and 0.4 percent, meaning that 125, 77, and 250 people would need to be treated for one individual over 4.4 years to not die, have a heart attack, or have a stroke, respectively. However, the numbers are lower when only looking at primary prevention, where the ARR was 0.6 percent, 0.7 percent, and 0.3 percent. Thus, 167, 143, and 333 people would need to be treated for one individual over 4.4 years to not die, have a heart attack, or have a stroke, respectively. Ultimately, the researchers concluded, "our analysis found that when considering the ARR of statins, the benefits are quite modest, and most trial participants who took statins derived no clinical benefit."

At the same time, their analysis did not disaggregate data on the effect of statins for primary prevention in individuals with low risk of developing cardiovascular disease. Thus, the small benefit may be larger than the actual benefit for this low-risk population. Additionally, the researchers themselves noted the limitation that they did not have access to the individual patient data, meaning they had to rely on unvetted data from published studies. Also, the data came from industry-sponsored studies rather than a base of independent trials. Yet, given these limitations, the authors found that their results were "inconsistent and inconclusive" regarding the widespread belief underlying clinical guideline recommendations for statin therapy that more LDL cholesterol reduction from statin therapy reduces all-cause mortality, heart attacks, or strokes.[40]

Like all treatments, statins are not free of risk; but, they are largely not severe. The most commonly cited adverse effects of statins are muscle pain and fatigue.[41] A 2016 review of observational data revealed that up to 10 percent of statin users may experience muscle-related side effects.[42] A 2012 *JAMA Internal Medicine* letter reported the results of an RCT, finding that generally healthy adults who received modest statin doses experienced worsening of energy or exertional fatigue compared to placebo.[43] Given that lifestyle factors account for roughly 80 percent of cardiovascular disease, side effects that make it more difficult to adopt healthy behaviors like exercise can be significant.[44]

Accordingly, statins may dissuade statin users from adopting healthy habits, such as healthy eating, which are recognized as optimal methods to reduce the risk of cardiovascular disease. A 2020 *Journal of the American Heart Association* cohort study examined 41,225 Finnish adults above the age of forty across four-year time intervals in 2000–13, finding that people who initiated antihypertensive and statin medications were more likely to become obese and physically inactive compared to those who did not.[45] At the same time, medication users were more likely to stop smoking and reduce drinking. A 2014 *JAMA Internal Medicine* study examined a national sample of almost 28,000 US adults aged twenty years and older from 1999 to 2010.[46] While caloric and fat intake was smaller for statin users compared to nonusers initially, statin users consumed significantly more calories (9.6 percent increase) and fat (14.4 percent increase) by 2009–10 while nonusers' intake stagnated. Statin users also experienced a statistically significant larger increase in their body mass index (BMI). These results show an association rather than alone proving causality. However, numerous scholarly analyses suggest a substitution effect where drug usage can replace more effective lifestyle changes.[47]

There are other much rarer harms of statins, such as diabetes and cognitive impairment; however, the data on adverse events with statins overall is highly lacking. Almost all statin trials are industry-funded, and the data is not available publicly or to researchers.[48] For example, the CTT has kept secret the IPD from twenty-four trials of statins since 1995, significantly limiting the ability for researchers to vet the published data.[49] Along with withholding data, industry control over design has distorted the extent to which trials find adverse events. The 2012 CTT meta-analysis results report that the excess risks of developing myopathy and diabetes by taking statins compared to placebo was one per 2,000 and five per 1,000, meaning that 2000 and 200 people would need to receive statin therapy over five years for one excess case of myopathy (a disease that weakens muscles) and diabetes.[50] However, these numbers, namely those for muscle pain and weakness, are at significant odds with observational findings and the views of many physicians.[51] For example, a 2008 examination of the CDC's

National Health and Nutrition Examination Survey found that the absolute risk of myopathy was one hundred times greater than shown in the CTT meta-analysis, where nineteen people would need to receive therapy for one excess myopathy case to occur.[52] The American Heart Association even recognizes muscle symptoms as the most statin-related adverse side effect.[53]

Why is there such a discrepancy? The CTT meta-analysis defined myopathy as muscle weakness or pain where blood creatine kinase levels are more than ten times the upper limits of the standard range.[54] By examining such a high value, the study did not actually examine the true extent of muscle-related adverse events. In fact, a 2016 *JAMA* article revealed that a review of forty-four RCTs showed that only one directly asked patients about muscle-related symptoms.[55] The one RCT focused on a disproportionately healthy and young (average age was forty-four) participant population and found that statin users experienced 4.8 percent more muscle symptoms than those using placebo. As Chapter 1 discusses, industry control of trials biased the reported outcomes by not asking the questions that could reveal bad effects from their products.

While the risk of side effects from statins are rarely severe, they are especially relevant given little to no clinical benefit for most patients, potential substitution for healthy lifestyle changes, side effects making it more difficult to adopt such changes, lifestyle factors accounting for 80 percent of cardiovascular disease, and health care costs. For the latter, the United States spent an estimated $24.5 billion on average annually from 2002 to 2018 on statins.[56] While generic statins are often relatively cheap for individual patients—monthly costs often range from $5 to $25—Americans paid high prices before patent expirations.[57] For example, Lipitor cost up to around $160 a month ($1,920 annually) out of pocket (OOP) as generic competitors entered the market in December 2011.[58] Overall, presenting nuanced information unreflected in guidelines to clinicians and patients about true benefits and risks can allow for informed choices. Transparency is especially important when other treatment options like lifestyle modifications exist, which address the predominant causes of cardiovascular disease and can become more difficult for statin users.

Based on 2005–12 data, the CDC found that 78.1 million Americans were eligible for statin therapy among which 43.3 million (55.5 percent) reported taking statins.[59] Following the 2013 ACC/AHA guidelines, national survey data showed that the number of individuals reporting taking a statin dramatically increased. Using survey results, in 2008–09, researchers estimated 31 million Americans took statins, climbing to 37 million in 2012–13 and then 92 million in 2018–19.[60] Annual prescriptions for statins shot up from 461 million in 2008 to 818 million in 2019. While most statin usage is for secondary prevention, survey results published in *Annals of Internal Medicine* revealed that 35.6 percent of statin indications were for primary prevention as of 2017–18, representing 76.7 million adults.[61] Roughly a third of the eligible adults actually took statins, meaning an estimated 24.9 million were primary-prevention users. However, there were around 33 million primary-prevention users if applying the 35.6 percent to the estimated 92 million 2018–19 statin takers. In either case, there was a significant increase, as national survey data estimated that 19.4 million Americans took statins for primary prevention before the 2013 guidelines.[62]

Updated guidelines continue to recommend statin therapy to millions of Americans for primary prevention. The updated 2018/2019 ACC/AHA guidelines recommend statin therapy for many adults with between 7.5 percent and 20 percent risk of cardiovascular events.[63] They also push a risk discussion about potential treatments like statins between clinicians and their patients for those at borderline risk (between 5 percent and 7.5 percent risk over ten years). In 2022, the US Preventive Services Task Force (USPSTF) slightly updated its previous 2016 recommendations, directing physicians to prescribe a statin to all American adults between the ages of forty and seventy-five if they have at least one risk factor for cardiovascular disease and their risk of having a cardiovascular event is at least 10 percent over ten years.[64]

In a 2022 commentary on the updated USPSTF guidelines, *JAMA* editor-in-chief Rita Redberg and her coauthors highlighted how the guideline authors did not have access to the IPD for many of the trials.[65] In particular, the CTT blocked access to all its twenty-four industry-sponsored trials comparing statin use with a control group. Redberg and her colleagues warned:

> There are further reasons to curb our enthusiasm about the use of statins for primary prevention of CVD. There is a difference between statistically significant and clinically meaningful benefit … the absolute benefit for those in lower-risk categories is likely small given that their baseline absolute risk is low, while the chance of adverse effects is constant across risk categories.

With the United States spending $24.5 billion on statins on average annually from 2002 to 2018 and many nonmedical factors causing cardiovascular disease, the authors reasoned that lowering individuals' LDL cholesterol is less effective for preventing poor health outcomes compared to the more widespread benefits of healthy eating and physical activity.[66] Thus, they cautioned against extolling "the marginal, likely small, and uncertain absolute benefits of statins for the few in primary CVD prevention."[67]

## Financial Ties with Industry

Along with lacking access to underlying clinical data and relying on unvetted industry manuscripts and study results to develop guidelines, key individuals involved in the production of CPGs have significant COIs with industry. Thus, along with varied and poor evaluation of evidence and the inability to access underlying clinical trial data, COIs may corrupt the interpretations of existing evidence to the benefit of industry and detriment of patients.

A 2002 *JAMA* study sent surveys to 192 authors of forty-four different CPGs published from 1991 to July 1999 that were endorsed by North American and European societies on common adult diseases.[68] They received responses from just 100 (52.1 percent) of the authors for thirty-seven CPGs, finding that 87.0 percent of authors had some form of relationship with pharmaceutical companies. These relationships included speaker honorarium/payment (64.0 percent), research support (58.0 percent), travel funding/honorarium (53.0 percent), educational program support (51.0 percent), service as an employee or consultant (38.0 percent), and equity (6.0 percent). On average, 81.0 percent of authors per CPG had interactions with the pharmaceutical industry, and 59.0 percent of authors had relationships with companies whose products were mentioned in the guidelines they wrote. The study results may have been conservative, as 47.9 percent of authors the researchers sent a survey to did not respond, and more conflicted authors could simply choose not to disclose their ties.

One example of such COIs is how the creators of previously described statin guidelines had ties to the statin-producing drug companies. Of the nine panel members who drafted the 2004 NCEP guidelines, eight had financial ties to statin makers.[69] Six had financial ties to at least three of the five relevant statin manufacturers through research grants, speaking honorariums, or consulting fees.[70] Two owned stock in the companies and two others left to work for drug companies after producing the guidelines.[71] One of the guideline developers who worked at NIH got $114,000 in consulting fees from statin manufacturers from 2001 to 2003.[72]

In 2004, Eli Lilly provided more than 90 percent of the funding for clinical guidelines about treating sepsis shock called the Surviving Sepsis Campaign (SSC).[73] These guidelines recommended the usage of activated protein C, otherwise known by Eli Lilly's brand name Xigris.[74] The basis for this guideline recommendation was a trial conducted at a single research center with results disproven by future trials.[75] Yet, the 2008 SSC guidelines continued to recommend Xigris, and eleven of the twenty-four guideline authors had financial ties to Eli Lilly. In 2011, Eli Lilly pulled Xigris from the market because its PROWESS-SHOCK trial failed to show a statistically significant reduction in all-cause mortality.[76]

In 2009, the IOM published a report entitled *Conflict of Interest in Medical Research, Education, and Practice*.[77] The report broadly covered issues with COIs across sectors—including biomedical research, medical education, medical practice, CPGs, and institutional COIs. Overall, the authors summarize:

> Widespread relationships with industry have created significant risks that individual and institutional financial interests may unduly influence professionals' judgments about the primary interests or goals of medicine. Such conflicts of interest threaten the integrity of scientific investigations, the objectivity of medical education, and the quality of patient care. They may also jeopardize public trust in medicine.[78]

The report acknowledges that the greatest impediment to "the development of sound clinical practice guidelines" is the lack of quality research and evidence.[79] This situation creates a need for "expert judgement based on clinical experience" that can be corrupted through COIs. Ultimately, "the risk of undue industry influence on clinical practice guidelines is significant."[80]

The IOM made several recommendations, like that guideline developers should "generally exclude" panel members with COIs and not accept direct funding from "medical product companies or company foundations."[81] Although general exclusion was not an explicit call for the lack of any conflicted members, the report further specified that the chair of a guideline panel along with a majority of members should not have a COI. The report also called for no panel members with COIs to engage in "deliberating, drafting, or voting on specific recommendations" in addition to public disclosure of such conflicts.

The 2011 IOM report entitled *Clinical Practice Guidelines We Can Trust* reaffirmed and expanded on both the findings and conclusions of the 2009 report. While CPG developing organizations had improved in disclosing members with COIs, "many experts are skeptical that disclosure alone minimizes the impact of conflicts."[82] As disclosures do not get rid of the actual integrity-compromising relationships between scientists and industry, scholars Daylian Cain, George Loewenstein, and Don Moore argue, "the most effective antidote for the problems caused by conflicts of interest is not to disclose them but to eliminate them."[83] Accordingly, the IOM recommended that guidelines avoid having conflicted authors "whenever possible," a majority of authors should never have conflicts, and both chairs and cochairs of guideline panels should not have conflicts.[84] The report also recommended that guideline panel members divest themselves of financial investments held by themselves or their family, and that they not participate in the marketing or advisory boards of entities that may be affected by guideline recommendations.

However, both IOM reports did not result in significant reductions in COIs plaguing guideline authors. The aforementioned 2012 *JAMA Internal Medicine* study that found that just 49.1 percent of 114 randomly selected guidelines published on the NGC website met a majority of IOM standards also examined adherence to COI standards.[85] The researchers found that a majority (53.2 percent) of guidelines did not disclose COIs, and that among the guidelines that did, 71.4 percent and 90.5 percent had chairs and cochairs with conflicts, respectively.

Reflecting these findings, seven of the fifteen experts on the panel who created the 2013 ACC/AHA guidelines that expanded the number of Americans recommended to receive statin therapy had disclosed financial COIs during the guideline development process.[86] One of the two cochairs, Dr. Jennifer Robinson, received over $100,000 in industry funding for statin research in 2013, and she had connections to over nine drug companies at the time of creating the guidelines.[87] Dr. Robinson received more than $3 million over the three years after the 2013 guidelines. Not included among the seven members with disclosed COIs was the chair of the committee, Dr. Neil Stone, who had financial connections with six companies as of May 2008, but he ended those relationships to lead the panel.[88]

Multiple studies over the last decade have confirmed the prevalence of COIs among CPG organizations and their authoring committee members. In a 2016 study published in *PLOS Medicine*, researchers examined the websites of ninety-five US and international medical organizations that produced 290 CPGs published in the NGC in 2012.[89] They also sent surveys to the selected organizations to obtain further characteristic information. Sixty (63.2 percent) out of the ninety-five guideline developing organizations received funding from biomedical companies, and sixty-four (67.4 percent) openly solicited funds on their websites. Among the thirty-eight organizations that responded to the survey, twenty (52.6 percent) disclosed receiving donations from for-profit companies compared to just nine (23.7 percent) from government sources and twelve (31.6 percent) from not-for-profit companies. Only 4 (1.4 percent) out of the 290 CPGs themselves had disclosure statements revealing the financial relationships of the organizations producing the guidelines. One hundred and forty-three (49.3 percent) or nearly half of the guidelines provided no disclosure statement regarding the financial relationships of committee members with biomedical companies. By contrast, 117 (40.3 percent) disclosed the existence of such financial ties compared to 30 (10.3 percent) reporting no ties. Thus, among the 147 guidelines with disclosure statements, 79.6 percent disclosed having members with financial ties with biomedical companies. Amid the 2,040 committee members behind the guidelines that had disclosure statements, 773 members (37.9 percent) disclosed financial ties.

A 2021 *Mayo Clinic Proceedings: Innovations, Quality & Outcomes* systematic review looked at studies from 2001 to 2019 that analyzed financial COIs among authors of CPGs published from 1980 to March 2019.[90] Among thirty-seven studies looking at 14,764 guideline authors, 6,589 authors (44.6 percent) had known financial COIs. Yet, nineteen of the studies relied on author disclosures from surveys or within a guideline's disclosure section, and seven studies relied on external searches such as disclosures in academic publications or peer-reviewed conferences. These studies revealed lower rates of author conflicts (43.3 percent and 34.7 percent, respectively) compared to the eleven studies relying on national databases (52.5 percent). Thus, disclosed conflicts may be a conservative reflection of actual financial ties. Accordingly, ten studies tracking undisclosed financial COIs found that 31.9 percent of authors had unreported conflicts, including 36.2 percent and 24.4 percent of authors with undisclosed general payments and research funds, respectively. Among the nine studies measuring the size of financial ties, median and mean payments ranged from $522 to $3,233 and $67,547 to $242,300, respectively. Therefore, many authors got relatively smaller payments compared to fewer who got incredible sums.

Within the large 2010 Affordable Care Act was the Physician Payment Sunshine Act that became federal law in 2012.[91] This law requires that all drug, device, biological, or medical supply manufacturers operating within the United States report payments to physicians and teaching hospitals. Manufacturers and group purchasing organizations—entities that negotiate medical products purchases collectively for multiple organizations—must also report ownership and investment interests held by physicians and teaching hospitals.[92] Additionally, the law mandated that HHS make the payments publicly available, and CMS started making such information available in September 2014 via the Open Payments Program (OPP).

Capitalizing on the OPP, researchers in *BMJ Open* investigated financial ties between 270 guideline authors and industry for twenty CPGs published in 2020.[93] The organizations that developed these guidelines were members of the Council of Medical Specialty Societies (CMSS), which is populated by major physician organizations such as the American College of Physicians, American College of Cardiology, and American Psychiatric Association.[94] All these organizations have disclosure policies for COIs. Yet, the researchers found that while 101 physician authors (37.4 percent) disclosed financial ties to industry within guidelines, the true number of COIs was far greater.

They found 199 authors (73.7 percent) to have received industry payments when searching through the OPP database. Thus, not only did three quarters of guideline authors have financial ties to industry, but disclosures only represented half of the true number of conflicts within the major physician organizations. Comparing guideline disclosures with the OPP database, they also found that just 26.7 percent of authors accurately disclosed their COIs: while 37.4 percent failed to disclose their conflicts, 8.5 percent underreported industry payments, 5.2 percent overreported payments, and 22.2 percent both underreported and overreported.

Violating IOM recommendations, only 25.0 percent of guidelines had panels with a minority of authors having financial ties to industry. Additionally, while seven (31.8 percent) of twenty-two panel chairs declared COIs, the OPP database revealed that eighteen (81.8 percent) had such conflicts, none of whom accurately disclosed them. Overall, the OPP documented over $98.7 million in total financial ties to industry with roughly $24.0 million (24.3 percent) being undisclosed. Around 80.8 percent of financial ties related to industry funding of a research institution or entity for research where the guideline author was a principal investigator. In comparison, 19.2 percent constituted direct payments, including payments for research, food and beverages, consulting, honoraria, royalties/licenses, education, gifts, travel, and lodging.

Researchers have not failed to identify more COIs among guideline authors. A 2023 *JAMA Network Open* analysis examined COIs among Infectious Diseases Society of America (IDSA) guideline authors.[95] Searching from June 2007 through March 2022, the authors identified ten IDSA guidelines with 149 authors that made drug-related recommendations. Seventy-one authors (47.7 percent) disclosed relationships with industry. Forty-eight (32.2 percent) disclosed such relationships where the pharmaceutical company produced a guideline-recommended drug at the time of guideline publication. The latter smaller cohort fit the author's strict definition of COI. Four of the ten guidelines had a majority of panel members with these narrowly defined COIs, and one guideline had a chair with such a conflict. Along with using a strict definition, the authors also only examined disclosed conflicts. As reflected by the *BMJ Open* study, disclosures may only be a fraction of the true number of financial ties.

Ultimately, the guidelines that physicians rely on for recommended standards of care suffer from COIs with industry among both the guideline-developing organizations and authors. These ties compound on the reality that guidelines often fail to evaluate and make recommendations on high-quality evidence. Instead, subjective author opinions and interpretations can direct their recommendations for clinicians. Even when guidelines are based on evidence from RCTs, the authors lack access to underlying clinical trial data, compromising them in the same manner as journal peer reviewers through their inability to vet the data.

## Weight-Loss Drugs

In recent years, large numbers of American adults have begun to use drugs to lose weight. According to a KFF poll from May 2024, around one in eight US adults reported ever taking a GLP-1 agonist: a type of drug used to treat type 2 diabetes and obesity through mimicking a hormone that the body naturally releases after eating.[96] For individuals with diabetes, these drugs help manage blood sugar levels. For obesity, they essentially make users feel less desire to eat. The percentage of Americans who reported ever using these drugs increased when looking at those told by a doctor that they had diabetes (43 percent), were overweight or obese in the last five years (22 percent), or had heart disease (26 percent). Among those who took GLP-1 agonists, slightly more than six in ten (62 percent) used the drugs to treat diabetes or heart disease and roughly four in ten (38 percent) utilized them only to lose weight.

The FDA approved the first GLP-1 drug—exenatide (Byetta)—produced by Amylin Pharmaceuticals and Eli Lilly in 2005.[97] However, the agency approved likely the most widely reported and known GLP-1 drug—semaglutide (Ozempic)—from Novo Nordisk in 2017. The FDA approved Byetta, Ozempic, and six of the seven drugs approved in between them for the treatment of type 2 diabetes, while it approved liraglutide (Saxenda) in 2014 for weight loss. Before the Ozempic approval, around one million people took liraglutide.[98] However, Ozempic's approval caused prescription volumes for GLP-1 medications to skyrocket, increasing by around 300 percent from 2020 to 2022 and accounting for around six million (65.4 percent) of all GLP-1 prescriptions by the end of 2022. Based on commercial insurance claims, GLP-1s surpassed other medications as the most dispensed weight-loss drug by 2023.[99]

While the FDA only approved Ozempic to treat type 2 diabetes, much of its vast uptake was due to off-label usage for weight loss. Its clinical trials showed that it significantly reduced body weight.[100] For example, the SUSTAIN 1 trial published in 2017 showed that, over thirty weeks, patients given placebo lost 1.0 kg (2.4 lbs) compared to nearly four times as much (3.7 kg or 8.2 lbs) and five times as much (4.5 kg or 9.9 lbs) with 0.5 mg and 1.0 mg doses of Ozempic, respectively.[101]

In the 2023 annual meeting of the Academy of Managed Care Pharmacy (AMCP), researchers presented findings from their study of a commercial health plan representing 20,000 members.[102] In 2008, only 6 percent of GLP-1 users did not have diabetes; this figure grew four and a half times over to 27 percent by 2022. Several news articles in 2023 and 2024 reported that diabetics were struggling to get ahold of their GLP-1 drugs, namely Ozempic, due to the significant off-label demand for a weight loss medication.[103] The FDA approved another Novo Nordisk semaglutide treatment, Wegovy, in 2021 specifically for weight loss.[104] However, immense popularity caused demand to far exceed the supply of the drug, resulting in many people taking other GLP-1s like Ozempic off label.[105]

With the rise of GLP-1s for weight loss, major clinical guidelines have recommended their usage for millions of Americans. In 2022, the American Gastroenterology Association (AGA) released its CPG recommending usage of weight-loss medications like semaglutide and liraglutide in combination with lifestyle modifications for Americans who were obese (BMI that is greater than 30 $kg/m^2$) along with those who were overweight (BMI that is greater than 27 $kg/m^2$) with weight-related complications like type 2 diabetes or heart disease.[106] This recommendation applied to those "who have an inadequate response to lifestyle interventions." In 2023, the American Academy of Pediatrics (AAP) released guidelines recommending that doctors "should offer" obese children—defined as those with a BMI at or greater than the ninety-fifth percentile for those of the same age and sex—who are at least twelve years old weight-loss medications like GLP-1s.[107] On June 20, 2025, the American College of Cardiology issued a consensus statement (discussed next in this chapter) recommending clinicians prescribe weight-loss drugs like GLP-1s as front-line treatments for obesity, meaning without first attempting lifestyle interventions.[108]

Yet, while weight-loss drugs reduce body weight, the contemporary evidence behind their long-term safety and effectiveness is highly lacking. In 2024, the USPSTF released guidelines concluding that "the totality of the evidence was found to be inadequate" for using weight-loss medications in obese children and adolescents.[109] There was a "small number of studies and limited evidence on long-term treatment harms." While the USPSTF has not released similar guidelines for adults, 2018 guidelines on behavioral interventions included studies on weight-loss medications, similarly finding that they have numerous "potential harms" like anxiety, nausea, mood disorders, and elevated heart rate that "have not been well studied."[110]

Furthermore, the studies on obesity drugs and consequent FDA approvals and clinical guidelines have focused on how they reduce overall body weight, which does not factor in fat versus muscle loss. Drugs like semaglutide have resulted in significant losses in lean muscle mass that yield consequences like weakening and worse metabolisms.[111] The 2021 clinical trial behind Wegovy analyzed the type of weight lost for a small subset of participants, finding that 40.0 percent of the reduction in BMI came from muscle rather than fat.[112] Over sixty-eight weeks, the placebo group lost 1.48 kg (3.3 lbs) of lean mass compared to almost five times as much (6.92 kg or 15.3 lbs) in the Wegovy group.

These results may understate potential muscle loss as the researchers provided counseling sessions over four weeks to help participants adhere to a healthy diet and exercise regime. This may not reflect the actual patient population, especially those who are overweight and obese and are inherently less likely to maintain a healthy lifestyle.[113] A 2023 CDC analysis of 2020 survey data found that not more than 28 percent of US adults got enough exercise.[114] A 2022 CDC study used 2019 national survey data to find that 87.7 percent and 90.0 percent of American adults failed to meet fruit and vegetable intake recommendations, respectively.[115] Exercise, especially resistance training, and proper diet are not just generally essential to build muscle, but they are key to minimizing muscle loss when losing weight.[116]

Weight-loss medications are also meant for long-term and even lifelong usage upon starting.[117] According to the codirector of the NIH's Office of Obesity Research in 2023, Susan Yanovski, "we wouldn't say, 'Well, great, your blood pressure is now down to normal, so stop the medication and we expect your blood pressure to stay down.'"[118] Yanovski told Axios that most people who stop taking these drugs regain their lost weight. The STEP 1 trial of semaglutide found that participants regained two-thirds of the weight they initially lost after stopping treatment within fifty-two weeks or one year after their sixty-eight weeks of treatment.[119] This trial was not unique, as numerous other studies have found similar results for a variety of weight-loss medications.[120]

Given the long-term nature of pharmacological treatment for weight reduction, the downsides of muscle loss are likely even more severe due to the negative outcomes of such weakness in old age. Harvard Medical School describes how muscle loss makes it harder to do daily activities, deal with and recover from illnesses and injuries, and can even cause dangerous or fatal falls.[121] A 2019 *Frontiers in Nutrition* review of the published literature notes how loss of strength and muscle function increases the risk of "falls, fractures, hospitalization, and reduced mobility in older persons."[122] According to Dr. Mitchell Steiner, the chief executive of biopharmaceutical company Veru and conductor of a trial involving semaglutide, "these weight loss drugs, they basically cause the development of frailty in older patients in months instead of years."[123]

With guidance from premier organizations like the ACC and AAP pushing clinicians to prescribe weight-loss medications to treat obesity for adults and children, the current directives make it so that most Americans take such medications under the direction of their doctors.[124] The 2024 KFF poll found that almost eight in ten US adults (79 percent) taking GLP-1 drugs say that they have got them from their primary care doctor or a specialist.[125] In May 2024, mainstream health information website *Healthline* quoted Dr. Katrina Mattingly who is the chief medical officer at Options Medical Weight Loss—an organization selling weight-loss treatment plans including through medications like GLP 1 agonists.[126] She stated that GLP-1 drugs are "grossly underutilized for overweight and obese populations." Dr. Mattingly is not alone in expressing this view; in 2020, the *Cleveland Clinic Journal of Medicine* published a commentary entitled "Overcoming Obesity: Weight-Loss Drugs Are Underused."[127]

Ultimately, the primary causes of weight gain and obesity are poor diet and lack of exercise, and weight-loss medications do not directly address either of these root causes.[128] There is a lack of evidence on long-term consequences even though medical professionals present them as potentially lifelong treatments. Adherence to such therapy results in overall weight loss, including a significant decline in lean muscle mass. As of July 2025, individual cartons of Ozempic and Wegovy cost around $1,000 and $1,300–$1,400, respectively, in the United States.[129] Around four in ten US adults and around one in five children are obese, and, pre-pandemic, almost three quarters of adults were overweight or obese.[130] Thus, according to the AGA and AAP guidelines, tens of millions of Americans are recommended weight-loss medications like semaglutide. While both guidelines also recommend lifestyle modifications, there is not quality evidence that weight-loss medication users adhere to such recommendations.

## Consensus Statements

Another source of medical knowledge that can direct physicians' behaviors is consensus statements. While clinical practice guidelines are ideally developed from a thorough systematic review of the available evidence to provide recommended standards of care, consensus statements are more specific to a certain point in time and disparate in their development.[131] Consensus statements are produced by a panel of experts who review currently and often newly available information to generate statements of fact rather than a thorough list of recommendations based on a consideration of benefits and harms.[132] However, consensus statements can also include recommendations and serve as forms of clinical guidance. Statements are often created when the collection of evidence for a more thorough clinical guideline has not finished.[133]

Inherent in the name, consensus statements are meant to "deduce perceived consensus" among relevant experts in particular fields.[134] When experts come together to produce a consensus statement, they are telling medical practitioners generally to listen to what a group of those with the best collective knowledge have deemed correct. Yet, consensus statements do not necessarily reflect an actual consensus in the scientific community, and they generally suffer from a low quality of evidence evaluation.[135] Following the IOM's 2011 report that called to raise the quality of guidelines, the American College of Foot and Ankle Surgeons switched to producing consensus statements due to not wanting to spend the money on rigorous CPGs.[136]

In 2014, *PLOS One* published an analysis of the quality of consensus statements in comparison to clinical guidelines published between January 2005 and September 2013 in three oncology-specific journals.[137] The researchers found that among the thirty-four consensus statements and sixty-seven CPGs, the score reflecting rigorous development for the statements was half that of the guidelines (32 percent compared to 64 percent). Only six (17.6 percent) of the statements referenced or conducted a systematic review of the evidence compared to 83.6 percent of the clinical guidelines. Regarding editorial independence—which includes whether the funders have influenced content—guidelines scored significantly higher (68 percent) compared to statements (53 percent).

The substandard rigor of consensus-based guidance is not limited to oncology. In 2021, the *BMJ* published an examination of twelve guidelines developed by the American College of Cardiology and American Heart Association that explicitly distinguished between consensus-based and evidence-based guideline recommendations.[138] The guidelines made 1,234 evidence-based recommendations, 304 (24.6 percent) of which were derived from low-quality evidence, while all consensus-based recommendations were rooted in low-quality evidence. The majority (58 percent) of the consensus-based guidance strongly made recommendations from such low-quality evidence, and the likelihood of making weakly substantiated recommendations was more than twice as likely compared to evidence-based guidance. Compared to evidence-based guidelines, the consensus-based approach was 2.6 times more likely to issue inappropriate discordant recommendations—where guidance was not warranted with the lacking evidence—and most (56 percent) were inappropriate. The authors also examined sixty-nine guidelines from the American Society of Clinical Oncology (ASCO), finding similar types of weak, discordant, and inappropriate consensus-based recommendations.

Researchers have not conducted the same level of widespread analysis to assess whether statements are affected by financial ties with industry; but, the *PLOS One* study documents a significant lack of disclosure.[139] Additionally, prominent organizations behind consensus statements have and continue to have significant COIs. For example, the American Association of Clinical Endocrinologists (AACE) produces consensus statements "to assist with clinical decision-making" regarding the management of type

2 diabetes patients.[140] AACE publicly boasts its Corporate AACE Partnership program, where it thanks companies that make diabetes-related products.[141] For example, the AACE website thanks companies like Novo Nordisk, Eli Lilly, Amgen, Bayer, Abbott, and Medtronic for being gold sponsors. As of July 2025, AACE publicly lists and thanks twenty-six corporate funders.

The 2023 AACE consensus statement that promotes numerous diabetes medications lists twelve authors, of whom ten disclosed financial ties with industry.[142] Illustrating the level of COI, one author got research funding from Abbott and AbbVie, actively served as a consultant to three companies including Novo Nordisk, actively was a speaker for seven companies like Eli Lilly, Bayer, and Novo Nordisk, was a national principal investigator for a diabetes trial funded by Gan & Lee Pharmaceuticals that tested the company's insulin injection product, owns her own private practice Endocrinology Associates, and co-owns the MediZen Institute that prescribes medications for weight loss.[143] The other nine author disclosures likewise revealed COIs often with multiple companies (see Figure 5). Previous AACE statement have similar levels of conflicts, as nineteen of the twenty authors of its 2018 consensus statement disclosed ties to industry.[144] Even the acknowledged individual who gave editorial support and writing assistance disclosed that she was a consultant for Lexicon Pharmaceuticals.

AACE's ties to industry are especially relevant considering that its recommendations helped push doctors to recommend expensive insulin treatments that provided little to no added clinical benefit for patients compared to cheaper alternatives.[145] The Cochrane Collaboration produced three reviews between 2006 and 2008, finding that insulin analogs were not more effective for type 2 diabetes patients compared to recombinant human insulin and only provided clinically insignificant benefits in terms of controlling blood sugar.[146] Yet, pharmaceutical companies pushed insulin analogs as far better products for types I and II diabetes patients and priced them accordingly.[147] In 2019, insulin analogs cost more than ten times the price of recombinant human insulin annually ($5,224 compared to $468).[148] Only 18.9 percent of US adults using insulin filled prescriptions for insulin analogs in 2000; this increased to 91.5 percent by 2010.[149] At the same time, AACE recommended insulin analog treatments through 2017. The organization's 2016 consensus statement said that "insulin analogs are preferred" and did not make any mention of the lack of significant benefit over cheaper recombinant insulin.[150] In 2018, AACE still pushed the superiority of insulin analogs, but it injected the following: "For those who find the more costly analog insulins unaffordable, human regular insulin or premixed human insulin for T2D are effective and less expensive options."[151] The 2023 consensus statement similarly prefers insulin analogs with a cost disclaimer.[152]

Furthermore, consensus statements can also mislead the public by stacking its members with those who conform to similar ideological stances. In a June 2024 commentary published in the *Journal of Clinical Epidemiology* entitled "Panel Stacking Is a Threat to Consensus Statement Validity," twenty-one medical researchers identify such "a major threat" where consensus statements become de facto forms of advocacy or lobbying.[153] They examine the specific case of a November 2022 consensus statement published in *Nature* that provided forty-one consensus statements and fifty-seven

| Author | Disclosed Conflict(s) of Interest |
|---|---|
| *Susan L. Samson* | • Member of the AACE Board of Directors and Executive Committee<br>• Research support to Mayo Clinic from Corcept Therapeutics<br>• Steering committee service<br>• National/overall Principal Investigator for Chiasma and Novartis<br>• American Board Of Internal Medicine Chair for the Longitudinal Knowledge Assessment Approval Committee for Endocrinology, Diabetes, and Metabolism |
| *Priyathama Vellanki* | • Consultant for Takeda Pharmaceutical Company<br>• National/overall principal investigator for NIH grant (number: K23 DK 11324-01A1) |
| *Lawrence Blonde* | • Consultant for Corcept Therapeutics, Merck, Novo Nordisk, Salix Pharmaceuticals, and Sanofi (paid through Ochsner Health) |
| *Elena A. Christofides* | • Research support from Abbott and AbbVie<br>• Consultant for Ascendis, Boehringer Ingelheim, and Novo Nordisk<br>• Speaker for Amryt, AstraZeneca, Bayer, Corcept, Eli Lilly, Boehringer Ingelheim, and Novo Nordisk<br>• Study protocol designer and national principal investigator for Gan & Lee pharmaceuticals' GLITTER1 diabetes mellitus trial<br>• Owner of Endocrinology Associates, Inc<br>• Part-owner of MediZen |
| *Rodolfo J. Galindo* | • Consultant for Bayer, Boehringer Ingelheim, Eli Lilly and Company, Novo Nordisk, Pfizer, Sanofi, and Weight Watchers<br>• Research support to Emory University for investigator-initiated studies<br>• National/overall principal investigator for Dexcom, Eli Lilly and Company, and Novo Nordisk<br>• Partially supported by the NIH's National Institute of Diabetes and Digestive and Kidney Diseases (numbers: P30DK111024-04S & 1K23DK123384) |
| *Irl B. Hirsch* | • Advisory board member for Abbott, Bigfoot, GWave, and Roche<br>• Research support from Beta Bionics, Insulet, and Medtronic Diabetes Care<br>• Consensus report developer regarding the Management of Type 1 Diabetes in Adults for the American Diabetes Association and European Association for the Study of Diabetes and an Endocrine Society guideline on inpatient diabetes management |
| *Scott D. Isaacs* | • AACE Board of Directors and Executive Committee member<br>• Unpaid consultant for Myovant Sciences, Madrigal Pharmaceuticals, Siemens, and Novo Nordisk |
| *Kenneth E. Izuora* | • AACE Board of Directors member<br>• Research support from Novo Nordisk<br>• Board member of the Nevada Clinical Endocrinologists Association |
| *Cecilia C. Low Wang* | • Research support to Jaeb Coordinating Center and the University of Colorado for investigator-initiated studies from Dexcom, Inc<br>• Treasurer of the American College of Diabetology<br>• Secretary of the Clinical Diabetes and Endocrine Institute<br>• Advisory Committee chair for the FDA on Endocrinologic and Metabolic Drugs |
| *Christine L. Twining* | None disclosed |
| *Guillermo E. Umpierrez* | • Research support and been a national/overall principal investigator for AstraZeneca, Dexcom, and Novo Nordisk<br>• President, Medicine & Science, for the American Diabetes Association<br>• Guideline developer regarding the Endocrine Society hospital diabetes guideline and Society of Critical Care CU diabetes guideline |
| *Willy Marcos Valencia* | None disclosed |

*These are only disclosed conflicts, meaning that the individuals could have undisclosed industry connections.*

**Figure 5** A table documenting disclosed conflicts of interest from the authors of the 2023 AACE consensus statement on managing type 2 diabetes. *Source*: Susan L. Samson et al., "American Association of Clinical Endocrinology Consensus Statement: Comprehensive Type 2 Diabetes Management Algorithm—2023 Update," *Endocrine Practice* 29, no. 5 (2023): 305–40, https://doi.org/10.1016/j.eprac.2023.02.001.

recommendations "to end the COVID-19 public health threat."[154] The statement had 386 listed authors with 40 core authors identified by the cochairs. The researchers found that at least 14 (35.0 percent) of the 40 core authors and 73 (18.9 percent) of all listed authors were directly "named in influential and highly visible Zero-COVID advocacy/activism" initiatives in North America and Europe. Zero-COVID refers to the policy, as occurred in China, of eliminating COVID-19 through preventing transmission and strictly controlling all outbreaks. Nineteen authors were anonymous; thus, 19.9 percent of all named authors were tied to Zero-COVID advocacy. Only 2 of the 73 authors disclosed their previous activism and advocacy in the paper's competing interests section. Overall, the commentary authors reasoned that the ideological balance of the consensus statement was extremely weighed toward Zero-COVID, as such policies had been widely abandoned by the time of publication, and the WHO director-general had stated that China's Zero-COVID policy was unsustainable.[155]

Additionally, the consensus statement did not conduct any systematic review of the evidence or take public comments, allowing for strongly opinionated experts to guide the drafting process with little checks. As the 2021 *BMJ* study found, consensus-based recommendations backed without quality evidence were several times more likely to produce inappropriate and discordant guidances compared to those rooted in thorough reviews of the evidence.[156] In a separate commentary, several of the *BMJ* authors advocated the abandonment of consensus-based guidelines generally to ensure trustworthy guidance.[157]

Given the severe issues with CPGs documented by the IOM and various research articles, the fact that consensus statements are significantly less evidence-based by comparison reveals the extreme extent to which they are not reliable, evidence-based forms of guidance that medical professionals can trust. Rather, consensus statements serve for groups of experts to argue their opinions in the name of a supposed consensus. Despite the weaknesses of clinical guidelines and consensus statements that undermine the medical community's ability to self-regulate, the American people ideally should be able to trust the basic safety and effectiveness of recommended treatments because they received FDA approval. Yet, as the next chapter discusses, weakening standards over the last several decades have greatly undermined the ability for Americans to do so.

5

# Faster Approvals and Weaker Evidence

What about the FDA? The previous several chapters have shown that industry controls most of the medical research behind the drugs and devices that Americans use. Their domination has not only prevented outside observers from independently analyzing and vetting clinical trial results, but it also includes significant financial entanglements with medical journals and clinical guidelines. Yet, the FDA stands as the guardian deciding whether medical products are safe and effective enough to be on the market. It has access to the underlying study data to make such decisions. Thus, if the agency is doing its job well, Americans can at least know that the treatments they receive are reasonably safe and effective, albeit for FDA-approved indications. However, is the FDA approval process a stalwart of public health?

According to Dr. Jonathan Darrow—a Harvard Medical School researcher—"there has been a gradual erosion of the evidence that's required for FDA approval."[1] Over the last several decades, changes in the US regulatory environment have fed industries' desire for faster approvals at the expense of thorough evaluations. For example, during the period from 1995 to 1997, more than four in five FDA approvals for new drugs were based on at least two pivotal trials: the most important trials for FDA approval decisions.[2] By 2015–17, this number had shrunk to 52.8 percent, meaning that nearly half of new drug approvals were mainly supported by one clinical trial. At the same time, the median time that the FDA took to review applications for approval fell by more than 67 percent from 1983 to 2018 even though the total time from authorization of clinical testing to approval remained relatively stagnant. The number of new drugs approved increased but not dramatically, rising from an annual average of thirty-four in the 1990s to forty-one from 2010 to 2018.

Since the passage of the Prescription Drug User Fee Act (PDUFA) in 1992, the FDA has formally become more intertwined with manufacturers and the pharmaceutical industry while prioritizing faster review times for product approvals under weaker standards of evidence. The FDA relies on industry for around half of all its funding for its operations, and this dependence is around 70 percent for human drugs specifically.[3] The agency directly negotiates with industry for what it recommends Congress pass in each five-year PDUFA reauthorization, and it regularly collaborates with sponsors during product development and review periods. Under congressional and industry pressure, the FDA has transitioned toward relying more on postmarketing surveillance rather than rigorous premarket review, granting power to manufacturers to market unproven products and control standards of safety and efficacy.

## Thirty Years of Decreased Standards and Industry Funding

In 1992, Congress passed the PDUFA, amending the Federal Food, Drug, and Cosmetic Act (FD&C Act) and transforming the relationship between pharmaceutical companies and the FDA through how the agency is funded.[4] Like other federal agencies, the FDA was almost entirely (over 95 percent) funded via congressionally appropriated funds from the US Treasury.[5] However, suffering from a lack of resources and understaffing, the agency did not review new drug applications in a timely manner. This issue was exacerbated by inflation-adjusted flat funding for the FDA under the Reagan administration through the 1980s.[6] By the late 1980s, the average time for the FDA to review a new drug application was twenty-nine months or nearly two and a half years.[7] Political support for expediting the FDA review process especially grew due to the AIDS epidemic and the search for an effective treatment, as one FDA official described the disease as "the poster child for rapid drug development."[8]

Rather than directly increase funding to the FDA, Congress passed the PDUFA—otherwise known as PDUFA I—creating a user fee program where pharmaceutical companies would directly negotiate with the FDA and fund the agency.[9] Companies that sought FDA approval for their products would pay the agency to help finance its operations.[10] The central purpose of the user fees under PDUFA I was to expedite the review of human drug and biologic applications. However, this was not officially codified into the FD&C Act until PDUFA II in 1997. In 1995, FDA spokesman Jim O'Hara stated that "protecting the public health does mean getting drugs to patients quickly."[11] The PDUFA is a living piece of legislation in the sense that Congress has to reauthorize the PDUFA every five years to continue providing user fee funding, and it has done so six times in 1997 (PDUFA II), 2002 (PDUFA III), 2007 (PDUFA IV), 2012 (PDUFA V), 2017 (PDUFA VI), and 2022 (PDUFA VII).

PDUFA I and its first reauthorization reduced review times in exchange for greater user fee funding. PDUFA I restricted the FDA to only use user fees for the "process for the review of human drug applications," and subsequent regulatory decisions committed the FDA to review 90 percent of standard applications within twelve months and 90 percent of priority applications within six months of submission by 1997.[12] According to a 1996 FDA policy, these priority reviews are reserved for products with "the potential for providing significant preventative or diagnostic therapeutic advance as compared to 'standard' applications."[13] For standard and priority supplements—applications to make changes to a product after it has already been approved—the FDA similarly set out to review 90 percent in twelve and six months, respectively.[14] PDUFA I did not allow the FDA to use user fee revenue to conduct postmarketing safety activities and monitoring, meaning it could not use the money to check the safety of products after approval.

In December 1992, the FDA finalized regulations for another mechanism: accelerated approval.[15] To qualify for accelerated approval, a drug must "have been studied for their safety and effectiveness in treating serious or life-threatening illnesses," and they must provide a "meaningful therapeutic benefit to patients over existing treatments." The program allowed the FDA to approve drugs whose clinical trials tested surrogate endpoints: measurements that predict a clinical benefit but do not themselves constitute such benefit. For example, many studies use cholesterol levels as a surrogate for cardiovascular disease risk. The regulations also allowed the FDA to approve a drug where evidence only shows efficacy and safety in very restricted circumstances. In this situation, the agency would limit distribution and prescription of the product along with requiring postmarketing efficacy and safety studies. Due to receiving accelerated approval based on surrogate endpoints, drug companies must conduct post-approval confirmatory trials "to verify and describe its clinical benefit." If a drug's confirmatory trial shows a clinical benefit, the FDA grants traditional approval. If the trial fails to show a benefit, the agency states on its website that it "has regulatory procedures in place that could lead to removing the drug from the market."[16]

PDUFA II (part of the FDAMA) set shorter performance goals, directing the FDA to review 90 percent of standard and priority applications and efficacy supplements in ten and six months, respectively, by the end of fiscal year 2002.[17] The reauthorization also created another expedited avenue: fast-track approval for drugs that are "intended for the treatment of a serious or life-threatening condition and … [demonstrate] the potential to address unmet medical needs for such a condition."[18] Receival of this designation can come from laboratory data rather than clinical trials.[19] The Fast Track designation for a drug allows the sponsor to frequently meet with regulators during the drug development process and prior to submission of an application for marketing approval. Rather than having to submit a complete application, sponsors can also get rolling approval from the FDA for the various sections of a complete application as they are ready. A Fast Track designation does not preclude a drug from also getting priority review and/or accelerated approval. Generally for all approved products, PDUFA II allowed the FDA to use user fee revenues to consult with manufacturers during clinical development, covering the period from the investigational new drug application submission that requests FDA approval to allow human testing through the agency's marketing approval decision.

Moreover, PDUFA II lowered the threshold for regulatory approval so that sponsors only need to submit one clinical trial to qualify for regulatory approval rather than two.[20] Thus, manufacturers often needed only to produce one trial with favorable results. The legislation also mandated that FDA officials meet with sponsors upon a sponsor's reasonable written request to discuss the design and size of a trial testing effectiveness. According to legal scholars Michael Malinowski and Grant Gautreaux, the PDUFA provided industry with "tremendous ongoing negotiation leverage" because user fee funding sunset every five years, meaning that the FDA would lose the funding it required for key operations and hundreds of staff if it failed to get support for reauthorization.[21] For the 1997 bill, the agency preferred a clean reauthorization of PDUFA I, but it accepted congressional and industry desires for further changes out of fear of budget cuts.[22]

Additionally, PDUFA II required the HHS secretary to create scientific advisory panels—now known as FDA advisory committees—to provide recommendations regarding a clinical trial and/or regulatory approval of a drug. These panels would include not just individuals with relevant expertise but also "a representative of consumer interests, and a representative of interests of the drug manufacturing industry not directly affected by the matter to be brought before the panel."[23] While the law requires panel members to disclose conflicts of interest and prevents anyone from voting "on any matter where the member or the immediate family of such member could gain financially from the advice given," it also allows the HHS secretary to grant a COI waiver to a member if they have "essential expertise."[24]

While PDUFA III did not shorten the application performance goals, it did expand industry influence over PDUFA reauthorizations and the FDA's ability to use user fees.[25] The legislation required the HHS secretary—and thus the FDA—to consult directly with "the regulated industry" (i.e., pharmaceutical companies) when developing its recommendations to Congress for what to include in subsequent reauthorizations.[26] The law also mandated the FDA to consult representatives of patient and consumer advocacy groups; yet, these organizations are also widely and significantly funded by industry.[27] Between 2010 and 2022, PhRMA and member companies gave over $6 billion in grants to over 20,000 organizations, including top patient advocacy groups like the American Heart Association and the American Cancer Society, which received $64 million and $23 million, respectively.[28] Results of a 2013–14 national survey of patient advocacy groups published in *JAMA Internal Medicine* found that 67.3 percent received industry funding.[29]

The legislation also allowed sponsors, during a product's development period, to request the FDA choose an independent consultant to help review the protocol for clinical studies. Furthermore, PDUFA III expanded the period when the FDA could use user fee revenue, beginning during preclinical development all the way through three years after regulatory approval for postmarket safety activities. Postmarketing activities could include the collection, development, and review of safety information.

Revealing the existence or perception of industry influence, PDUFA IV—part of the FDAAA—increased the opportunities for the public to see the FDA's recommendations for future reauthorizations following negotiation with industry.[30] It also mandated that HHS hold meetings at least once a month with patient and consumer advocacy groups to discuss their views on reauthorization during the period when government negotiates with industry. Congress's decision to make this requirement demonstrates the dominance of industry in negotiating the terms of PDUFA reauthorizations compared to other actors.

PDUFA IV also included a mandate to enhance the FDA's postmarketing authorities as a result of increased congressional and public scrutiny over the agency's ability to guarantee the safety of drugs.[31] In light of the Vioxx debacle that killed an estimated 30–60 thousand Americans and other worrying trends—such as increased risk of suicidal thoughts among children taking antidepressant medications like Paxil and Zoloft—Congress commissioned the Institute of Medicine in 2004 to evaluate the FDA's capacity to evaluate and ensure drug safety postmarketing. In its 2007 report, the

IOM found that contrary to its public health mission, the FDA failed to "consistently demonstrate accountability and transparency to the public by communicating safety concerns in a timely and effective fashion."[32]

Thus, the legislation bolstered the FDA's postmarketing activities by creating the Risk Evaluation and Mitigation Strategy (REMS) program, where the FDA can require drugmakers to implement a REMS—meaning "a structured plan ... intended to manage specific serious safety concerns" for certain drugs.[33] Strategies can include elements like ensuring a drug is only given in high-quality health facilities. PDUFA IV also expanded the FDA's ability to direct user fee revenue to postmarketing activities by eliminating the three-year postapproval limitation.[34] Thus, the FDA could use user fees to conduct such actions indefinitely over the life of a product. Additionally, PDUFA IV broadened the range of postmarketing activities that the FDA could direct user fee revenue toward, such as the collection and review of adverse event data, development and maintenance of adverse-event reporting systems, creation of better analytical tools to assess potential safety issues, and the enforcement of FDA requirements like those relating to postmarketing studies, labeling changes, and clinical trials. The legislation also created user fees for direct-to-consumer advertisements, where companies must pay a fee when submitting an advertisement for FDA advisory review.

In 2012, PDUFA V decreased the threshold for acceptable evidence for marketing approval, encouraged the increased use of accelerated approval, and created a new expedited Breakthrough Therapy designation.[35] Section 901 of the legislation "encouraged" the FDA to further expedite the development and review of new medicines, including to use "a broad range of surrogate or clinical endpoints and modern scientific tools earlier in the drug development cycle when appropriate."[36] The language explicitly revealed that doing so could "result in fewer, smaller, or shorter clinical trials."[37] Thus, while the 1992 regulations regarding accelerated approval already allowed the FDA to approve products based on surrogate endpoints, Congress gave the FDA a directive to expand this practice more broadly.

Moreover, the Breakthrough Therapy designation applies to drugs meant "to treat a serious or life-threatening disease or condition and preliminary clinical evidence indicates that the drug may demonstrate substantial improvement over existing therapies" based on at least one "clinically significant" endpoint.[38] The FDA currently includes surrogate endpoints that are potentially clinically significant but not firmly accepted as such.[39] Drugs with the Breakthrough Therapy designation receive all features of a Fast Track designation, the benefits of priority review, and other actions like intensive guidance from the FDA on drug development and clinical trial design along with the agency's organizational commitment.[40]

PDUFA VI in 2017 did not include many significant policy changes like past reauthorizations due to the passage of the 21st Century Cures Act in 2016. But, it directed the FDA to take actions relating to expanded access along with expediting review of generic drugs.[41] Expanded access refers to the pathway for patients with serious or immediately life-threatening medical conditions to access unapproved products still in the investigational period of development. The legislation also required the FDA to convene a public meeting within 270 days of the Act's enactment—including relevant stakeholders such as drug sponsors, health care providers, and patients—to discuss clinical trial inclusion and exclusion criteria, such as alternative trial designs. PDUFA VI encouraged participants to discuss collecting data from the expanded access programs as part of evidence of effectiveness. Congress mandated that the US Comptroller General produce a report on the state of the Expanded Access Program, including to what extent it reduced burdens of entry into the program and improved access to investigational, unapproved products.

Furthermore, PDUFA VI expedited the approval of certain generic drugs by granting priority review for generic drugs where there are less than three approved products without patent/exclusivity protections and for those that are on the FDA's shortage list.[42] For drugs with only one version (brand or generic) on the market, the legislation directed the FDA to expedite the development and review of competitive generic therapies through increased and intensified interactions between the FDA and the drugmaker.[43] Expediting generic drug approvals contrasts with PDUFA II and PDUFA V, which respectively granted and made permanent a six-month market exclusivity extension for drug companies that conducted studies in pediatric populations.

Unlike PDUFA VI, the 21st Century Cures Act (Cures Act) both expedited drug approval and reduced the quality of evidence required for approval among other industry-friendly reforms, like allowing drug companies to promote health care economic information supporting off-label uses if they include a disclaimer.[44] The legislation created an accelerated approval pathway for regenerative advanced therapies, meaning regenerative medicine therapies that treat serious or life-threatening medical conditions and where preclinical evidence suggests "that the drug has the potential to address unmet medical needs" for the respective condition(s).[45] Within this pathway, Congress allows the FDA to approve regenerative advanced therapies based on surrogate and intermediate endpoints along with potential postapproval study requirements that do not include using clinical data. These therapies are also eligible for priority review.

Regarding tools used for drug development and regulatory review—such as biomarkers and clinical outcomes assessments—the Cures Act made it optional for the FDA to accept submitted data based on scientific merit. Additionally, the legislation directed the FDA to allow approval of new indications/uses for drugs based on "real world evidence."[46] Rather than requiring the highest quality evidence from randomized clinical trials, the Cures Act allowed data from "ongoing safety surveillance, observational studies, registries, claims, and patient-centered outcomes research activities" to form the basis for approvals of new indications.[47] When establishing this program, Congress directed the FDA to consult with stakeholders including the "regulated industry" along with patient advocacy organizations that industry funds.[48] Along with real world evidence, the Cures Act permitted the FDA to "rely upon qualified data summaries to support the approval of a supplemental application" for a new indication, meaning that summaries of clinical data rather than the actual underlying data could form the basis for proving safety and efficacy.[49]

In 2017, Congress passed the Right to Try Act, easing federal law to allow the usage of unapproved, investigational drugs for terminally ill patients.[50] Patients are eligible if diagnosed with life-threatening diseases/conditions, have exhausted approved treatment options, cannot participate in a clinical trial for the particular drug, and provide written informed consent to their treating physician.[51] The drugs and biologics included in the Right to Try program have had a phase I clinical trial but have not been approved by the FDA. The agency has made clear that it has not determined if Right to Try drugs are safe, could cause serious adverse events, or lead to any clinically meaningful improvement.[52] The program produces a process of eligible patients and their physicians working with drug companies directly without FDA involvement or review of requests.

In contrast, the Expanded Access program—formalized in 1987—permits the FDA to allow usage of investigational drugs, biologics, and medical devices that it has not yet approved when a patient meets similar eligibility criteria to Right to Try in addition to determining if the potential benefit of treatment "justifies the potential risks."[53] Physician requests on behalf of patients for investigational drugs are approved by an Institutional Review Board (IRB), an administrative body with the purpose of protecting the welfare and rights of people. The FDA has approved around 99 percent of requests in this program, the vast majority of which in a few days; thus, critics of Right to Try question its need and removal of FDA oversight.[54]

The most recent authorization—PDUFA VII—did not significantly change application review speeds, evidence quality requirements, or industry influence over the reauthorization process.[55] This "clean reauthorization" of PDUFA came as a result of negotiations between differing House and Senate versions of the bill at the same time as Congress was working to fund the federal government.[56] Still, the performance goals

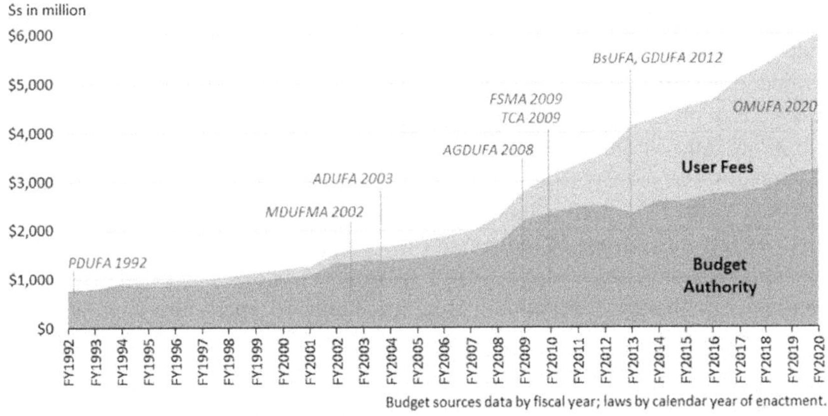


**Figure 6** A chart showing the FDA's growing reliance on user fees for its funding since the 1992 PDUFA. *Source*: Amanda K. Sarata, "The Food and Drug Administration (FDA) Budget: Fact Sheet," Congressional Research Service, December 9, 2022, https://crsreports.congress.gov/product/pdf/R/R44576.

of the FDA reflect its commitment to the expedited programs and lower evidentiary standards from past reauthorizations and the Cures Act.

As PDUFA and its reauthorizations created avenues for expedited development and review, they also significantly increased the FDA's reliance on user fees to fund its activities (see Figure 6).[57] In 1992, the FDA's budget was under $1 billion, and it has increased more than sixfold over the last thirty years. While user fees represented a very small portion of agency funding during the 1990s, they began to grow faster following PDUFA III, increased further by the late 2000s, and exploded during the 2010s.

For FY 2024, $3.3 billion or nearly half (47.8 percent) of the entire FDA budget came from industry user fees.[58] However, when looking at the budget for human drugs specifically—which constituted over $2.3 billion and is the largest FDA program—more than $1.6 billion (69.2 percent) of the funding came from industry user fees. The numbers are relatively much lower but still significant for the smaller biologics and medical devices/radiological health programs—representing 8.3 percent and 11.5 percent of the total FDA budget—where user fees comprised 53.1 percent and 43.7 percent of funding, respectively.

## Consequences and the Limits of Transparency

The original 1992 PDUFA grew out of the demands for faster drug review and approval during the AIDS epidemic.[59] Advocates argued that those suffering from serious and life-threatening conditions and diseases should be able to access potentially life-saving treatments, as the risks for not getting new treatments could outweigh the risks of receiving them. However, the various pathways and designations for faster product development and review have applied to an increasingly broad range of treatments and produced augmented risks of adverse events. Additionally, lower standards of evidence have allowed the FDA to approve products based on poor evidence, such as surrogate endpoints that do not actually reflect relevant clinical outcomes.

Since 1992, review times for products have significantly decreased. The median review time of new drugs and biologics fell from 26.6 months prior to PDUFA I to 8.1 months by PDUFA VI in 2017.[60] Standard review times fell from 33.5 to 12.0 months, and priority review times fell from 21.6 to 8.0 months. Most novel drugs approved by the FDA used at least one of the expedited programs. In 2024, the FDA approved fifty novel drugs, of which thirty-three (66.0 percent) used at least one of the following programs: accelerated approval, priority review, Fast Track designation, and Breakthrough Therapy designation.[61] More specifically, 56.0 percent of approved novel drugs went through priority review, 44.0 percent had Fast Track status, 36.0 percent were given Breakthrough Therapy recognition, and 14.0 percent went through accelerated approval. The year 2024 was not an outlier, as 60–74 percent of approved novel drugs in 2023 back through 2015 used at least one of the four programs, with an average of around two-thirds.[62]

Several studies have found that faster review times resulting from PDUFA yield greater safety problems and adverse events that can lead to the FDA removing a product off the market or mandating a black box warning on its labeling. The FDA gives black box warnings when deemed necessary to warn the public that a product can cause serious adverse reactions leading to injury or death.[63] A 2008 *NEJM* article tracked all approved new molecular entities (NMEs) between 1993 and 2005, finding that the novel drugs approved within two months before their PDUFA deadline were significantly more likely to be withdrawn from the market over safety concerns, receive a black box warning, and have dosage forms discontinued by the manufacturer compared to drugs approved at later times. Greater safety issues for drugs approved close to the PDUFA-expedited review deadlines were potentially due to pressures to approve products on time despite unresolved or under-scrutinized safety issues.[64] For NMEs submitted from January 1993 through December 2004, drugs were 3.4 times as likely to receive FDA approval in the relevant period—the two months prior to the PDUFA deadline—compared to all other periods for NMEs under both standard and priority review. Thus, in the years following PDUFA I, II, and III, the expedited drug review process had a likely consequence of significantly increased safety risks.

Additionally, a 2017 *JAMA* investigation involved a cohort study of the 222 novel therapeutics that received FDA approval from January 2001 through December 2010.[65] The authors tracked this cohort through February 28, 2017, finding that therapeutics that were approved within the sixty days prior to the statutory FDA decision deadline and those that underwent accelerated approval were statistically more likely to have had a postmarket safety event. These events included withdrawals due to safety concerns, FDA-added black box warnings, and FDA-issued safety communications. Priority review was not associated with more safety events. Another 2017 analysis in *Drug Safety* examined 219 NMEs submitted to the FDA from November 1997 through December 2009, finding that drugs that underwent priority review were 3.51 times more likely to receive a black box warning postmarketing.[66] Interestingly, it did not share findings surrounding safety and review time windows.

Moreover, a 2017 cohort study in *BMJ* examined the 382 novel therapeutics—not including vaccines and diagnostics—that the FDA approved between 1997 and 2014, including 135 drugs that went through at least one of the priority review, Fast Track, and accelerated approval programs.[67] They matched the expedited drugs with similar therapeutics that went through the standard pathway, finding that the expedited drugs were significantly more likely to receive safety-related labeling changes. Less than 5 percent of these labeling changes lessened the risk language, meaning that they predominantly indicated more risk. The authors highlighted that the two most clinically important types of changes—black box warnings and contraindications—occurred at a 48 percent higher rate in expedited drugs compared to standard pathway drugs. A less sophisticated 2016 *Health Affairs* examination of FDA-approved drugs in the sixteen years following the 1992 PDUFA found a significant correlation where drugs approved after the legislation were more likely to get withdrawn from the market or receive a black box warning compared to those approved beforehand.[68]

Theoretically, enhanced clinical trial transparency could help researchers, medical professionals, and doctors identify safety risks from products benefitting from expedited development and FDA review. Disclosure of underlying clinical trial data could allow outside actors to add extra eyes and increased scrutiny that FDA reviewers may have trouble applying, especially with the constant demand for faster reviews and decisions since 1992. Additionally, independent researchers and organizations may not face the same pressure from industry and Congress as the FDA does to approve more treatments. However, in the vast majority of circumstances, transparency would not be able to prevent or properly limit FDA approval of a dangerous treatment, as that would require sharing of clinical data prior to approval. While such early sharing of data has occurred, such as in the case of muraglitazar, this is extremely rare and currently up to the discretion of trial sponsors.

Another significant obstacle for enhanced transparency to yield better results is the decreased quality of clinical trial evidence that the FDA relies upon for approval decisions. Clinical trial data is useful insofar as the information is relevant to the medical uses being tested for. However, if the evidence itself is low quality, then revealing more data may not provide much public benefit. While lower standards can be a practical necessity for rare or life-threatening conditions without alternative treatment options (e.g., insufficient

| Four Criteria | |
|---|---|
| **The drug was compared to a control (placebo or another treatment).** | *A control group is necessary to contextualize measured outcomes from a treatment. Outcomes from participants under the same conditions in a trial except the different treatments can reveal causal differences or lack thereof from a tested product. Without any control, any measured change in outcomes could be from factors wholly unrelated to the tested treatment.* |
| **The study measured a clinical endpoint rather than a surrogate.** | *Surrogate endpoints are meant to predict a clinical benefit like survival but do not themselves measure such a benefit. Surrogate validity relies on a strong association with a relevant clinical outcome, which may still not show causality. Relying on surrogates can fail to measure harms outside of a trial's focus, such as a trial measuring a cardiovascular drug's effect on cholesterol missing an increase in non-cardiovascular mortality.* |
| **At least two "well-controlled" trials demonstrated effectiveness.** | *Having multiple studies showing a drug's safety and effectiveness is critical to show one trial's results are replicable and not due to chance. Trials' statistical analyses rely on probabilities, and there is always some chance an outcome is due to chance.* |
| **The participants and investigators were blinded.** | *Blinding is critical to prevent bias – such as the placebo effect – from both trial participants and those administering/conducting the trial. A participant's or researcher's knowledge of whether someone received a treatment or control can alter their behavior, corrupting trial results.* |

**Figure 7** Details of four critical components for high-quality clinical trials that can produce the most reliable results. *Sources*: The Lever and McGraw Center for Business Journalism, "Do Your Drugs Work? A Searchable Database," The Lever, accessed June 13, 2025, https://www.levernews.com/do-your-drugs-work-a-searchable-database/; Jeanne Lenzer and Shannon Brownlee, "Should Regulatory Authorities Approve Drugs Based on Surrogate Endpoints?," *BMJ* 374, no. 8306 (September 16, 2021): n2059, https://doi.org/10.1136/bmj.n2059.

patients for a randomized trial for an extremely rare disease), real-life applications have been much broader. Among 427 FDA drug approvals from 2013 to 2022, 71.9 percent did not meet one or more of four critical criteria for high-quality trials (see Figure 7).[69]

A majority (51.8 percent) of the approvals relied on surrogate endpoints, nearly half (48.9 percent) did not have at least two well-controlled studies, three in ten (30.2 percent) relied on studies that were not blinded, and almost one-fifth (18.5 percent) relied on studies with no control group. Additionally, 122 drugs (28.6 percent) received a boxed warning (25.3 percent), were discontinued (2.1 percent), or underwent some form of withdrawal (1.2 percent). The investigators themselves noted that these numbers are "purposefully biased" in favor of industry.[70] For example, they listed drug approvals as depending on clinical outcomes even when actually relying on surrogate endpoints because the trial also tested and failed to show a clinical outcome benefit. They counted a study as blinded when it was partially blinded or if a blinded third party evaluated results when the actual participants and investigators were unblinded.

A 2020 *JAMA* investigation scrutinizing the quality of clinical trial evidence supporting FDA approval examined the pivotal trials behind 273 novel therapeutic approvals for 339 indications across three distinct periods: 1995–97, 2005–07, and 2015–17.[71] The percentage of approved drugs and biologics using at least one expedited program increased over time from 34.6 percent during 1995–97 to 57.9 percent during 2005–07 to 64.2 percent during 2015–17. The number of randomized trials fell from 93.6 percent during 1995–97 to 82.2 percent in 2015–17. Over the same periods, the percentage of double-blinded trials—blinding of both the participants and researchers to treatment status—fell from 79.4 percent to 67.6 percent. While 44.1 percent of pivotal trials during 1995–97 used an active comparator—another treatment for the tested indication—only 29.2 percent did in 2015–17. The percentages of trials using placebos and no comparison group increased: 47.4 percent to 53.0 percent and 8.5 percent to 17.8 percent, respectively. While 43.8 percent and 48.3 percent of 1995–97 pivotal trials relied on clinical and surrogate endpoints, respectively, the percentage of trials relying on surrogate endpoints increased to 59.3 percent and those using clinical endpoints fell to 23.3 percent during 2015–17. Interestingly, for therapeutic trials involved in an expedited program, the percentage using clinical endpoints stayed relatively constant while those relying on surrogates fell from 75.3 percent to a smaller 67.2 percent majority; but, the decrease was not statistically significant. This result may reflect both the increase in surrogate reliance from traditionally approved therapeutics (41.3 percent to 51.2 percent) and the overall larger usage of expedited programs.

Furthermore, PDUFA II's allowing of sponsors to submit one clinical trial to qualify for regulatory approval rather than two had a significant effect. The percentage of indication approvals relying on at least two pivotal trials fell from 80.6 percent during 1995–97 to 60.3 percent in 2005–07 and 52.8 percent in 2015–17. This decrease is likely driven by therapeutics in expedited programs, as the percentage of those indication approvals relying on at least two pivotal trials decreased from 75.0 percent to 38.1 percent. The drop for traditionally approved indications was 8.3 percent and not statistically significant. While the percentage of indication approvals that relied on trials using only surrogate endpoints did not significantly change across the periods, a significant percentage

(45.3 percent) were in this category during 2015–17, including a majority (55.6 percent) of those involved in expedited programs and 30.2 percent of those traditionally approved. Additionally, the number of indication approvals that relied on at least one trial with any comparator fell from 96.0 percent during 1995–97 to 83.0 percent in the 2015–17 period. One metric that shows a potential strengthening of rigor is that the duration of trials increased from 1995–97 to 2015–17. The percentage of indications approved based on at least one trial of a duration of six months or more increased from 25.8 percent to 46.2 percent and a duration of twelve months or more from 18.5 percent to 35.8 percent.

A 2020 *JAMA* paper examining all FDA-approved novel therapeutic drugs in 2020 corroborates key findings from the previous analysis.[72] Over half (57.1 percent) of all drug approvals relied on a single pivotal trial for approval. Only 76.0 percent of pivotal trials had at least partial randomization, meaning that nearly a quarter of pivotal trials forming the basis of FDA approvals were not randomized at all. Trials were not randomized for 26.5 percent of drug approvals. Additionally, nearly four in ten pivotal trials (38.7 percent) did not blind both researchers and participants, and 42.9 percent of approved drugs relied on pivotal trials that were not double-blinded. Surrogate measures were the primary endpoints for 45.3 percent of pivotal trials—meaning the main result—and most (57.1 percent) of the drug approvals relied on at least one pivotal trial with a surrogate as the primary endpoint. A majority (52.0 percent) of the pivotal trials used a placebo or vehicle control rather than an active control as the comparator (17.3 percent). Additionally, only 2.7 percent of trials used both an active control and placebo to both compare the drug with an existing treatment while controlling for the placebo effect on safety and efficacy. Twenty-eight percent of pivotal trials used historical, external, or other controls, and this category includes single-group trials with no comparator. The authors also divided the data by whether they pertained to oncology or nononcology approvals, and each measure showing weak scientific rigor was significantly more prevalent among oncology approvals.

## Invalid Surrogates

As FDA approvals have increasingly depended on pivotal trials relying on surrogate endpoints, evidence suggests many of these measures are not strongly tied to relevant clinical outcomes. An April 2024 *JAMA* investigation examined meta-analyses—including systematic reviews and pooled analyses—of clinical trials relating to nononcologic chronic disease treatments where researchers used surrogate measures as the primary endpoints.[73] They identified thirty-seven different surrogate measures relating to thirty-two nononcologic chronic diseases that were posted on the FDA's Surrogate Endpoint Table. This table—by the mandate of the Cures Act—includes the "surrogate endpoints which were the basis of approval or licensure (as applicable) of a drug or biological product" for both accelerated and traditional approval.[74] The FDA officially states that endpoints listed in the table "should facilitate consideration of potential surrogate endpoints when developers are designing their drug development programs." Officially, surrogates to support traditional approval must be "known to predict clinical benefit" while only needing to be "reasonably likely to predict clinical benefit" for accelerated approval.

For 59.5 percent of the surrogate measures backing approvals, there were no meta-analyses of clinical trials examining the connection between the surrogate and the relevant clinical outcome. Among the remaining 40.5 percent of measures with at least one meta-analysis, the authors identified fifty-four of such analyses looking at 109 surrogate measure–clinical outcome pairs. Fifty-nine of the pairs measured the strength of the correlation between the surrogate measure and clinical outcome via an $r$ or $R^2$ value, finding that only 16.9 percent of these pairs were justified based on strong correlations. The remaining fifty pairs had different statistical analyses of which almost half (48.0 percent) reported no statistically significant relationship between surrogate measures and respective clinical outcomes.

Furthermore, as oncology drugs are more likely to undergo some form of expedited development and review—especially accelerated approval—relevant trials have disproportionately relied on surrogate endpoints compared to other therapeutic classes. Several analyses have specifically examined the strength of surrogate measures in relation to relevant clinical outcomes for the approval of oncology drugs. In a 2016 study published in *Mayo Clinic Proceedings*, medical researchers analyzed all FDA approvals for oncology drugs between 2009 and 2014, finding that fifty-five (66.3 percent) of the eighty-three FDA-approved oncologic indications had marketing applications that relied upon surrogate endpoints.[75] All twenty-five applications that underwent accelerated approval used surrogate endpoints while thirty traditional applications (51.7 percent) relied on surrogates. Most accelerated approvals (56.0 percent) and 36.7 percent of the traditional approvals relied upon surrogate endpoints where the authors could find no formal analysis of the correlation between the surrogate and the most important oncologic clinical outcome: overall survival. The researchers only found level 1 analyses—the highest quality method to evaluate a surrogate measure—for four (16.0 percent) of the accelerated approvals, all of which yielded relatively weak correlations that undermined the validity of the surrogates. Half of traditional approvals had a corresponding level 1 analysis, of which the majority (53.3 percent) had low correlations, 26.7 percent had medium correlations, and 20.0 percent had high correlations.

A 2020 *JAMA Internal Medicine* research article looked at all 194 unique FDA approvals based on surrogate endpoints for 132 cancer drugs between 1992 and 2019.[76] One hundred and five (54.1 percent) of the 194 approvals were regular/traditional while 89 (45.9 percent) were accelerated. A surrogate endpoint was used for the first time in roughly one-third (32.9 percent) of all approvals compared to two-thirds (67.0 percent) for subsequent uses. Among the approvals where a surrogate endpoint was used in relation to a particular cancer where it had previously never been used, 60.9 percent (thirty-nine) had no documented correlation with overall survival, 15.6 percent (ten) had low correlations, 1.6 percent (one) had medium correlations, 4.7 percent (three) had high correlations, and 17.2 percent (eleven) had differing levels of correlation across multiple analyses. In the 76.6 percent of approvals relying upon surrogates with unknown or low correlations with overall survival, a majority (53.1 percent) were traditional approvals while 46.9 percent were accelerated approvals.

A subsequent 2022 *Journal of Cancer Policy* article buttressed the aforementioned research by reviewing the FDA's own analyses of surrogate outcomes and their correlation with overall survival for oncologic drugs between 2014 and 2022.[77] While seeking to find all analyses between 2005 and 2022, the authors could not locate any that occurred from 2005 to 2013. Thus, while the FDA approved drugs based on surrogate measures, the agency had not actually conducted analyses—at least ones that are publicly available—to gauge their validity. From 2014 to 2022, the FDA conducted fifteen analyses examining one or more surrogate measures, and only one study identified a surrogate marker—event-free survival—with a strong correlation with overall survival.

A previous 2015 *JAMA Internal Medicine* research letter examined approved cancer drugs in the years after approval, finding that reliance on surrogate measures was not reliable for improving overall survival.[78] The authors analyzed all FDA marketing approvals for oncology drugs from 2008 to 2012, identifying that surrogate endpoints backed thirty-six (66.7 percent) of the fifty-four identified approvals. Of these surrogate-based approvals, twenty-one (58.3 percent) were traditional and fifteen (41.7 percent) were accelerated. All accelerated approvals relied on surrogate measures compared to 53.8 percent for traditional approvals. Within a median 4.4-year follow-up, only five (13.9 percent) of the thirty-six approved drugs had randomization studies showing that they improved overall survival. In comparison, half failed to show an improvement in overall survival and thirteen (36.1 percent) had unknown effects on survival due to a lack of testing or no reported overall survival results as primary or secondary outcomes. While traditionally approved drugs were more likely to have shown an improvement in overall survival compared to accelerated approvals, both percentages were low: 19.0 percent and 6.7 percent, respectively. Additionally, 57.1 percent of traditional approvals failed to show an improvement in overall survival compared to 40.0 percent of accelerated approvals. Accelerated approvals were more likely to have unknown effects on overall survival compared to traditional approvals (53.3 percent compared to 23.8 percent).

Ultimately, the available evidence shows that the FDA's increasing acceptance and reliance on surrogate endpoints to approve treatments is not based on scientific rigor and often fails to reflect the actual safety and effectiveness of products. Even though surrogate endpoints are more publicly attributed to accelerated approvals, significant percentages of traditional approvals also rely on surrogates. While surrogates for traditional approvals should meet a higher standard of validation than accelerated approval, many of the supposedly validated surrogate measures are not actually valid. Many surrogate measures do not have rigorous tests demonstrating a connection to relevant clinical outcomes. Thus, clinical trial transparency might help outside researchers and peer reviewers identify weak evidence, but it would not change the strength of the evidence itself.

Even when clinical trials fail to show benefits, single individuals within FDA leadership can unilaterally provide approval. On June 20, 2024, the FDA expanded the label of Sarepta's gene therapy product Elevidys so that it was approved for all people above the age of four to treat Duchenne muscular dystrophy (DMD). DMD is a progressive genetic disorder of muscle weakening and degeneration.[79] Previously, the FDA had licensed Elevidys under the accelerated approval pathway to treat DMD only in four- to five-year-old children with DMD. The only randomized, placebo-controlled trial for the drug failed to show that it improved function.[80] While it did affect a surrogate measure, that surrogate did not actually correlate with the study's functional outcome.

Both FDA reviewers and advisory committee members admitted that they did not know that the surrogate measure met the statutory standard of being reasonably likely to predict clinical benefit. The FDA's Cellular, Tissue, and Gene Therapies Advisory Committee voted 8–6 to recommend accelerated approval.[81] One of the expert members who voted in favor remarked that while "there were pluses and minuses in the study," he was convinced by compelling evidence such as company-provided videos showing patients running and playing on a playground after taking the therapy.

By receiving accelerated approval, Sarepta had to conduct a confirmatory trial. Yet, the trial failed to show that Elevidys met the primary clinical endpoint of improving muscle function.[82] Three FDA review teams opposed fully approving the drug. The integrated review from the clinical and clinical pharmacology team stated that "the totality of the data does not provide substantial evidence of effectiveness of ELEVIDYS for treatment of ambulatory DMD patients of any age."[83] However, Center for Biologics Evaluation and Research (CBER) director Dr. Peter Marks overrode all the teams and two high-level staffers to push approval through.[84] According to former FDA acting chief scientist Luciana Borio:

> I don't know what to say. Peter Marks makes a mockery of scientific reasoning and approval standards that have served patients well over decades ... This type of action also promotes the growing mistrust in scientific institutions like the FDA.[85]

Marks made his decision based on determining that Elevidys improved the trial's secondary endpoints, such as how long it takes patients to rise from the floor or walk 10 meters. Yet, the director of the Office of Clinical Evaluation and the super office director of the Office of Therapeutic Products found the evidence for these endpoints to be inconclusive and even "conflicting."[86] Not only did Dr. Marks use his authority to override FDA review teams and approve Elevidys without evidence that the drug improved muscle function, he expanded the indicated population far beyond the initial accelerated approval. Rather than just treat four- and five-year-olds with DMD, Marks approved Elevidys for everyone above the age of four with DMD. As of June 2025, over 900 patients used Elevidys with two reported deaths—a fifteen- and sixteen-year-old—from liver failure following usage.[87]

## Orphan Drugs

The PDUFA expanded upon the 1983 Orphan Drug Act, which Congress passed to encourage and expedite the development of drugs for rare diseases with relatively small patient populations otherwise known as orphan drugs.[88] According to FDA historian Dr. John Swann, 20–25 million Americans were affected by around 5,000 rare diseases by the early 1980s.[89] To incentivize orphan drug development, the law provides seven years of marketing exclusivity for the drug and its use in treating a rare disease/condition. Orphan drug manufacturers also are exempt from user fees and can get a tax credit for up to 50 percent of the costs of qualified clinical research in addition to receiving grants from the FDA's Office of Orphan Products Development (OOPD).[90]

The original legislation defined relevant rare diseases as diseases or conditions that occur "so infrequently in the United States that there is no reasonable expectation that the cost of developing and making available" a drug in the country "will be recovered" from its nationwide sales.[91] Therefore, when manufacturers requested to the OOPD that their drug get an orphan drug designation, they had to prove that their drug would be unprofitable. However, in 1984, Congress amended the law through the Health Promotion and Disease Prevention Amendments of 1984, changing the definition so that the unprofitability requirement only applied to drugs treating rare diseases with a patient population of more than 200,000 people.[92] If a manufacturer produced a drug for a rare disease that affected fewer than 200,000 patients, there was no requirement to show no reasonable expectation of profitability. Almost all 2,000-plus orphan drug designations obtained between 1983 and 2011 utilized the definition of targeting fewer than 200,000 patients.[93]

Consequently, orphan drugs have been disproportionately profitable for pharmaceutical companies and have larger price tags for consumers compared to other treatments. In the journal *Healthcare*, researchers examined the prices of the 242 orphan and nonorphan drugs approved by the FDA from 2017 to 2021 that were marketed in the United States by the end of March 2022.[94] They found that slightly under half (48.8 percent) of new drugs and biological products were orphan drugs, and their median cost was nearly $219,000 compared to almost $13,000 for the nonorphan drugs. The Congressional Research Service (CRS), thus, noted that such disproportionately high costs can lead to the "misalignment of incentives" for manufacturers to pursue orphan drug designations for their products.[95]

Meanwhile, the FDA has approved orphan drugs via expedited approval pathways and based on weaker evidence through surrogate endpoints. From 2015 to 2024, a slight majority, 234 (50.3 percent), of the 465 total novel drug approvals were for orphan drugs.[96] Of these 234 orphan drugs, 203 (86.8 percent) used at least one of the four following expedited pathways: accelerated approval, priority review, Fast Track designation, and Breakthrough Therapy designation. This percentage is higher than the two-thirds of all approved novel drugs that used an expedited pathway over the same period. A 2023 *BMJ* analysis comparing 170 orphan and nonorphan cancer drugs for 455 indications that the FDA approved between 2000 and 2022 similarly found greater usage of expedited pathways for orphan drugs.[97]

The study authors also noted that clinical trials for orphan drugs employed smaller participant populations, were less likely to be randomized, and more likely to rely upon surrogate endpoints. A previous 2011 *JAMA* analysis produced similar results, comparing the traits of clinical trials supporting orphan versus nonorphan cancer drugs that the FDA approved between 2004 and 2010.[98] Orphan drug trials relied on significantly lower quality evidence, as the vast majority (69.6 percent) of the twenty-three orphan cancer drug trials used no comparator (neither active nor placebo), 69.6 percent were not randomized, 91.3 percent were not blinded, 82.6 percent relied on surrogate endpoints, and the median number of trial enrollees was 96. Similarly, a 2023 *Perspectives in Clinical Research* study compared clinical trials of orphan versus nonorphan drugs for infectious diseases that the FDA approved between 2010 and 2020.[99] Among thirty-five orphan drug trials, 57.1 percent were not randomized,

62.9 percent had no blinding, 45.7 percent did not use an active comparator, and the median number of participants was 89. Nonorphan drug trials were significantly more frequently randomized (87.0 percent), double blinded (60.0 percent), and done with an active comparator (59.1 percent) while enrolling more participants (median of 452).

Along with weaker evidence backing their approvals, a 2022 *Orphanet Journal of Rare Diseases* study examined all FDA approved orphan drugs from 1999 to 2018, finding that around seven in ten orphan drugs had safety-related changes to their labeling after approval by the end of 2019.[100] Of the 214 approved drugs with orphan designations, 83.6 percent utilized an expedited program and 29.4 percent had black box warnings upon approval. Within a median time of over 6.7 years following approval, 69.2 percent of the orphan drugs had at least one postmarketing safety event, meaning that there were safety-related changes to their label. Of the 641 events, 443 (69.1 percent) involved adverse reactions and 453 (70.7 percent) introduced new warnings and precautions. Forty-nine severe postmarketing safety events occurred in 14.5 percent of the drugs, including forty-eight new or reinforced black box warnings and one temporary marketing suspension.

## The Failure of Postmarketing Surveillance

While the FDA has increasingly approved treatments through both traditional and accelerated pathways based on weaker standards of evidence—like the usage of surrogate endpoints—the agency has justified this based on lifecycle regulation.[101] In exchange for the approval of more treatments, especially for serious and life-threatening conditions and diseases, the FDA relies on postmarketing requirements (PMRs) and postmarketing commitments (PMCs). The central difference between PMRs and PMCs is that the former refers to studies and clinical trials that sponsors are legally required to conduct while the latter refers to those that sponsors have committed to conduct but are not legally required to do so.[102] However, the FDA's oversight and enforcement of PMRs and PMCs has been significantly lacking, leading to many postmarket studies not occurring and the FDA not pulling some treatments from the market that fail to show benefits. Additionally, the shift from rigorous standards of evidence for initial review toward lifecycle regulation grants significant power to industry to influence physician behavior while under less regulatory scrutiny.

There are four general areas where the FDA requires postmarketing studies and clinical trials. Before the 2007 FDAAA, the FDA could require postmarketing studies to determine clinical efficacy and safety for drugs approved via accelerated approval, deferred submissions for pediatric uses in line with the 2003 Pediatric Research Equity Act (PREA), and for products approved based on effectiveness data from animal studies.[103] Consequently, sponsors largely voluntarily conducted postmarket studies if they chose to do them at all considering that most approvals came outside of the accelerated approval process along with the other highly specific areas. Yet, the 2007 FDAAA greatly expanded the FDA's authority to require postmarketing clinical trials and studies. The legislation allowed the agency to issue PMRs to any drug/biologic sponsor "to [1] assess a known serious risk related to the use of the drug involved ... [2] assess signals of serious risk related to the use of the drug ... [and 3] identify an unexpected serious risk when available data indicates the potential for a serious risk."[104] Following the FDAAA, the number of PMRs that the FDA issued swelled, as there were 221 PMRs from 1990 to 2004 compared to 1,256 from 2008 to 2014.[105]

While the FDAAA expanded FDA authority and increased the number of PMRs issued, PMRs and FDA-requested/voluntary PMCs have failed to ensure the efficacy and safety of products on the market. A 2023 analysis in the *Journal of Clinical Pharmacology* found that around 43 percent of clinical pharmacology–related PMRs and PMCs for NMEs approved between 2009 and 2020 were not fulfilled by the time of their investigation.[106] In 2018, *BMJ* published an analysis of all FDA-approved drugs and biologics—excluding generics, reformulations, and combination treatments of nonnovel therapeutics—from 2009 to 2012, with follow-ups up to mid-November 2017.[107] Of the 110 drugs approved for 120 indications, 97 drugs (88.1 percent) approved for 106 indications (88.3 percent) had a total of 437 PMRs. Of these 97 drugs, only 28 (28.9 percent) and 9 (9.3 percent) underwent priority review and accelerated approval, respectively, indicating many PMRs for drugs and biologics that went through standard pathways. FDAAA authority backed 344 (78.7 percent) of the required studies. Along with not being able to find up-to-date progress information on 30.0 percent of PMRs, the researchers found that only 38.0 percent of the PMRs were fulfilled according to FDA and sponsor data. The researchers noted that the PMRs had largely very short public descriptions and lacked sufficient information to properly describe most of the study designs.

A 2017 *JAMA* investigation examined the FDA-required postapproval trials for drugs that underwent accelerated approval between 2009 and 2013.[108] The FDA approved twenty-two drugs for twenty-four indications and required thirty-eight postapproval confirmatory trials. While 65.8 percent of the postapproval trials were RCTs, the remaining 34.2 percent were for single-group trials, meaning that there was no comparator. At a minimum of three years following the PMRs, only half of the postapproval trials had been completed, and eighteen of these nineteen trials had published reports available for the researchers to review. Of these eighteen completed trials, just ten (55.6 percent) and one (5.6 percent) were randomized and double-blind, respectively, while seventeen (94.4 percent) relied on surrogate measures as primary endpoints. Therefore, the postapproval trials completed to prove safety and efficacy relied on similarly weak evidence that drove the FDA to require additional study. Of the twenty-four approved indications, ten (41.7 percent) had fulfilled their PMRs and demonstrated efficacy, but all the studies used to show clinical benefit and update drug labeling relied on surrogate measures. While the ten indications related to cancer, none tested for overall survival, and only one of the eighteen studies with published reports listed overall survival as a primary endpoint.

A 2019 *JAMA Pediatrics* cohort study tracked the characteristics of postmarketing studies required by the PREA for new FDA-approved drugs and indications from 2007 to 2014 with follow-up on their status through December 1, 2017.[109] Only 75 (33.8 percent) of the required 228 studies were completed as of December 2017. Completeness was particularly lacking for trials testing efficacy (28.8 percent) and safety (32.1 percent) compared to studies that focus on how bodies process the product (55.9 percent). Information on several key aspects of the trial designs were available for 162–188 (71.1 percent to 82.5 percent) of the 228 studies. Among these transparent studies, 48.9 percent were not randomized, 53.5 percent had no blinding (57.2 percent were not double-blinded), 54.9 percent had no comparator, and 75.3 percent relied on surrogate endpoints. Just 13.0 percent directly measured clinical outcomes. The percentages were less severe but still significant for efficacy-only studies: 22.8 percent were not randomized, 28.3 percent had no blinding (33.8 percent were not double-blinded), 28.4 percent had no comparator, and 55.6 percent relied on surrogate endpoints. Only 23.3 percent directly measured clinical outcomes. Active comparators existed for 20.9 percent and 32.1 percent of all trials and efficacy-only trials, respectively, compared to 24.2 percent and 39.4 percent using placebo.

The researchers also tracked whether the sponsors of the seventy-five completed postmarketing trials complied with federal law requiring public reporting of trial results on ClinicalTrials.gov and/or whether they submitted the information elsewhere. They found that eighteen (24.0 percent) of the studies were not posted on ClinicalTrials.gov, submitted to a peer-reviewed journal, or available in an FDA review summary. More specifically, 72.0 percent were not posted in a trial registry and 54.7 percent were not submitted to a journal. Furthermore, the labeling for the approved products was additionally lacking. At the time of each approval, 84.2 percent of 114 drug labels lacked any efficacy, safety, or dosing information for pediatric use. Lack of disclosure improved to just 58.9 percent by December 2017, including 61.4 percent lacking information on pediatric efficacy or safety and 64.9 percent not having information on pediatric dosing or pharmacokinetics and pharmacodynamics properties—meaning how the body affects a drug and how a drug impacts the body, respectively.[110]

In September 2022, the HHS Office of Inspector General published a report on confirmatory, postmarketing trials for drugs that underwent accelerated approval.[111] The report found that the number of accelerated approvals had grown over time since the program's inception in 1992. Out of the 278 accelerated approvals between 1992 and 2021, 70 (25.2 percent) came from just 2020 and 2021. At the same time, 104 or 37.8 percent of the accelerated approvals still had incomplete confirmatory trials. Of these accelerated approvals with incomplete trials, 35 (33.7 percent) had one trial that was late, meaning that the trial was not completed by its agreed-upon completion date with the FDA.

Four drugs were at least sixty-four months—over five years—late: Makena (hydroxy-progesterone caproate), Folotyn (pralatrexate), Proamatine (midodrine hydrochloride), and Sulfamylon (mafenide acetate). The situation has changed since the HHS report. The FDA approved Makena in 2011, yet it took until April 2023—sixty-four months after the agreed-upon completion date—for the FDA to remove it from the market.[112] Sulfamylon came onto the market in 1998 and its completion date was in 2010; the FDA only removed it from the market in November 2022 after the parent company of the sponsor requested withdrawal, deeming it too difficult to conduct the confirmatory study.[113] The FDA approved Proamatine in 1996, and while the FDA proposed withdrawing it from the market in 2010 for failing to complete its postmarketing requirements, it decided against doing so as the manufacturer agreed to fulfill the PMR by 2014—which was extended to 2015.[114] Information via a published article in a peer-reviewed journal only became available in 2016, two decades following its approval onto the market. Folotyn—which was approved in 2009—is still on the market where it is around nine years late in completing its confirmatory trial as of July 2025.

Moreover, HHS conservatively estimated that Medicare and Medicaid spent around $18 billion from 2018 to 2021 on covering products that underwent accelerated approval and of which still had incomplete confirmatory trials that were late. This spending particularly fell on Medicare Part B, which spent around $12.6 billion compared to $1.7 billion and $3.6 billion for Part D and Medicaid, respectively. Medicare Part C/ Medicare Advantage additionally spent $5.9 billion. For the four extremely late drugs, Medicare and Medicaid spent $978.4 million over the three-year period.

Furthermore, tracking the status of PMCs inherently differs from PMRs because the latter is legally required while the former is voluntary for sponsors. However, existing examinations of these commitments reveal significant limitations in the extent to which industry voluntarily conducts rigorous postmarketing efficacy and safety testing. A 2019 *BMC Medicine* analysis examined PMCs for drugs and biologics that the FDA approved from 2009 to 2012.[115] Of the 110 drugs/biologics approved for 120 different indications, 61 (55.5 percent) had at least one postmarketing commitment. Of these 61 products, the significant majority neither went through priority review (65.6 percent) nor accelerated approval (88.5 percent). In total, there were 331 PMCs; however, the vast majority of 271 (81.9 percent) pertained to studies regarding the production and quality of products. Only 49 (14.8 percent) described clinical trials, including 33 (10.0 percent) for new clinical trials and 16 (4.8 percent) referring to the submission of final reports/data from ongoing trials.

FDA approval letters contained extremely limited information on the characteristics of the thirty-three PMCs for new clinical trials; however, twenty-eight had information listed on ClinicalTrials.gov. Of these limited new trials, almost all (92.9 percent) were randomized and most (78.6 percent) were double-blind. However, just 14.3 percent of trials used an active comparator while 64.3 percent used placebo and 21.4 percent had no comparator. Only 17.9 percent directly measured clinical outcomes while 21.4 percent relied on surrogate measures and 60.7 percent used clinical scales (a standardized and less rigorous measurement tool compared to clinical outcomes). The trials were also short, being only 1.6 months on average in duration. ClinicalTrials.gov classified twenty-three (82.1 percent) of these twenty-eight trials as either completed or terminated, and all but one of these reported results. Yet, eighteen (81.8 percent) were late with a median reporting of thirteen months after scheduled submission. The characteristics of the sixteen ongoing trials revealed less scientific rigor, as 37.5 percent were not randomized, 62.5 percent were open label rather than blind, 37.5 percent used no comparator rather than placebo (37.5 percent) or an active comparator (25.0 percent), and 62.5 percent relied on surrogate endpoints. But, these trials were longer (5.6 months).

Significant analyses of PMCs are lacking likely due to their voluntary nature. For example, a 2022 *JAMA Internal Medicine* study identified 387 PMRs and 328 PMCs for 135 newly approved drugs between 2013 and 2016.[116] However, only 87 (26.5 percent) of the PMCs were reportable, meaning that the authors could not investigate their characteristics. The authors did not provide data stratified by PMR/PMC status; collectively, more than seven in ten of the 330 PMRs and PMCs expected to be completed by the fourth quarter of 2020 were late. Regardless of late status, the reality that almost three quarters of PMCs were not reportable reflects their limited value in providing safety and efficacy information to physicians and patients. On top of the potential issues surrounding trial design and evidence quality, relevant stakeholders are unlikely to know the results of many voluntary postmarketing studies.

Overall, the existing evidence shows that a significant number of postmarketing studies are not fulfilled for many years, are late regarding their agreed-upon completion date with the FDA, and rely upon weak evidence—namely surrogate endpoints. This reality may be a consequence of the FDA's approach regarding PMRs and PMCs. In 2019, *The Milbank Quarterly* published an investigation by Matthew Herder who conducted a policy and legal analysis of FDA documents along with interviews with twenty-three former FDA officials.[117] Herder documented how as the FDA has faced pressure from Congress—through legislation like the Cures Act—to continuously expedite the approval process for treatments, it has also sought to abide by user fee arrangements with industry to meet deadlines for premarket reviews. Consequently, the FDA has shifted much of the burden of designing postmarket studies to industry. While the FDA can use user fee funding for postmarketing surveillance, most funding still goes toward premarket activities. Concurrently, according to a 2015 GAO report, the agency "lacks reliable, readily accessible data on tracked safety issues and postmarket studies needed to meet certain postmarket safety reporting responsibilities and to conduct systematic oversight."[118] Thus, the incentives of these circumstances naturally push the agency toward greater focus on premarket review rather than postmarket surveillance even as it increasingly relies on the latter.

Additionally, existing penalties for industry failure to comply with PMRs have been limited.[119] Penalties can include issuances of warnings or untitled letters and civil monetary penalties.[120] While penalties can be up to $250,000 per violation, the total fine cannot exceed $1 million for the first month of a proceeding and, if violations continue, $10 million for all violations in a single proceeding. The FDA can withdraw approval; however, the existing evidence shows that failure to complete PMRs has not resulted in such a punishment for many products. The FDA also has the authority to charge companies for violating the FD&C Act; but, this is reserved for if other actions have been exhausted and is not an avenue the FDA has seriously employed.

Furthermore, the current regulatory environment prioritizes the premarket approval process and getting more drugs on the market over the postmarket monitoring of safety and effectiveness. The system set up by the PDUFA and its numerous reauthorizations has led to fast deadlines with increasing levels of funding. A 2017 *NEJM* article notes the contrast between the "slow, irregular pace of postapproval studies ... [and] the short, rigid deadlines and other shortcuts used to speed marketing approval."[121] Ultimately, there is significantly more political pressure pushing for the approval of more treatments compared to postmarket activities, as the former has the backing of the multibillion dollar pharmaceutical industry, patient advocacy organizations, and Congress.

In September 2020, the HHS OIG released a report on the FDA's REMS requirements for drug manufacturers in light of the opioid epidemic.[122] The report highlights how a key consequence of the shift to life cycle regulation is that industry can market drugs that "would otherwise be unavailable due to known serious risks."[123] While REMS relies on educating prescribers on the risks of drugs, the report acknowledged that pharmaceutical marketing campaigns can counter such education "to increase prescribing." Ultimately, the OIG found that the FDA struggled to use REMS successfully to mitigate the "misuse of opioids" and protect public health.[124]

The shift toward increasing reliance on postmarketing surveillance to justify expedited approvals of products has further consequences on physician behavior. Regulatory approval and initial publication in primary sources of medical knowledge—namely peer-reviewed medical journals—have the most influence on physician behavior through first impacting what information is available. Industry then capitalizes on approval and supporting materials from journals to conduct extensive marketing campaigns (as the following section "Aduhelm" describes). In contrast, postmarketing surveillance and findings can only secondarily impact physicians. While the FDA has the power to withdraw products when necessary, the agency more commonly changes product labels in accordance with new evidence along with adding black box warnings in more severe cases. Such actions can reduce physician prescribing of ineffective or unsafe treatments.[125] However, the impact of postmarketing actions has to compete with past understandings, already-formed opinions, and industry efforts to maintain as much profit as possible.

## Aduhelm: Special Scrutiny, Standard Behavior

The impetus for the September 2022 HHS report was the FDA's 2021 approval of Biogen's Alzheimer's drug aducanumab (Aduhelm).[126] In November 2020, Biogen presented its clinical evidence to the FDA's Peripheral and Central Nervous Systems Drugs Advisory Committee (PCNS Advisory Committee), where the committee nearly unanimously voted against recommending traditional approval with just one member voting uncertain.[127] Biogen had stopped its two central clinical trials of Aduhelm, EMERGE and ENGAGE, in March 2019 due to interim analyses showing the low probability of the trials producing statistically significant results of clinical benefit.[128] However, post hoc reanalysis of EMERGE data identified statistically significant but clinically insignificant effects of high-dose Aduhelm on a surrogate measure.[129] At the same time, Biogen's clinical data showed that 41.3 percent of patients treated with Aduhelm experienced amyloid-related imaging abnormalities or brain swelling compared to just 10.3 percent of patients treated with placebo.[130]

Following the PCNS Advisory Committee's rejection of traditional approval for Aduhelm, the FDA overrode their recommendation and granted accelerated approval. Three of the committee members subsequently resigned.[131] In an opinion piece for *The New York Times*, one former committee member, Dr. Aaron Kesselheim, wrote that the careful FDA review process that Americans could rely upon to know the drugs they take are safe and effective "has been eroded, and it reached a low point" with the Aduhelm approval.[132] The basis for this statement, according to Kesselheim, was the progressive lowering of "its standards of effectiveness and safety required for drug approvals" at the same time as the FDA approved drugs based on "fewer studies and less adequate clinical trial designs." Kesselheim also claimed that most FDA drug approvals relied on surrogate endpoints that "may not reflect clinical benefit."

While the FDA allowed Biogen to market Aduhelm through the accelerated approval process, CMS restricted coverage for the drug only to those who enrolled in qualifying clinical trials, principally meaning the FDA-required confirmatory studies.[133] Biogen withdrew its marketing application for Aduhelm with the European Union in April 2022 and announced it would discontinue the drug overall in January 2024.[134] Thus, the company ended its postapproval trial for the drug as well.[135]

The FDA's decision to overrule the PCNS Advisory Committee and provide accelerated approval for Aduhelm resulted in significant outside scrutiny and prompted an eighteen-month investigation by the US House Committees on Oversight & Reform and Energy & Commerce that was published in December 2022.[136] The report documented extensive and significant interaction and coordination between the FDA and Biogen that the Committees deemed atypical and improper. For example, Biogen and FDA officials met at least 115 times over a twelve-month period between July 2019 and 2020, and many of the meetings were not properly documented according to agency protocol. In fact, the FDA decided to proactively work with Biogen on pushing Aduhelm through the regulatory process before they had conducted analyses of Biogen's "incomplete, complicated, and partially discordant data set" essential to understanding the overall results.[137] The FDA also recommended that Biogen seek approval for the broad label indication of treating "people with Alzheimer's disease" even though this did not represent the actual population included in the Aduhelm clinical trials.[138] Biogen recognized this and, while holding internal reservations about the lack of data, accepted the FDA's recommendation, which became the indication that received accelerated approval.

Furthermore, the FDA collaborated with Biogen on the joint briefing document prepared for the PCNS Advisory Committee's review of Aduhelm at the same time as there was significant dissent among different agency offices over the drug's efficacy. This document blended the analyses of the FDA and Biogen, making it difficult to distinguish between the two. Additionally, the House Committees found that the FDA decided to abruptly change from considering Aduhelm under traditional approval—which it did for nine months—to accelerated approval only after an FDA expert council meeting involved "unfavorable feedback" for traditional approval.[139] The FDA did not seek the guidance of any advisory committee for accelerated approval. At the time of the accelerated approval, the agency's own guidance document stated that "no sufficiently reliable evidence [exists] that any observed treatment effect on such biomarker measures [including the beta-amyloid surrogate endpoint with Aduhelm] would be reasonably likely to predict clinical benefit."

While the Committees' report documented potentially troubling behavior on the part of the FDA, it more so reflected, at most, a more blatant representation of normal behavior. Extensive collaboration between the FDA and industry is legally encouraged, and the FDA has increasingly seen granting more approvals as an achievement rather than rigorously vetting every product so that they are backed by robust evidence. Although the broad approved indication for Aduhelm may be particularly extreme due to the FDA's central role in pushing it on Biogen, it is standard for industry to seek to expand and increase indications so that there are more potential patients. As previously described, the FDA has approved many treatments based on surrogate endpoints for both accelerated and traditional approvals when there is not quality evidence proving that the surrogates are strongly correlated with relevant clinical outcomes.

Moreover, the Committees' report dedicated an entire section to the fact that Biogen planned to spend billions on marketing Aduhelm to providers, patients, policymakers, payers, and patient advocacy groups.[140] Specifically, company documents revealed that Biogen sought to engage in an aggressive marketing campaign that would cost $3.3 billion between 2020 and 2024. This planned spending was more than 2.5 times the amount the company had spent developing the drug over its lifetime from 2007 through its approval in June 2021. The spending included $500 million–$600 million toward building its salesforce to primarily target primary care physicians. Biogen aimed to reach over 16,000 health care providers by using 300 medical experts for education and engagement and acting as Aduhelm advocates. In addition, Biogen planned to work closely with Alzheimer's patient advocacy groups as part of an engagement campaign to influence stakeholders including government agencies. Specific company language included using patient groups to "leverage Biogen-provided materials to communicate to their membership" and capitalizing on the organizations' support to show that Aduhelm provides "value to patients, caregivers and society at large."[141]

Biogen's marketing campaign included manipulating the media and promoting Aduhelm based on racial equity. Media outreach efforts included educating over fifty journalists and directing them toward chosen medical experts to "shape the narrative" regarding Aduhelm. To target racial minorities, Biogen developed a strategy to target Black and Latino patients and work with patient advocacy organizations that specifically represent minority groups. The Committees' report highlights how the "comprehensive health equity offering" Biogen sought to provide significantly contradicted Aduhelm's clinical trials, as the phase III trials only included patient populations with 3.0 percent Hispanics, 0.6 percent Blacks, and 0.03 percent Native Americans.[142]

The report described Biogen's extensive planned marketing campaign as one of the harmful consequences of the Aduhelm approval because Biogen knew that the product would be very financially straining on both patients and the Medicare program. Among their recommendations, the Committees proposed that "Biogen and other drug sponsors should consider value and patient access when setting prices" as extremely high prices for products, especially drugs "with unproven benefit, without consideration of patient access and affordability, are an abuse of the public trust."[143]

While the Committees' report suggests Aduhelm as a special case, Biogen's marketing campaign—including its manipulation of doctors, advocacy groups, patients, and the media—is reflective of standard pharmaceutical company behavior. While the exact levels of spending may vary depending on patents and the projected profitability of a product, the industry's standard method of maximizing profit is to get as many physicians to prescribe their product, get the support of patient advocacy groups for legitimacy when applicable, get as many patients asking their doctors for their product, and get the media to report favorably on their product. Additionally, as the available evidence shows that pharmaceutical marketing is not associated with the actual added clinical benefit of a drug, and many drugs are approved based on weak surrogate endpoints, Aduhelm is not a unique case.[144]

In key aspects, Aduhelm reveals the limits of transparency reform; however, it also demonstrates its potential effectiveness. Regarding limits, the FDA had access to Biogen's underlying clinical data, and it actively chose to work with the company to ensure its approval even at the expense of overriding the PCNS Advisory Committee and abruptly switching from traditional to accelerated approval. The FDA's priorities rather than a lack of data access led it to granting accelerated approval based on a surrogate endpoint deemed not "sufficiently reliable" by its own guidance document.[145] However, CMS' knowledge of the limited evidence behind Aduhelm led it to heavily restrict coverage, and the public attention and scrutiny over the FDA's decision to grant accelerated approval to Aduhelm may have led to its low sales and Biogen's decision to discontinue it. Therefore, in the many potential cases of products with far less public attention, clinical trial data transparency can allow independent analyses to reveal flaws, weak evidence, and potential safety concerns that impact physician prescribing and payer coverage behavior.

## Chevron Deference

On June 28, 2024, the Supreme Court published its 6–3 decision in *Loper Bright Enterprises v. Raimondo*, overruling a previous 1984 decision: *Chevron U.S.A. Inc. v. Natural Resources Defense Council*.[146] The consequences of this decision may significantly affect the FDA's capacity to regulate medical products through greatly empowering companies to challenge industry decisions in court, including determinations on whether to approve a drug or device. A pharmaceutical company may be able to sue the FDA over declining to approve its product and successfully convince a judge that the highly technical clinical evidence actually supports approval.

Generally, the role of the executive branch—including agencies like the FDA—is to enforce the laws that Congress passes. However, many provisions within pieces of legislation are not highly specific; rather, they are ambiguous and leave room for significant interpretation. For example, the FD&C Act allows the FDA to reject an application for a new drug if there is "a lack of substantial evidence that the drug will have the effect it purports or is represented to have under the conditions of use prescribed, recommended, or suggested" within the drug's proposed labeling.[147] The law defines such substantial evidence as "evidence consisting of adequate and well-controlled investigations" that are conducted by qualified experts and where "it could fairly and responsibly be concluded by such experts" that the drug produces the intended effect.

The law does not define what adequate and well-controlled investigations are or how such studies reasonably show that the drug indeed produces the intended effect. Thus, the FDA has produced various technical regulations to direct industry on what it will consider to meet such standards. Under what legal experts have dubbed the *Chevron* doctrine created by the 1984 decision, if someone sues an agency for a particular regulation or rule based on a statute that is ambiguous—meaning that it does not clearly and directly provide the agency with the authority to make such a decision—a court will defer to the agency if its position is reasonable. For example, the FDA has rejected drug applications on the basis that the results of a clinical trial are not clinically or therapeutically meaningful—that is, the drug does not positively affect "how an individual feels, functions, or survives"—even if the results are statistically significant.[148] While this standard is not explicitly outlined in the FD&C Act, courts have found that the agency's interpretation of their authority is reasonable even if particular court judges would not have reached the same conclusion on what the law allowed.

In *Loper*, Justice John Roberts wrote the majority opinion, arguing that the *Chevron* deference violated the Administrative Procedures Act that explicitly delegated the power of reviewing the legality of agency decisions to the courts without mention of anything representing *Chevron* deference.[149] Based on the decision, judges will no longer defer to agencies' interpretations of ambiguous law if they seem reasonable; rather, they will conduct their own investigations to determine the legal legitimacy of agency regulations. These investigations can still include significant input from agencies, but courts have far greater control.

Courts will not necessarily strike down FDA regulations; *Loper*'s impact remains to be seen. However, the decision may empower regulated entities like pharmaceutical companies to challenge FDA decisions as often as possible to increase the chances that they can market their products. Industry has multibillion-dollar resources to engage in such frequent litigation. Numerous lawsuits could discourage the agency from issuing regulations that challenge industry interests and thus bring lawsuits that strain FDA resources.[150] But ultimately, courts may or may not side with the FDA. Relying on *Loper* in April 2025, a federal court struck down an FDA rule defining laboratory developed tests as medical devices subject to regulation.[151]

Congress can pass legislation to solidify the FDA's ability to make regulations. However, the likelihood of such action is currently questionable given that Congress has sided with industry to erode FDA evidence standards over the last several decades and more than two-thirds of members received campaign support from pharmaceutical companies in 2020.[152]

Whether or not *Loper* turns out to be consequential, over the last several decades the priorities of the FDA have shifted away from guaranteeing safety and effectiveness of pharmaceuticals and toward increasing the speed at which they are reviewed and let onto the market. Meanwhile, FDA collaboration and ties with industry have grown stronger through user fee funding and de facto teamwork during drug development and review processes. Congress has also weakened the standards of evidence that the FDA requires to approve products through several pieces of legislation. Yet, as the next chapter delves into, FDA regulation of drugs is by no means weaker than medical devices.

6

# It Gets Worse: Medical Devices

While the PDUFA pertained to human drug and biological products, Congress also passed similar laws for medical devices known as the Medical Device User Fee Amendments (MDUFA) beginning in 2002 with its fifth reauthorization, MDUFA V, passing in 2022.[1] These pieces of legislation have also made industry a significant funder of the FDA's medical devices and radiological health program (43.7 percent in FY 2024).[2] Congress has passed other user fee laws with reauthorizations, such as the Biosimilar User Fee Act (BsUFA), Generic Drug User Fee Amendments (GDUFA), Animal Drug User Fee Act (ADUFA), and more.[3] While the PDUFA continuously weakened evidence standards for approved drugs, the primary means of expedited approval with little evidence for medical devices relies less on the MDUFA and more on a specific regulatory loophole: the 510(k) pathway.

The 1938 FD&C Act is the primary statute providing the FDA authority to regulate medical devices.[4] These devices include instruments, apparatuses, implements, machines, contrivances, implants, in vitro reagents, or other similar or related articles.[5] While all FDA-regulated products conceptually meet the definition of a drug under the law, a key way devices are legally distinct is that they do not achieve their "primary intended purposes through chemical action within or on the body of man or other animals" and are not "dependent upon being metabolized for the achievement" of their primary purpose.[6]

The FDA's current class- and risk-based classification system for devices comes from the 1976 Medical Device Amendments (MDA).[7] The FDA reported at the end of 2017 that 47 percent, 43 percent, and 10 percent of devices were Class I, II, and III, respectively.[8] When the agency categorizes a device as Class I—such as elastic bandages and oxygen masks—it deems that device to be low-risk and not meant for use in supporting or sustaining life, not to be important in preventing impairment to human life, and not presenting a potential unreasonable risk of illness or injury.[9] The FDA uses general controls—like device registration and good manufacturing practices—to "provide reasonable assurance of effectiveness and safety" of Class I devices. Around 95 percent of Class I devices are exempt from the regulatory process, meaning they don't need premarket approval or clearance.[10]

Class II devices—such as MRI scanners and syringes—are considered to be moderate-risk and "cannot be classified as a class I device because the general controls by themselves are insufficient to provide reasonable assurance of the safety and effectiveness."[11] These devices are subject to special controls in addition to general controls, such as postmarket surveillance, patient registries, and guideline development and dissemination. Class III medical devices are high-risk—such as prosthetics and pacemakers—and largely sustain or support life, are implanted, or present unreasonable risk of injury or illness. Class III devices are subject to general controls, and manufacturers must apply for Premarket Approval (PMA) to market their products. The PMA process is like the regulatory process for new drugs in that it requires clinical trial data for safety and effectiveness along with laboratory studies.

## The 510(k) Pathway

The FDA considers every new device introduced after the MDA intended for human use to be a Class III device requiring a PMA application regardless of the risk it poses unless the device is "substantially equivalent" to a pre-MDA device type or another device type classified as Class I or II.[12] Thus, the most commonly utilized regulatory avenue for all medical devices to reach the market is the Premarket Notification 510(k) pathway. Of the more than 155,000 medical devices that the FDA approved or cleared from 1976 through 2020, around 99 percent used the 510(k) pathway.[13] Through the pathway, a device manufacturer demonstrates substantial equivalence to a predicate device, meaning one that is already on the market. Manufacturers must submit a notification to the FDA at least ninety days prior to marketing the device. If successful, a new device receives the same classification as the predicate device.

To prove substantial equivalence, the manufacturer must show the device has the same intended use as the predicate device and either the same technological traits, such as "materials, design, energy source, or other features," or different technological characteristics that do not "raise different questions of safety and effectiveness" from the predicate device.[14] A manufacturer can use multiple predicate devices as part of their 510(k) submission; a 2023 *JAMA* investigation found that the mean number of predicate devices for FDA-cleared devices from 2003 to 2018 was 2.6.[15] For only a small minority of 510(k)-cleared medical devices, the FDA requires some clinical data. One 2022 estimate from a consulting firm puts this at 10–15 percent of 510(k)s.[16] Due to the 1997 FDAMA, the FDA must take the least burdensome approach when conducting premarket evaluations.[17]

The substantial equivalence standard for cleared medical devices differs from generic drug approvals. Generic drug manufacturers must prove to the FDA that a drug has the same active ingredient and is overall pharmaceutically equivalent to the brand-name drug it is based on.[18] A manufacturer must conduct studies to show bioequivalence: the active ingredient has an equal rate and extent of absorption as the brand-name drug. FDA scientists analyze test results to determine if the drug would produce the same results as the branded drug. In contrast, the 510(k) pathway often does not involve testing if the new device produces the same results as the predicate device unless the FDA sees significant technological differences. These studies often are not clinical, meaning they do not observe human participants.[19] Additionally, generic drugs are based on a brand-name drug that received FDA approval for safety and effectiveness, while the 510(k) pathway allows new medical devices to get clearance based off predicate devices that were similarly cleared rather than approved.

Along with less testing to get market access, device manufacturers benefit from significant cost savings by using the 510(k) pathway. For FY 2025, the FDA's standard user fee for a 510(k) application was $24,335 compared to $540,783 for a PMA, meaning that companies get to pay twenty-two times less per application for using premarket notification rather than approval.[20] These cost savings are likely trivial compared to savings from not having to run clinical trials testing safety and efficacy, as manufacturers can save potentially more than $63 million overall by using the 510(k) pathway compared to PMA for a device.[21]

The widespread usage of the 510(k) program means that most medical devices for human use on the market have not proven safety and effectiveness to the FDA, leading to harm and injury to the public. In 2019, the FDA cleared the JET 7 Reperfusion Catheter with Xtra Flex Technology (JET 7)—created by the medical device company Penumbra—as a Class II device, sharing the class designation with powered wheelchairs.[22] JET 7's purpose was to help individuals experiencing ischemic strokes through breaking down and eliminating blood clots.[23] Penumbra did not need to prove safety and effectiveness to the FDA, as the company filed a premarket notification claiming substantial equivalence to a predicate device. Instead, Penumbra proved equivalence by providing the FDA with a literature review and preexisting animal data.[24]

In fact, Penumbra used the 510(k) pathway for several devices all the way back to 2007, when the FDA cleared the Penumbra System: the second mechanical device meant to treat ischemic strokes.[25] The Penumbra System also did not need to prove safety and efficacy, as Penumbra successfully claimed substantial equivalence to Concentric Medical's Merci Retriever, which the FDA also cleared based on a predicate device. The FDA cleared the Merci Retriever via the 510(k) pathway based on a predicate device with a different approved indication from treating stroke. Clearance for the Penumbra System relied on a nonrandomized pivotal trial of 125 participants with no comparator.[26] If the product caused one significant adverse event or even death for every 126 patients using the product, the trial was not powered to detect this.

Penumbra initially dominated the market for aspiration catheters treating ischemic stroke; however, by 2019, the company began to lose market share to competitors.[27] Thus, Penumbra launched JET 7 in July 2019, highlighting its greater flexibility (hence the "Xtra Flex" title). Four months after the FDA clearance and three months after the product launch, the FDA's Manufacturer and User Facility Device Experience (MAUDE) database recorded the first death associated with JET 7. In June 2020, Penumbra's distributor in Japan, Hirata, issued a warning to hospital providers about JET 7 that stated that the "catheter inflated into a balloon … [damaging] the patient's blood vessel."[28] In July, Penumbra similarly warned providers in the United States. In the eighteen months following FDA clearance, the MAUDE database listed over 200 adverse events, and eighteen deaths were linked to JET 7 by December 2020.[29] Penumbra voluntarily recalled the device in December, and the FDA followed suit by announcing a Class I recall—the most severe type of recall for issues that can reasonably cause serious health consequences or death—in January 2021.

The 510(k) pathway allowed Penumbra to market JET 7 without conducting randomized trials to prove safety and efficacy, leading to numerous deaths and adverse events.[30] The 200 adverse events figure is likely an underestimate, as the MAUDE database is based on voluntary reporting from patients and physicians. Ultimately, JET 7 is not an isolated case among blood clot–removing devices. The FDA announced Class I recalls for the Penumbra 3D Revascularization Device (used in combination with JET 7), the Micro Therapeutics' Mindframe Capture Revascularization Device, and Stryker's Trevo XP ProVue Retriever in 2017, 2018, and 2020, respectively.

A 2024 *Annals of Internal Medicine* study tracked the 137 Class I recalls for 157 cardiovascular devices from 2013 to 2022, with 71.3 percent being 510(k) devices compared to 28.7 percent being FDA-approved Class III devices.[31] Only seven 510(k) devices (6.3 percent) underwent premarket clinical testing, none had required postmarket surveillance, and twenty-six (23.2 percent) had multiple Class I recalls. A 2023 *JAMA* study examined 35,176 medical devices cleared by the FDA through the 510(k) pathway from 2003 to 2018, finding that 11.4 percent of devices were recalled, and these devices were associated with nearly *25,000 deaths* between 2003 and 2020.[32] Clearances based on newer or more predicate devices, especially three or more, were significantly more likely to be recalled. Similarly, a 2021 *JAMA* investigation revealed that 10.7 percent of 28,246 510(k) devices cleared from 2008 to 2017 were recalled; but, only 0.8 percent of devices had a Class I recall.[33]

In 2011, the IOM published a report on the 510(k) approval process based on concerns raised across the US government about its questionable effect on public health. The authors concluded that the pathway "is not intended to evaluate the safety and effectiveness of medical devices with some exceptions" and that it cannot turn into a "premarket evaluation of safety and effectiveness as long as the standard for clearance is substantial equivalence."[34] Not only are devices themselves not proven safe and effective through the 510(k) pathway, but often the predicate devices that they were substantially equivalent to also did not need to show safety and effectiveness.

This loop of lacking safety and effectiveness data has allowed for severely unsafe devices to serve as the basis for future dangerous device clearances. A 2023 *JAMA* study showed almost half of 510(k) medical devices that received Class I recalls used predicates that also received Class I recalls (see Figure 8).[35] Among the 127 out of 156 devices subject to Class I recalls from 2017 to 2021 with available predicate data, 44.1 percent used predicate devices with Class I recalls. For the 156 total devices subject to Class I recalls, two-thirds served as predicates for future devices, and 48.1 percent of these future devices were also subject to Class I recalls.

Furthermore, the FDA has placed responsibility of postmarketing surveillance for medical devices largely into the hands of device manufacturers. According to the 2011 IOM report, manufacturers are responsible for collecting information, investigating, and making mandatory reports that the FDA's surveillance system relies upon.[36] Voluntary reporting of adverse events, such as the 200 events reported for JET 7, rely on patients and physicians identifying issues, connecting issues with medical devices,

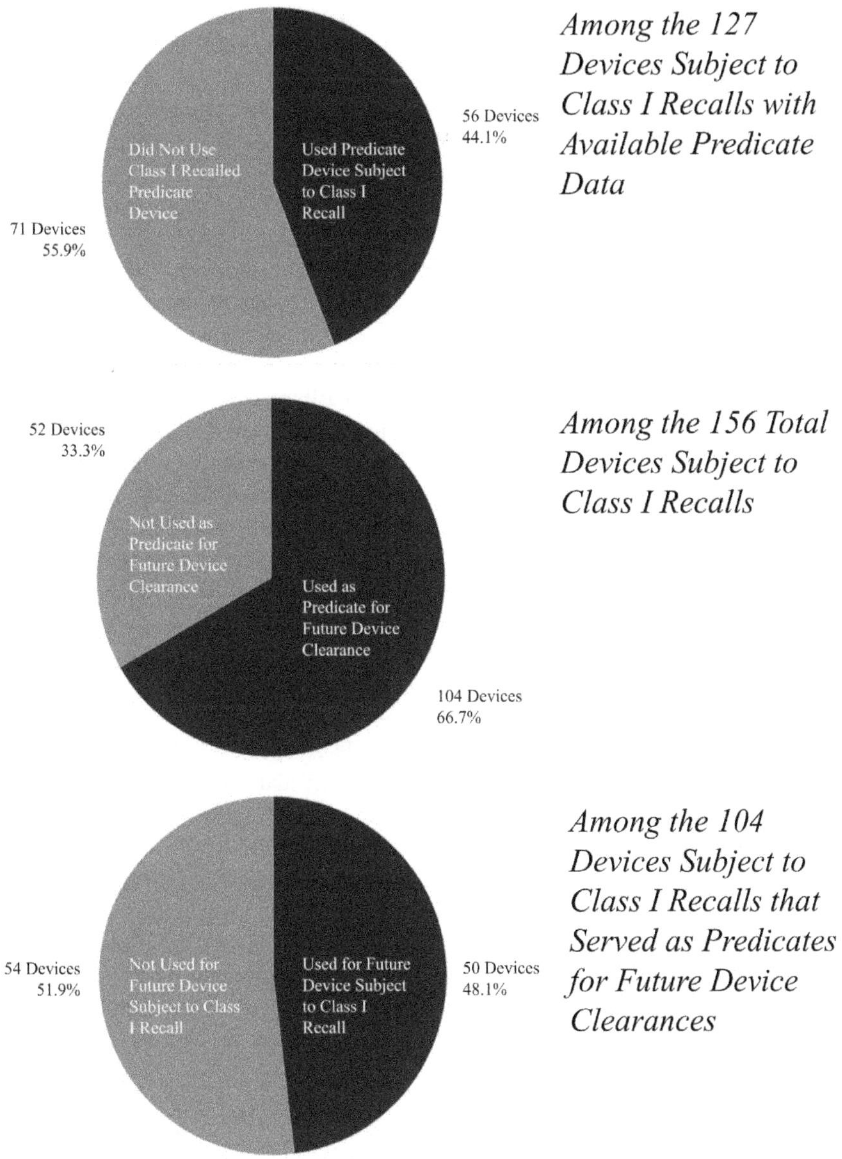


**Figure 8** Study results showing how the 510(k)-clearance process has allowed devices recalled for the most severe safety issues to serve as predicates that the FDA used to clear other dangerous devices. *Source*: Kushal T. Kadakia et al., "Use of Recalled Devices in New Device Authorizations Under the US Food and Drug Administration's 510(k) Pathway and Risk of Subsequent Recalls," *JAMA* 329, no. 2 (January 10, 2023): 136–43, https://doi.org/10.1001/jama.2022.23279.

and then filing reports. As a result, the system's inadequacy and lack of data "make it impossible to confidently draw broad conclusions about the safety and effectiveness of products that are on the market."[37]

Adverse event reporting is inherently passive. A 2012 report on hospitals' incident reporting from the HHS inspector general found that only an estimated 14 percent of events experienced by a national sample of Medicare beneficiaries in October 2008 were reported.[38] Noting over 1.7 million injuries and 83,000 deaths from medical devices from 2007 to 2018, a 2024 GAO report documented that the FDA began to create an active postmarket surveillance system by partnering with industry to coalesce and analyze patient data.[39] Yet, the planned system is limited with actively surveilled devices increasing from two in 2024 to six in 2025, ten in 2026, fourteen in 2027, and eighteen or more in 2028.

The FDA even admits that manufacturers voluntarily recall devices more often than the FDA forces them to do so, and recalls do not always mean the device is taken off the market.[40] Recalls include when a manufacturer doesn't remove a device from the market but corrects it through repairing, modifying, adjusting, relabeling, or inspecting a device to address the problem making it unsafe.[41] From 2019 to 2023, 164 or nearly half (48.5 percent) of Class I device recalls were corrections rather than removals.[42]

Additionally, as nearly 99 percent of approved or cleared medical devices used the 510(k) pathway from 1976 to 2020, the FDA allowed many high-risk Class III devices on the market through premarket notification and, thus, without proving safety and effectiveness.[43] According to a 2009 GAO report, the FDA received more 510(k) submissions from Class III device manufacturers than original PMA submissions, and 228 or two-thirds of 342 510(k) submissions to the FDA for Class III devices successfully obtained clearance based on substantial equivalence.[44] Out of the 10,670 premarket notifications for Class II devices that the FDA cleared, the GAO found that one quarter pertained to devices that could have been Class III by being "implantable ... life sustaining; or ... [presenting] significant risk to the health, safety, or welfare of a patient."[45]

Congress directed the FDA to use the PMA process for medical devices or otherwise reclassify them in the 1990 Safe Medical Devices Act.[46] However, the FDA cleared 24 different types of Class III devices via premarket notification during FYs 2003–07.[47] From April 2009 to July 2012, the FDA cleared 263 devices substantially equivalent to Class III devices.[48] It ultimately took twenty-nine years in 2019 for the FDA to reclassify all preamendment devices.[49]

## Premarket Approval

Although the vast majority of devices use the 510(k) pathway, the remaining fraction that go through the stricter PMA process still face less stringent requirements than the FDA drug approval process.[50] Clinical trials for medical devices often employ weak designs, such as smaller participant groups not representative of the intended patient populations, lack of any comparators, no randomization, poor blinding, and reliance on surrogate endpoints.

In December 2009, *JAMA* systematically reviewed 123 summaries of safety and effectiveness data for seventy-eight PMAs for Class III cardiovascular devices that the FDA approved between 2000 and 2007.[51] Of the 123 studies backing the approvals, 73.2 percent were not randomized and 86.2 percent had no blinding. Of the seventy-eight approvals, 65.4 percent were based on a single study. Out of the studies' 213 primary endpoints, 187 (87.8 percent) were surrogate measures, and 77.7 percent of relevant primary endpoints analyzed a different number of patients than were actually enrolled in the study. Nearly half (47.9 percent) of primary endpoints for patients using medical devices were not compared to results from a control group, and 30.6 percent of controls were retrospective, meaning the treatment group results were compared with previously existing data. According to the lead author and then editor-in-chief of *JAMA Internal Medicine*, Dr. Rita Redberg, "the majority of these high-risk implanted devices were approved without the support of high quality data on safety and effectiveness."[52]

The FDA has approved many high-risk medical devices without comparative effectiveness data from clinical trials. A 2012 *JAMA* study examined all publicly available FDA summaries of safety and effectiveness data for Class III cardiovascular devices approved from 2000 to 2011.[53] Among 121 summaries based on 203 clinical studies, there were 353 primary endpoints among which 39.7 percent used an active comparator, 25.5 percent used numeric performance benchmarks derived from previous studies or expert opinion, 22.1 percent had no control group, and 12.7 percent used historical controls, meaning data from control groups in previous studies. Thus, the FDA approved most high-risk cardiovascular devices for over a decade without direct comparative effectiveness data against other standard treatments.

Furthermore, manufacturers often modify medical devices, requiring the submission of PMA supplement applications. The clinical trials backing these supplement applications have also suffered from significant limitations. A 2017 *JAMA* paper looked at eighty-three clinical studies backing seventy-eight panel-track supplements—those involving significant changes to a medical device—that the FDA approved between 2006 and 2015.[54] Nearly all applications (91.0 percent) were backed by a lone study. Of the eighty-three studies, 55.4 percent were not randomized, 69.9 percent were not blinded, 89.1 percent were not double-blinded, and the median number of participants in each study was 185 with the researchers keeping track of participants for roughly half a year. Four of every five primary endpoints (80.7 percent) were surrogates, and 62.0 percent had no control group comparison. Additionally, 39.8 percent of studies did not disclose the age of participants, and 30.1 percent did not report sex. The FDA required that manufacturers conduct postapproval studies for twenty-nine (37.2 percent) of the supplements.

The 2016 Cures Act created the Breakthrough Devices Program for medical devices, superseding the existing Priority Review and Expedited Access Pathway programs.[55] This program similarly expedites the development and review process for eligible medical devices and encourages greater collaboration between the FDA and industry. Eligible devices provide "more effective treatment or diagnosis of life-threatening or irreversibly debilitating human disease or condition," represent breakthrough technologies, and their usage is in the best interest of patients. Additionally, these devices either have no approved/cleared alternative or the FDA determines that these devices "offer significant advantages" over existing alternatives.

The program also reduces the evidence standards for eligible medical devices. According to the current FDA guidance, the agency "may accept a greater extent of uncertainty of the benefit-risk profile for these devices."[56] The FDA works to make the design of clinical trials more "flexible," like allowing for greater use of surrogate endpoints.[57] A 2025 *JAMA Internal Medicine* study examined seventy-five breakthrough-designated therapeutic devices the FDA approved from 2016 to 2024, of which sixty-seven (89.3 percent) underwent premarket clinical testing.[58] Among seventy-five pivotal studies, 48.0 percent were not randomized, 54.7 percent had no blinding, 81.3 percent were not double-blinded, 49.4 percent used surrogate endpoints, and 18.5 percent of all primary effectiveness endpoints were not statistically tested. Thirty devices had FDA-required postmarket studies, where 60.0 percent of measured endpoints were surrogates. Nine devices (12.0 percent) were ultimately recalled, including one Class I recall.

Evidence for devices approved under priority review before the Cures Act's weakening of standards was already limited. In a 2018 *JAMA Internal Medicine* letter, researchers examined the pivotal trials behind Class III cardiovascular device priority approvals from 2007 to 2017.[59] Eighteen trials supported fourteen approved cardiovascular devices, of which 50.0 percent were randomized, 83.3 percent had no blinding, 100 percent were not double-blinded, 72.2 percent used surrogate endpoints, and the mean number of participants was 499. A plurality (44.4 percent) of trials used an active comparator, while one-third used retrospective controls and 22.2 percent had no comparator. Additionally, half of the studies used a noninferiority hypothesis for at least one primary endpoint, meaning that they were studying whether the device was at least no worse than a comparator. Also, FDA expert advisory committees reviewed ten of the fourteen devices, resulting in four of nine votes determining that the devices were not effective. The FDA ultimately mandated postapproval clinical studies for thirteen devices (92.9 percent). By May 23, 2018, there were two Class I and thirteen Class II recalls for six devices.

Accordingly, priority-reviewed Class III medical devices have often been recalled. A 2020 *JAMA Internal Medicine* study examined Class III medical devices granted PMA between 2005 and 2015.[60] While most devices (87.4 percent) underwent standard review, those that received priority review were significantly more likely to get recalled. Most priority-reviewed devices (62.1 percent) were recalled compared to 29.9 percent of standard-reviewed devices. Significant majorities of priority- and standard-reviewed device recalls (80.6 percent and 74.8 percent, respectively) were Class II, meaning that use or exposure to the device could cause "temporary or medically reversible adverse health consequences or … the probability of serious adverse health consequences is remote."[61] A fifth of priority- and standard-reviewed device recalls (19.4 percent and 20.0 percent, respectively) were Class I, indicating the most severe and potentially deadly safety issues.

Inside Health Policy (IHP) reporting on December 10, 2015 revealed that the device provisions of the Cures Act came from direct collaboration between the medical device industry and senior FDA officials.[62] One such official was Dr. Robert

Califf, who served as FDA commissioner from 2016 to 2017 and from 2022 to 2025. On August 7, 2015, FDA acting commissioner Stephen Ostroff, Deputy Commissioner Califf, and Center for Devices and Radiological Health (CDRH) director Jeff Shuren met with representatives from the lobbying group Advanced Medical Technology Association (AdvaMed). Among these representatives was AdvaMed president Stephen Ubl (who currently is the president and chief executive officer [CEO] of PhRMA). Other industry attendees represented companies like J&J and device maker CVRx. A background document shared to members before the meeting stated, "CDRH representatives and AdvaMed worked together on proposed language for most of the device provisions in 21st Century Cures." These provisions included the priority review for breakthrough devices and the later-to-be-discussed humanitarian device exemption. During the meeting, AdvaMed thanked Dr. Shuren and CDRH "for meeting with AdvaMed regularly during the legislative process for getting the 21st Century Cures Act passed."

In response to IHP outreach, the FDA defended the extensive collaboration with industry as being standard protocol. According to the senior executive vice president for government affairs at AdvaMed, the reality "that an association and an agency might discuss how a particular piece of legislation might be operationalized or might impact them is not uncommon." Indeed, FDA negotiating with industry has been a required aspect of user fee legislation reauthorizations. Such a regulator-industry partnership is a feature and not a bug of the current regulatory regime. However, Diana Zuckerman—who worked in Congress from 1984 to 1994 and for the Clinton administration from 1995 to 1996—argued this was not always the case:

> I worked in the House and Senate for a decade, and this would never have been considered acceptable. For years, there was a revolving door between CDRH leadership and the device industry, but this is even worse than a revolving door: It is a partnership that excludes public health and consumer advocates who do not have close ties to industry.[63]

Further reflecting industry interests, device manufacturers, like drugmakers, have not completed many postmarketing trials in a timely manner, even though such trials would buttress the passive reporting system for adverse events from medical devices. A 2015 *JAMA* article found that among the twenty-eight Class III therapeutic devices approved in 2010 and 2011, only 12.7 percent of postmarketing studies were completed in three to five years while 75.0 percent were ongoing and 12.3 percent were terminated or of unknown status.[64] Additionally, the FDA only required thirty-three (16.2 percent) of the studies. The manufacturer initiated the other 83.8 percent. Of the completed or ongoing trials, 56.4 percent were not randomized, 79.3 percent had no blinding, 94.4 percent were not double-blinded, and roughly half (48.0 percent) had no comparator. Median enrollment was 222 to 250 patients, and 43.6 percent of the studies relied on surrogate endpoints. Additionally, three quarters of the Class III devices were implantable, meaning that if they turned out to be unsafe or ineffective, it would be relatively difficult to stop using the device.

In a 2020 follow-up, the researchers examined the same postmarketing studies, finding that slightly over half (55.4 percent) were completed, while 26.0 percent were terminated or had an unknown status and 18.6 percent were still ongoing.[65] Only seventy-five studies (36.8 percent) were completed and reported results on ClinicalTrials.gov or journal publications. It ultimately took eight to ten years to complete and publicly report over a third of postmarketing studies. Additionally, only thirty-three trials (16.2 percent) were completed, published, and used a comparator. Just twenty-two (10.8 percent) of these studies tested if the device was superior to the comparator, of which twelve (54.5 percent) failed to demonstrate superiority.

## Humanitarian Device Exemption

In the 1990 Safe Medical Devices Act, Congress created an additional avenue for FDA approval that lessened evidentiary requirements.[66] Originally, the Humanitarian Device Exemption (HDE) allowed the FDA to approve medical devices missing data proving effectiveness if they benefitted a patient population of fewer than 4,000 people, lacked a comparable device not also under the exemption, did not post "an unreasonable or significant risk of illness or injury," and the risk of benefit probably outweighed the risk of harm taking into account potential alternatives. The 2016 Cures Act expanded the number of devices eligible to get FDA approval without proving effectiveness to devices for patient populations not exceeding 8,000 people.[67]

Additionally, the original law prohibited device makers from profiting from devices approved under the humanitarian device exemption; thus, companies were hardly incentivized to exploit the law. However, the 2007 FDAAA and 2012 FDASIA created large exceptions to the prohibition to incentivize greater use, especially in pediatric populations (defined as twenty-two years old or younger).[68] The profit ban currently does not apply for devices (1) intended and indicated to treat or diagnose diseases/conditions that occur in pediatric populations or (2) intended and indicated to treat diseases/conditions that occur only in adult populations or where developing the device to treat children "is impossible, highly impracticable, or unsafe."[69] But, the FDA still limits the profitability of exempted devices by determining the number of devices reasonably necessary for each patient and multiplying it by 8,000. Thus, if a patient needed to use three of a particular device, the company could sell up to 24,000 units per year.

Without having to prove effectiveness, the clinical evidence behind humanitarian devices can be significantly weak and consequently call into question their safety profiles.[70] In 2005, the FDA approved an intracranial stent—a small tube placed in the brain—produced by the device manufacturer Stryker called the Wingspan stent system.[71] The basis for this approval was a single-arm trial—meaning that all participants used the device without any comparison to placebo—with an initial total population of forty-five adults who had recurrent symptoms attributed to a condition called intracranial stenosis.[72] The individuals were enrolled at least a week following a stroke, were deemed to have at least a moderate disability, and had unsuccessful therapies previously. Within one month, two (4.5 percent) of the forty-four participants who had a successfully placed stent had a stroke, and, by the passage of six months, the total increased to three (6.8 percent) with one death (2.3 percent). While the study had no control group, the authors reasoned that historical controls from previous studies showed a higher risk of stroke. Thus, they deemed Wingspan as reasonably safe even though they had no actual comparative effectiveness data for the studied patient population.

The FDA accepted the use of historical controls by claiming that "no alternative standard therapy was readily available for this disease state"; however, a subsequent NIH-funded study on the Wingspan system did use a control group.[73] Additionally, the FDA approved the usage of the Wingspan system in a far larger group than was studied in the trial by not accounting for factors like patient age, time since last stroke, severity of previous stroke, and the location of the intracranial stenosis. Therefore, the FDA approved the device for a patient population that the trial did not test safety for. Under the HDE, manufacturers must produce annual reports following approval, including any updated information on the devices along with reported adverse events. However, the FDA did not require any actual postapproval studies for Wingspan.

The later NIH-funded trial occurred in 2008—three years after the FDA let Wingspan stents on the market—included a much larger population of 451 patients, and the *NEJM* published the results in 2011.[74] The study compared the Wingspan stent system to aggressive medical management in patients who suffered a transient ischemic stroke or stroke attributed to stenosis within thirty days prior to enrollment. The trial stopped enrolling patients prematurely after finding that the rate of stroke or death was two-and-a-half times higher in the Wingspan treatment group (14.7 percent) compared to the medical-management group (5.8 percent). For every eleven people treated with the Wingspan system, roughly one additional stroke or death occurred. These findings were only made possible by CMS' decision to only cover the cost of the device if patients using it were enrolled in the clinical trial.[75]

Even though HDEs are only legally allowed when there is no "unreasonable or significant risk of illness or injury," the FDA did not take the Wingspan stent system off the market.[76] Rather, in March 2012, the FDA convened the Neurological Devices Panel of its Medical Devices Advisory Committee to go over the new evidence. The transcript of the meeting reveals that "the majority of the Panel does not think the data ... support the probable benefit."[77] The committee especially raised concerns about off-label usage of the device. Consequently, the FDA tightened the indicated population for which the device was approved to patients below the age of eighty who did not have a stroke within the last week of usage, believing this better fit the population of the original trial compared to the NIH-funded study.[78] Additionally, the FDA required Stryker to complete a postmarketing study.

It took six years for the WEAVE trial to conclude, and the American Heart Association published its results in 2019.[79] The study did not include any control group to provide comparative safety data, and the researchers only followed up to see the incidence of stroke or death within seventy-two hours of device implantation. Among 152 patients who met the FDA-approved indication criteria, 4 people (2.6 percent) had a stroke or died. The study also looked at 46 patients outside the FDA-approved indication, 11 (23.9 percent) of whom had a stroke or died. The FDA used these results to add a black box warning to the Wingspan stent system label highlighting the danger of using the device outside of its FDA-approved indication.[80]

In 2022, *JAMA* published the results of the CASSISS trial funded by the Chinese government and in which several authors had financial ties to Stryker, including a "co-first" author and the author who had full access to the trial data and who took "responsibility for the integrity of the data and the accuracy of the data analysis."[81] The trial included 358 patients and analyzed the risk of stroke or death in patients with transient ischemic attack or stroke due to intracranial stenosis for those who just received medical therapy and those who received such therapy along with the Wingspan stent system. The stent group had a statistically insignificant marginal increase in the risk of death compared to the medical therapy group. Thus, the authors concluded that the results did not support usage of the device. A commentary in an AHA journal noted that the trial "failed to show a benefit of percutaneous angioplasty and stenting over medical therapy for the prevention of stroke due to intracranial atherosclerotic stenosis."[82]

The Wingspan saga reveals not just the weaknesses of the HDE but also the FDA oversight of medical devices overall. The exemption allowed Stryker to not prove that the device was actually effective, and the FDA actively chose to approve the device based on safety information derived from a low-quality trial with no comparator and for a broad indication not supported by the study. The device was on the market for three years until an NIH-funded trial exposed the danger of the device, resulting in the FDA advisory committee finding that the evidence did not show the Wingspan met the probable benefit standard for humanitarian devices. Yet, the FDA kept the product on the market and narrowed its indication, mandating a postapproval study that took not just six years to complete but thirteen years after initial approval. The FDA did not require the trial to get comparative safety data.

Seventeen years after the FDA approval letting Wingspan on the market, the CASSISS trial—made possible from foreign-government funding—showed that the device was not better than medical therapy. Thus, the Wingspan did not meet the criteria for humanitarian devices that they provide probable benefit in situations with no alternative treatment. The Wingspan case study may be severe regarding the poor quality of evidence. But, it reveals not just how the FDA makes evidence-lacking decisions, but how its reliance on postmarketing studies lets devices that can cause harm and not benefit patients stay on the market for many years before such trials are completed. As with the WEAVE trial, for all the years postmarketing trials take to finish, they can still employ low-quality designs.

Ultimately, while the evidence standards for drugs and biologics have been significantly weakened over the last several decades, they are higher than the very low medical device standards. Around 99 percent of medical devices did not have to prove safety and effectiveness to the FDA to reach patients from 1976 through 2020.[83] Among the remaining percent that had to conduct clinical trials, many of the trials were poor quality due to factors like lack of randomization, no blinding, use of surrogate endpoints, and small sample sizes. Additionally, many postmarketing trials are not completed or take many years to be completed, and they also lack high-quality designs. The FDA does not even publish approved labels—containing key, summary data underlying approval—in a publicly accessible and searchable database for devices like it does for drugs.[84] Unlike drugs, dangerous or ineffective devices can be extremely costly and difficult to remove, especially if implanted. Thus, the FDA does not actually determine the safety and effectiveness of the vast majority of medical devices based on quality evidence, and patients have significant barriers to adjust if a medical device they use is harmful or ineffective.

The weak standards of evidence for proving safety and effectiveness investigated in the last two chapters regarding both pharmaceuticals and devices evolved out of congressional policy directives that fundamentally shifted the FDA's processes and priorities. Yet, as the next chapter discusses, the FDA itself has not been an innocent bystander to these institutional changes. Rather, the agency has grown very close and intertwined with industry to the extent that it shares personnel, funding, and priorities.

7

# Regulatory Capture and Corruption of the FDA

The previous chapters detail how policymakers have altered the FDA's regulatory priorities at the FDA in favor of industry, such as pushing faster reviews for approval, weakening evidentiary standards, and embracing lifecycle regulation. However, the FDA has not been an unwilling participant in these changes, and the agency itself has significant ties to the companies that it regulates. There is significant evidence that the agency has fallen victim to regulatory capture: the process in which a regulatory entity—such as a federal agency—systemically identifies with and protects the interests of the industry the public has charged it with regulating over the public interest.[1]

A prominent example is the railroad-regulating Interstate Commerce Commission (ICC) in the late-nineteenth and early-twentieth centuries. Railroads supported the ICC to protect industry in the face of populist outrage, particularly from farmers over price discrimination.[2] Railroad-friendly individuals staffed the ICC, and the agency pushed industry-friendly policies.[3] In 1892, future attorney general Richard Olney described the ICC as "of great use to the railroads. It satisfies the popular clamor for a government supervision of railroads, at the same time that that supervision is almost entirely nominal ... [it] becomes a sort of barrier between the railroad corporations and the people and ... against hasty and crude legislation hostile to railroad interests."[4] With the FDA, similar entanglements demonstrate regulatory capture, including the revolving door between industry and government, financial ties within important advisory committees, user fee funding of the FDA, and agency officials adopting industry views.

## The Revolving Door

One key indication of regulatory agencies intertwining with industry is the extent to which the same people work on both sides. The revolving door refers to when individuals transition from working in the government to being employed by the industry they regulate, vice versa, or both. This dynamic creates an ethical dilemma where government policymakers and regulators may be incentivized to serve the special interests of their past and/or future employers at the expense of the public interest.

There is extensive evidence of federal government officials—both within Congress and executive departments/agencies—being a part of the revolving door. A 2016 *Interest Groups & Advocacy* study examined all members of Congress who left their position between 1970 and 2012, finding that while the number of annual retirees did not significantly change, the number of retiring members becoming lobbyists dramatically increased, namely starting in the 1990s.[5] By the 2012 election cycle, slightly below 40 percent and 60 percent of House and Senate retirees, respectively, registered as lobbyists. A 2019 Public Citizen analysis found that around two-thirds of former members of Congress from the 115th Congress (2017–19) entered jobs in industry for which they could influence policymaking.[6] Of these former members, 59.1 percent worked for lobbying/consulting firms (50.0 percent) or business/trade groups (9.1 percent) that worked to influence the federal government.

One notable congressional case of the revolving door is Representative Billy Tauzin (R-LA). Tauzin was one of the key architects of the Medicare Modernization Act (MMA) of 2003, and he helped ensure that the federal government could not negotiate drug prices as part of the newly created Medicare Part D program.[7] This prohibition was a key priority in PhRMA's multimillion-dollar lobbying and advocacy campaign surrounding the negotiations over the bill.[8] Following the MMA's passage, Tauzin declined to run for reelection, and he became the president and CEO of PhRMA immediately upon exiting Congress in January 2005.[9] Tauzin made millions at PhRMA, becoming the highest-paid health-law lobbyist in 2010, earning $11.6 million.[10]

Researchers and watchdogs have also tracked significant revolving door activity within the federal agencies. OpenSecrets—a nonprofit organization that tracks the influence of money in politics—maintains a database of federal agency employees who either entered government after working as a lobbyist or turned to lobbying following their public service.[11] OpenSecrets has identified eighty-seven revolving FDA employees since 1998; however, this number is limited as it just tracks those who became registered lobbyists or took lobbyist-adjacent positions and admittedly relies on "imperfect information."[12] A 2023 *Health Affairs* study examined the 766 (94.9 percent) of 807 HHS officials appointed between 2004 and 2020 with available pre- and post-employment data.[13] They found that 15 percent had worked in private industry—including biopharmaceutical, medical device, insurance, consulting, and law companies/firms—immediately prior to their government employment and 32 percent went to work for industry following their public service. The level of revolving door activity varied between HHS agencies. Most appointees at the Office of the Deputy Secretary (55 percent), CDC (54 percent), and CMS (53 percent) exited to industry. The FDA had an exit-to-industry rate of 38 percent.

The FDA's top leadership has a lengthy record of working for industry, particularly pharmaceutical companies. In 2019, the news organization *Quartz* reported that nine out of the last ten FDA commissioners, stretching back to 1981, had gone on to work for the pharmaceutical industry after leaving their position.[14] However, a year later, Ellodi Pharmaceuticals announced that the previously sole exception to the revolving door, David Kessler, joined its Board of Directors.[15] Since then, the situation has not changed: every subsequent FDA commissioner has gone on to work in some capacity for industry (see Figure 9). Even several temporary, acting commissioners have joined industry.[16] Ultimately, every FDA commissioner over more than the last four decades has gone on to work for industry after leaving government.

Shortly following the Vioxx debacle that killed an estimated 30 to 60 thousand Americans, Commissioner Lester Crawford resigned and became senior counsel for Policy Directions—the lobbying firm supporting Vioxx's owner Merck.[17] Crawford would later plead guilty to lying about owning stocks in FDA-regulated companies, ultimately receiving three years of probation and a $90,000 fine.[18] Among these companies was PepsiCo—which sells sodas and various ultra-processed foods. Crawford previously served as the USDA's Food Safety and Inspection Service administrator, Georgetown University's Center for Food and Nutrition Policy director, and the head of an FDA obesity working group.[19]

Despite federal ethics requirements for disclosure and divestment, one former commissioner, Margaret Hamburg, maintained financial ties during her 2009–15 tenure.[20] Hamburg's husband, Peter Brown, worked for the hedge fund Renaissance Technologies, becoming co-CEO in 2010. The Office of Government Ethics (OGE) allowed Hamburg and Brown to maintain their holdings in Renaissance's Medallion Fund, even though it held stock in FDA-regulated companies including Amgen, Novo Nordisk, and AstraZeneca at an average value of $518 million. The couple earned over $3 million from the fund from 2009 to 2010. Reportedly, the OGE allowed this financial tie to exist because the Medallion Fund based its decisions on programming

| FDA Commissioner (Term) | Industry Connection (Position) |
|---|---|
| *Arthur Hayes (1981-1983)* | E. M. Pharmaceuticals (President) |
| *Frank Young (1984-1989)* | Braeburn Pharmaceuticals (Executive vice President) |
| *David Kessler (1990-1997)* | Ellodi Pharmaceuticals (Board Member) |
| *Jane Henney (1999-2001)* | AmerisourceBergen Corp. (Board Member) |
| *Mark McClellan (2002-2004)* | Johnson and Johnson (Board Member) |
| *Lester Crawford (2005-2005)* | Bexion Pharmaceuticals (Board Member) |
| *Andrew von Eschenbach (2006-2009)* | Bausch Health (Board Member) |
| *Margaret Hamburg (2009-2015)* | Alnylam Pharmaceuticals (Board Member) |
| *Robert Califf (2016-2017)* | Verily (Advisor) |
| *Scott Gottlieb (2017-2019)* | Pfizer (Board Member) |
| *Stephen Hahn (2019-2021)* | Harbinger Health (CEO) and Flagship Pioneering (CEO-Partner) |
| *Robert Califf (2022-2025)* | Verily (Advisor) |
| *Marty Makary (2025-Present)* | N/A |

***These are not exhaustive, meaning that the individuals may have more connections with industry.***

**Figure 9** A table documenting how nearly every FDA commissioner after 1980 has gone on to work for the drug industry. *Sources*: Foley, "Trust Issues Deepen as yet Another FDA Commissioner Joins the Pharmaceutical Industry"; "Ellodi Pharmaceuticals Welcomes Dr. David Kessler and John Fraher to Its Board of Directors"; "Stephen M. Hahn," Flagship Pioneering, accessed July 10, 2024, https://web.archive.org/web/20240710200022/https://www.flagshippioneering.com/people/stephen-m-hahn-2.

predominantly without human input. Yet, 2014 Senate testimony by Brown explicitly contradicted this as he admitted significant human input in the programming. Ultimately, Hamburg's story is unique, but it demonstrates the limitations of government oversight, as OGE only had seventy-five employees in 2024 while covering agencies across the executive branch.[21] In 2018, Hamburg joined Alnylam Pharmaceuticals' board of directors, where she still resides as of July 2025.[22]

The revolving door culture spreads further down within the agency as well. In a 2016 *BMJ* letter, Drs. Vinay Prasad and Jeffrey Bien followed fifty-five hematology-oncology reviewers at the FDA from 2001 to 2010.[23] Among the twenty-six reviewers who left the agency over the decade, fifteen (57.7 percent) left to work or consult for the pharmaceutical industry, and an additional eight (30.8 percent) could not be identified.

In 2018, *Science* magazine identified not just FDA staffers who left the agency to join industry, but staffers who went to work for the same companies that manufactured the drugs they regulated.[24] Simple public web searches identified that eleven (68.8 percent) of sixteen examiners who worked on twenty-eight drug approvals left to work/consult for the companies that they previously regulated. The investigation identified several specific examples like the case of Thomas Laughren, who served as the agency's director of psychiatric products.

In 2009, federally funded researchers, including Dr. Wayne Ray, published the results of a cohort analysis of individuals on Tennessee's Medicaid records from 1990 to 2005 in *NEJM*.[25] This cohort included 44,218 and 46,089 users of typical and atypical antipsychotic drugs, respectively, along with 186,600 matched nonusers of antipsychotic drugs. Among the atypical drugs studied was AstraZeneca's Seroquel. Typical and atypical drugs, including Seroquel, doubled the risk for sudden cardiac death, especially for individuals taking higher doses. In 2009, Ray testified to the FDA's Psychopharmacologic Drugs Advisory Committee (PDAC), which included Dr. Laughren, describing his research and arguing against the approval of Seroquel. Laughren was among the committee members who were critical of Ray's research and who defended AstraZeneca's clinical trial findings supporting approval.[26] While PDAC unanimously voted to not recommend approval for Seroquel as a first-line therapy for depression and anxiety conditions, Laughren and five other members successfully voted to recommend the approval of Seroquel as a supplemental therapy for major depressive disorder.[27]

Two years later in 2011, the FDA mandated a label change for Seroquel validating the risk of sudden cardiac death that Dr. Ray warned of. In 2013, Dr. Laughren would go on to form Laughren Psychopharm Consulting that advised pharmaceutical companies on how to best approach and navigate FDA approvals.[28] Laughren's LinkedIn page states that one of the goals of his company is "planning and preparation for meetings with the Psychopharmacological Drugs Advisory Committee (PDAC)."[29] Laughren also has other industry ties, as he sits on the advisory board of drugmaker VistaGen Therapeutics.[30]

Furthermore, a 2023 *BMJ* investigation documented how two key FDA regulators went to work for Moderna after holding oversight roles over COVID-19 vaccines.[31]

Dr. Doran Fink began working for the FDA in 2010 as a clinical reviewer, and he was later promoted in 2013 to lead medical officer of the agency's Division of Vaccines and Related Product Applications (DVRPA) within CBER's Office of Vaccines Research and Review (OVRR). From 2018 to 2022, Fink served as the deputy director-clinical for DVRPA.[32] Fink had a significant role with the development and emergency use authorization (EUA) of COVID-19 vaccines. According to his personal LinkedIn, he served on the "senior leadership team for COVID-19 vaccine review and policy activities," worked with "vaccine manufacturers throughout the COVID-19 pandemic to advise on development of COVID-19 vaccines and to coordinate expedited review of regulatory submissions," and contributed "to FDA Guidance for Industry on development, licensure, and EUA of COVID-19 vaccines." He also appeared in several FDA and CDC advisory committee meetings discussing the vaccines. Fink contributed to the FDA's decision to grant EUAs for the Moderna and Pfizer vaccines. Just two months after leaving the FDA in December 2022, Fink began his new position working in a leadership role in Moderna's clinical development program for infectious diseases.

Dr. Jaya Goswami joined the FDA's CBER in 2020 as a medical officer.[33] According to herself, she had "broad oversight over vaccines and biologics clinical development," and she held responsibility for ensuring the clinical data underlying Moderna's vaccine met regulatory standards for approval.[34] In June 2022, five months after the FDA reissued licensure for the Moderna vaccine in January 2022, Goswami left the agency to join Moderna as director of clinical development in infectious diseases. The *BMJ* investigation also noted that Goswami played a role in trying to bring another Moderna mRNA vaccine for the respiratory syncytial virus (RSV) to market, and Fink and Goswami's former place of employment, the FDA's OVRR, was reviewing and determining its fate. At the end of May 2024, the FDA approved this vaccine—mRESVIA (mRNA-1345)—to protect against lower respiratory tract disease caused by RSV in adults older than sixty years.[35]

The revolving door relationship between the FDA and Moderna relating to COVID-19 vaccination is not limited to Fink and Goswami. Dr. Moncef Slaoui, President Donald Trump's appointee to lead Operation Warp Speed (OWS)—the federal program to work with industry to expedite the development of COVID-19 vaccine products—had served on Moderna's board of directors. Slaoui also worked for over thirty years at GlaxoSmithKline (GSK), leading efforts to develop several vaccines. To bypass federal regulations requiring officials to divest holdings related to their work, the administration hired Slaoui as a contractor.[36] While Slaoui agreed to sell his $12 million in Moderna stock, he successfully refused to give up $10 million in GSK stock, arguing that it was for his retirement. Slaoui agreed to donate the profits from the stocks to the NIH; however, this donation was only required upon the last death of either Slaoui or his wife. GSK received as much as $2.1 billion in federal funding as part of OWS.[37] Furthermore, the FDA commissioner during the beginning of the COVID-19 pandemic, Dr. Stephen Hahn, who oversaw the EUA for Moderna's vaccine, joined Flagship Pioneering in 2021 as chief medical officer (CMO). Flagship Pioneering is the venture fund that "birthed Moderna."[38] He is now the fund's CEO-partner.[39]

## Limited Regulation

Concerns surrounding the revolving door between government and the industries it regulates are not limited to outside observers, as federal and state laws and regulations aim to limit such conflicts of interest. However, these legal restrictions are very limited and fail to prevent the revolving door across government. For the FDA, current law does not sufficiently guard against the perverse incentives for employees to work for the drug, biologic, and/or device makers that they regulate.

Section 207 of Title 18 of the United States Code regulates the behavior of former federal employees, including officials of executive agencies.[40] Section 207(a)(1) institutes a lifetime ban for any former employee from making—with the intent to influence—a communication or appearance to any employee or entity of the US government on behalf of anyone who is not the United States in relation to matters they were personally and substantially involved in. The government also must be a party to any such matter or have a direct or substantial interest. For example, an FDA reviewer cannot leave the agency during the review process for a drug and then engage in talks with the FDA on behalf of their new pharmaceutical employer regarding the very review they were previously a part of. However, the DOJ has explicitly written that this restriction does not prevent former employees from giving "behind-the-scenes" aid.[41] Thus, the former FDA reviewer could aid the pharmaceutical company in navigating the review as long as they avoid communications/appearances with the government.

Section 207(a)(2) is very similar to Section 207(a)(1). The main difference is that it imposes a two-year ban rather than a lifetime restriction, and the prohibited behavior is more broad. While Section 207(a)(1) pertained to matters the former employee was personally and substantially involved in, this section regards matters *that were actually pending under their official responsibility* within one year of the end of their employment. Again, the US government must be a party or have a direct or substantial interest in such matters. Legally, having official responsibility means that the individual has "direct administrative or operating authority, whether intermediate or final … to approve, disapprove, or otherwise direct Government action," and this pertains to both sole and shared authority along with direct actions or authority through subordinates.[42] For example, an FDA official who had official responsibility over a pending review for a drug during the last year of their employment cannot afterward represent the pharmaceutical sponsor in communication with the FDA regarding the review even if this particular official was not personally and substantially involved. However, this restriction lasts just two years and again only pertains to communications and appearances before government employees or entities, so it does not prevent behind-the-scenes activities. Additionally, the DOJ clarified that the restriction does not apply if the former employee should not have reasonably known that the matter was under their official responsibility during their last year of service.

While Section 207(b) covers behind-the-scenes activities, it only concerns trade agreements and treaties and is not particularly relevant to most former FDA employees, especially those who go on to work for the industries they previously regulated. The law prevents former employees during the one-year period following termination of their employment from knowingly representing, aiding, or advising entities that are not the US government on ongoing trade/treaty negotiations that they personally and substantially participated in during their last year of employment. This restriction only applies if the employee represents or advises others based on confidential information. While this section is not particularly relevant to the FDA, it does show precedent that policymakers can ban behind-the-scenes behaviors that they deem to be against the public interest.

For the vast majority of FDA employees, only subsection (a) is relevant. However, Section 207(c) levies additional restrictions on senior personnel that are like Section 207(a)(1), but shorter lasting and farther reaching. For one year after service in their senior position, this section bars such employees from knowingly making communications or appearances before any person within the department/agency that they served in during the one-year period before the end of their employment. These communications must involve the intent to influence on matters where the former employee "seeks official action" from a current employee, and be made on behalf of a third party not counting the United States. Therefore, this restriction bars communications/appearances regardless of whether the senior employee had any involvement in the relevant matter. Additionally, it only bars such communications/appearances made to the department/agency and employees that they served with.

Importantly, 207(c) applies only to senior employees; thus, it does not affect anyone below them or the very senior employees above them. The definitions of senior employees and very senior employees depend on if a particular employee meets at least one of several conditions.[43] For the FDA, whether or not someone is a senior employee depends on their pay, as the other conditions relate to military service grades and if they were appointed by the president or vice president under specific statutes that do not include FDA officials. Senior employees include those who have fixed pay according to the Executive Schedule (ES), which is the payment system for higher ranked US government officials and has five levels: I–V. The FDA commissioner is a senior employee, as this position earns a base salary under Level IV of the ES.[44] Senior employees also include many individuals earning a basic annual pay of at least 86.5 percent of Level II of the ES, which was $191,943.50 in 2024.[45] In September 2024, 1,902 (9.1 percent) of 20,912 total FDA employees earned adjusted basic pay of over $200,000, increasing to 2,805 employees (13.4 percent) for those earning over $190,000.[46] Some of these senior employees included Drs. Peter Marks and Patrizia Cavazzoni, who were the directors of CBER and the Center for Drug Evaluation and Research (CDER), respectively, in the Biden administration.[47]

While Section 207(c) does not apply to very senior employees, no official at the FDA currently counts as a very senior employee.[48] This category includes the vice president, specific officials appointed by the president or vice president who earn basic pay precisely at Level I of the ES, and being employed in the Executive Office of the President at the rate of pay for Level II of the ES.[49] None of these concern anyone at the FDA. Rather than Section 207(c), very senior employees are subjected to slightly more stringent restrictions in Section 207(d). This restriction is the same as 207(c) except that it extends over two years after an individual leaves their very senior position.

207(d) also prohibits communications to and appearances before anyone serving in a position listed in the ES.

Like the previous subsections of Section 207, the restriction in 207(c) does not bar behind-the-scenes assistance. Therefore, when former FDA commissioner Scott Gottlieb joined Pfizer's board of directors just two months after resigning from the agency in April 2019, he could not have sent communications or appeared in front of any FDA entity or official on behalf of Pfizer regarding matters concerning an official action, like approval of a drug, up until April 2020.[50] Once April 2020 arrived, Gottlieb could engage in such activities. Beforehand, between April 2019 and April 2020, Gottlieb was legally cleared to aid and advise Pfizer on how to interact with the FDA as long as he did not make any communications or appearances himself. Additionally, the director of the US Office of Government Ethics can waive 207(c) if they determine that the restrictions would "create an undue hardship" for the government to hire qualified employees and that a "waiver would not create the potential for use of undue influence or unfair advantage."[51]

Along with statutory restrictions, appointed officials in executive agencies have traditionally been restricted by executive order pledges. On his inauguration day, President Joe Biden issued Executive Order 13989 titled "Ethics Commitments by Executive Branch Personnel."[52] Similar orders were issued by previous presidents, including his last two predecessors, Presidents Donald Trump and Barack Obama. Section 1 of the order detailed the nine listed elements to the ethical pledge that every executive agency appointee had to sign. Five of the elements—two through six—regard the "Revolving Door Ban."[53] For appointees entering government, element two stopped them from being involved in matters concerned with their former employer or clients, including regulations and contracts, for a period of two years after their appointment. Similarly, element three concerned appointees who served as lobbyists within two years before their appointment, preventing them from participating in particular matters and specific issue areas that they lobbied on for two years after their appointment. Element three also bans such appointees from seeking or accepting employment with any executive agency that they lobbied during the two years before their appointment. For appointees leaving government, element six banned lobbying of covered executive branch officials, including cabinet members and noncareer Senior Executive Service appointees, on behalf of foreign governments that would require an individual to register as a foreign agent under the Foreign Agents Registration Act (FARA).[54] This ban existed for whatever is later: two years past the appointment or through the remainder of the Biden administration.

Elements four and five regulated appointee behavior after leaving government service, but they specifically applied to senior officials covered under Section 207(c). Element five also covered very senior employees under Section 207(d). Element four extended Section 207(c)'s one-year restriction to two years. Under this pledge, Scott Gottlieb would have had to wait until April 2021 until he could have discussed FDA approval of a drug to FDA employees on behalf of Pfizer. However, this was not actually the case, as President Biden's Executive Order 13989 only applied to the executive agency officials appointed on or after January 20, 2021. President Trump's version of the same order in his first term did not extend Section 207(c) to two years.[55] Moreover, element five made appointees pledge to not assist lobbying activities or certain behind-the-scenes activities for one year following the end of their appointment.[56] They could not "materially assist others in making communications or appearances" that they are otherwise prohibited from doing under Sections 207(c) and 207(d).

Yet, President Donald Trump rescinded Biden's order at the beginning of his second term, and he has not issued his own ethics order as of July 2025.[57] Thus, Trump's political appointees are subject to no requirements other than under statute, and Biden appointees no longer must comply with their pledges. Even if President Trump did not rescind Executive Order 13989, the additional restrictions are limited in who they target. The order only pertained to appointed executive branch officials, who are higher-level appointees. Thus, the vast majority of FDA employees, including many medical reviewers, did not have to abide by the pledge. Elements four and five were further restricted to appointed officials who were senior and very senior employees covered under Sections 207(c) and 207(d), and the FDA does not have very senior employees.

Furthermore, the specifics of these pledges vary between administrations.[58] Trump's executive order in his first administration did not include the one-year ban on behind-the-scenes activities included in Biden's order. Conversely, Trump required appointees to agree to a five-year post-appointment ban on lobbying activities that Biden did not require, nor did President Obama. However, President Bill Clinton had a similar provision in his version of the executive order.

Both the statutory limitations detailed in Section 207 of Title 18 and the further restrictions in Executive Order 13989 are weak barriers to the revolving door between FDA officials and the companies they regulate. Only Sections 207(a)(1) and 207(a)(2) cover all agency officials, and these are very limited. Former FDA employees are free to use their experience to aid industry if they do not communicate with or appear in front of US government personnel and entities. Even if they do engage in such communications or appearances, the restrictions only apply if they regard particular matters that the former employees were personally and substantially involved in or that were pending while under their official responsibility. Regarding the latter, this restriction only holds for two years after their employment ends. Thus, a former FDA official can immediately provide behind-the-scenes aid to industry regarding a drug review they were personally involved in. If they just had an official responsibility during the drug development and review process, the official can engage in direct lobbying after two years.

Additionally, both restrictions only apply to situations that involve a specific party or specific parties either at the time of participation (207[a][1]) or while the matter was pending (207[a][2]). In a 2004 summary, the DOJ wrote that "it is quite possible that an employee who participated in a rulemaking while employed by the Government will, after leaving Government service, be able to appear before his former agency concerning the application of that rule to his new private sector employer without violating" the law.[59] The DOJ's rationale for this possibility was that rulemaking doesn't often involve specific parties. In theory, the government may adopt a different interpretation; however, the fact that this viewpoint has existed reveals a significant limitation.

All the restrictions except element five of Executive Order 13989 did not prevent behind-the-scenes activities not involving direct communications with or appearances in front of federal officials. Therefore, they did nothing to stop former agency officials from educating new industry employers on actions to take, who to reach out to, and any other beneficial information gleaned from their experience. In a 2019 report on the federal revolving door, Craig Holman and Caralyn Esser for Public Citizen bluntly described the situation:

> Such a narrow category of prohibited activity means that former public officials may immediately upon leaving government join a lobbying firm, design a lobbying campaign on behalf of paying clients, organize and direct the lobbying team—but simply avoid picking up the telephone and making the lobbying contact. Any and all strategic consulting activities are permitted, and in all likelihood the sitting lawmakers will even know that the former official is behind the lobbying campaign.[60]

Members of Congress have also recognized this significant limitation, as a key piece of legislation introduced by Democratic members in previous years—the For the People Act—redefines lobbying activities under the 1995 Lobbying Disclosure Act. In the 2021 version of the bill, lobbying activities are redefined to include "counseling in support of such preparation and planning activities, research, and other background work that is intended, at the time it is performed, for use in contacts, and coordination with the lobbying activities of others."[61] The bill adds that the law would consider anyone who knowingly counsels the lobbying contacts of others to have also made the same lobbying contacts.

Regarding element five of Biden's executive order, this restriction only applied to appointed FDA officials who were also senior employees under Section 207(c), and it lasted for one year. Additionally, unlike communications and appearances directly involving the government, it is questionable to what extent the Biden administration could realistically have enforced element five. To find a former appointee guilty of violating their pledge, the administration would need to obtain evidence that the individual materially aided others. Thus, if a former FDA appointee verbally provides a pharmaceutical lobbyist material support—defined as providing substantive assistance—in private, there is not a high likelihood of facing repercussions unless someone privy to the conversation told government enforcers or the administration got a hold of a written admission.[62] This limitation similarly applies to the For the People Act's proposed reform. Also, the order stipulated that material support did not include general or background education on matters of law or policy that are related to the individual's subject matter expertise.

Moreover, all the restrictions are time-limited except for Section 207(a)(1). These time limits are predominantly only for one year and at most two years, except for the foreign agent restriction in Biden's order (element six). This requirement lasted the remainder of his administration if that was over two years when the appointed official left their post. Thus, even if the restrictions covered all activities that allow former agency officials to capitalize on their government experience to the benefit of the regulated industry, they would only have been temporary. In practice, companies would still have had a readily available population of former FDA officials to recruit; they would have just waited a year or two.

Furthermore, all the restrictions focused on lobbying or lobbying-adjacent activities that concern former government employees capitalizing on their experience once outside of government. Aside from not robustly protecting against this behavior, they do not touch the potential corrupting financial incentives for employee behavior while they are in government. Government employees generally earn significantly less than their industry counterparts.[63] There is a potential financial incentive to not go against the interests of industry when they (1) may be future employers and (2) pay them larger salaries.[64]

This dynamic is reflected by a scandal in 1905 involving the three major life insurance companies—Equitable Life, Mutual Life, and New York Life.[65] New York state investigators uncovered that the companies kept secret, unreported bank accounts that they would use to contribute to political candidates and parties. As part of his testimony, the US Senator representing New York, T. C. Platt, rejected the notion that there was any *quid pro quo* (this for that) attached to company contributions to politicians. However, in response to the question of whether "the use of these contributions in the election of candidates to office puts the candidates under more or less of a moral obligation not to attack the interests supporting," Platt responded, "that is what would naturally be involved."[66]

Executive department and agency officials do not receive direct contributions reflecting the campaign donations that elected officials rely upon. Yet, the dynamic between these officials and the industries in which they regulate can include a similar reality of financial reward. Outside of government service, one of the most relevant uses of former agency employees' experiences is to apply their knowledge to companies within the regulated industries. Indeed, there is an existing and recognized market of former government employees and private employers. Companies view their experiences as extremely valuable, as they have unique knowledge of internal government processes and personnel along with connections to potentially key figures.

Several studies show that lobbyists with government experience are more effective. A 2012 *American Economic Review* analysis examined publicly available lobbyist disclosure reports from 1998 to 2008 in relation to Congress, finding that former congressional staffers are responsible for generating 56 percent of private lobbying firm revenues.[67] A 2016 *Academy of Management Journal* article examined the lobbying activities of firms in the S&P 500 Index between 2004 and 2009.[68] Higher levels of political connectedness, measured by "the number of revolving door lobbyists employed ... the number of board members with prior government experience ... and the number of congressional campaigns to which the firm donated," yielded significantly greater contract returns.

Thus, agency employees' knowledge that there is a possible future career with the industry they are regulating—where they can also earn more money—is a key dynamic of the revolving door problem. Then-FDA commissioner Gottlieb recognized this issue in a June 2018 report to Congress: "[FDA] employees are ... attractive to industry and other private entities, which are sometimes able to attract such employees

... with higher salary and benefit packages."[69] This knowledge can naturally incentivize individuals to not oppose the interests that will reward them. Here, the problem is not the potential for former government employees to directly engage with federal officials on behalf of industry, it is the possibility that they can work for the industries they used to regulate at all. This revolving door signifies agency capture through the embedding of industry-tied employees throughout the FDA during their employment and even afterward, particularly among high-ranking officials.

## Advisory Committee Conflicts of Interest

Although FDA employees are legally barred from receiving direct payments from the companies they regulate, the same does not hold true for the members of the advisory committees who significantly affect drug and device approvals. A 2023 *JAMA Health Forum* investigation into the voting behavior of the FDA's human drug advisory committees and the FDA's corresponding approval decisions examined 409 meetings held by eighteen different advisory committees between 2010 and 2021.[70] FDA decisions only differed from advisory committee votes in 36 (12.1 percent) of the relevant 298 instances, highlighting the importance of committee votes.

When Congress ordered the creation of scientific advisory panels to provide approval recommendations in PDUFA II, it required that panel members had to disclose conflicts of interest and prevented any member from voting on matters where they or their immediate family members could gain financially from the decision.[71] The FDA can waive this requirement if it deems an individual has essential expertise. Regardless, the current system at the FDA has failed to prevent the presence of significant financial COIs between advisory committee members and the companies whose products they are reviewing.

Title 18 Section 208 of the US Code regulates financial COIs for all federal government employees, including special government employees (SGEs) like FDA advisory committee members.[72] Section 208(a) bars any employee from participating in government matters where there is a financial interest tied to them or their spouse, child under the age of eighteen, general partner, organization where they are serving as an officer, director, trustee, general partner or employee, or any person/organization with which they are negotiating or have any arrangement regarding prospective employment. There are various exceptions to this prohibition. For advisory committees members, whoever appoints them can waive the ban after reviewing their financial disclosure and certifying "in writing that the need for the individual's services outweighs the potential for a COI created by the financial interest involved." Another exception that applies to all employees is that if an individual fully discloses their potential COI to the government official responsible for appointing them, the official can determine that their interest is "not so substantial" as to affect the integrity of their relevant services.

While the statute does not define such financial interests, HHS regulations define a financial interest as "anything of monetary value, whether or not the value is readily ascertainable."[73] In practice, the FDA and other agencies like the NIH consider examples of financial interests to include but not be limited to stocks, bonds, interests through ownerships, partnerships, LLCs, consulting arrangements, grants, contracts, or employment.[74] Prior to FDA advisory committee meetings, the committee members fill out a Form 3410 to disclose their own and associates' potential COIs that relate to the subject matter of the meeting, including both those tied to the company behind a product being examined and its competitors.[75] They must reveal their investments by type, owner, number of shares, current value, and percentage of net worth. They must disclose their full-time or part-time employment situation, regardless of whether it is current or under negotiation, along with their status as a consultant or advisor and if that is related to the committee meeting's issues. Other disclosures on the form relate to contracts, grants, patents, royalties, trademarks, appearances as an expert witness, speaking and writing financial interests, and other relevant involvements such as "involvement in a lawsuit, researcher initiated study, gift of research materials, etc."[76]

However, disclosure of any interests on this form does not mean the FDA determines that an advisory committee member has a COI worthy of prohibiting their involvement in a particular committee meeting. The agency follows procedures outlined in publicly available guidance documents.[77] Current FDA rules do not allow committee members to participate in a meeting if their personal or immediate family has COIs worth more than $50,000.[78] However, no such limit exists for "imputed" COIs that "are attributed to the individual through his employer (i.e., the employer has a relevant financial interest) or through his position as an officer, director, trustee, or general partner."[79] For example, a scientist whose research benefits from a grant of $500,000 that a pharmaceutical company provides to their employer could then participate in an advisory committee meeting relating to matters concerning the same company.

Ultimately, the FDA has significant discretion over whether disclosed COIs bar someone from serving on an advisory committee. The agency decides whether (1) disclosed financial interests would not cause a reasonable person to question the member's impartiality or—if they would—(2) if the government's interest in the individual's participation outweighs the concern that a reasonable person would question the FDA's integrity. Thus, current statutory law, regulations, and agency interpretations leave ample room for subjective interpretation.

During the five-year period between the 2007 FDAAA (PDUFA IV) and the 2012 FDASIA (PDUFA V), there was additional restriction of advisory committee members with COIs. The FDAAA imposed caps on the number of waivers that the FDA could issue to allow conflicted members to participate in committee meetings.[80] Originally, the percentage of members the agency could grant waivers to fell from 13 percent in 2009 to 11.5 percent by 2012. While the FDA never actually approached the cap, FDASIA repealed the cap entirely, allowing a potentially infinite number of granted waivers.[81] Additionally, FDASIA changed the selection criteria for advisory committee members to just prioritize expertise while it had previously included expertise and financial disclosures.

In 2011 testimony to the House Energy & Commerce Committee regarding the PDUFA V reauthorization, then-CDER director Janet Woodcock claimed that the FDA had trouble recruiting qualified individuals for their advisory panels due to the COI restrictions.[82] However, the FDA did not lack an abundance of unconflicted experts to choose from.[83] A 2009 *Health Affairs* study included a 2007 mailed survey of 3,028 life science researchers, finding that even though a majority (52.8 percent) had financial ties to industry, nearly half (47.2 percent) did not.[84] Similarly, while a 2011 *JAMA Internal Medicine* analysis of individuals who helped create cardiovascular clinical practice guidelines in 2008 found that a majority (55.6 percent) had COIs, there were still 44.4 percent of expert contributors who did not.[85] While this evidence indicates significant issues with conflicts in medical research and public health, it also shows many unconflicted experts who could serve on FDA advisory committees. Additionally, the FDA's own data revealed that—at the time of Woodcock's testimony—they had not granted COI waivers to more than 5 percent of advisory committee members in a given month, far below the cap.[86] Regardless of whether the percentage of waivers accurately reflects the number of members with COIs, the agency did not determine that more than 5 percent of authorized members had COIs necessitating waivers.

The lead author of a report in *Science*—Dr. Susan Wood—formerly worked in the FDA as assistant commissioner for Women's Health and director of the Office of Women's Health.[87] Wood and her coauthor, Dr. Jillian Mador, documented the lack of evidence that lifting the caps actually addressed a real recruitment issue.[88] Wood publicly explained that "panels top-heavy with experts who have financial ties to industry might be more likely to dismiss or ignore scientific evidence of risks or other problems." The report pointed to two different examples. In 2001, the FDA approved Bayer's contraceptives Yaz and Yasmin.[89] In December 2011, an advisory committee voted 15–11 to keep the drugs on the market, because the risk of blood clots from these treatments was outweighed by their benefits. This decision came after the drugs had been linked to one hundred deaths and consumers filed over 10,000 lawsuits against Bayer alleging harm. An October 2011 *BMJ* cohort study had found that the risk of blood clots was two times greater for Yaz and Yasmin compared to other contraceptives.[90] A *Washington Monthly* and *BMJ* investigation found that at least four of the voting committee members had financial ties to Bayer that the FDA had not publicly disclosed, representing enough votes to flip the committee's decision.[91]

In February 2005, the FDA held a joint meeting with the Arthritis Advisory Committee and the Drug Safety and Risk Management Advisory Committee to examine the cardiovascular risk posed by a group of COX-2-inhibiting nonsteroidal anti-inflammatory drugs: Vioxx, Bextra, and Celebrex.[92] The Center for Science in the Public Interest found that ten (31.3 percent) of the thirty-two scientific experts on the committee had financial ties to the makers of the drugs: Merck and Pfizer. Another seventeen (53.1 percent) had ties to drugmakers other than Merck and Pfizer. Thus, twenty-seven (84.4 percent) of the thirty-two committee members had financial ties to industry. The joint advisory committee voted that all three drugs should remain on the market: 17–15 (Vioxx), 17–13 (Bextra), and 31–1 (Celebrex).[93] The ten directly-conflicted members voted 9–1, 9–1, and 10–0 to keep Vioxx, Bextra, and Celebrex on the market, respectively. Thus, if their votes had not counted, the joint committee would have voted in favor of withdrawing Vioxx and Bextra from the market 14–8 and 12–8, respectively, while the Celebrex outcome would not have changed.[94] Overall, twenty-eight (93.3 percent) of the thirty votes made by the ten directly conflicted members supported the drugs' approval compared to thirty-seven (56.1 percent) out of the sixty-six votes made by the other committee members.

On April 7, 2005, Pfizer pulled Bextra off the market at the request of the FDA for increasing serious cardiovascular adverse events like heart attacks and strokes without offering therapeutic advantage over other comparable treatments.[95] Importantly, Merck had pulled Vioxx from the market in September 2004 due to cardiovascular adverse events, the company announced in 2007 that it would pay $4.85 billion in a settlement to end the thousands of lawsuits stemming from alleged injuries, and the drug killed an estimated 30 to 60 thousand Americans.[96] Thus, the FDA advisory committee voted to keep Vioxx on the market *after* Merck itself had pulled the product due to its known lethality.

Although the FDA can choose unconflicted advisory committee members, several different studies have consistently found significant portions of members holding COIs with the very companies whose products they are voting on over the last several decades. A 2006 *JAMA* investigation looked at all FDA drug advisory committee meetings from 2001 to 2004 listed on the agency's website.[97] Among 221 meetings, 146 (66.0 percent) had at least one committee member with a COI, and this grew to 162 meetings (73.3 percent) when also including voting consultants. Among all 1,957 advisory committee members, 564 (28.8 percent) had disclosed at least one COI, and 265 (26.8 percent) out of 990 voting consultants disclosed a COI.

The authors only identified a weak but statistically significant correlation between certain COIs and votes that would not have changed the outcome of any vote included in the study. However, they noted that COIs can impact voting patterns in numerous ways, like affecting the behavior of all voters or differently affecting close and nearly unanimous votes, which limited observational data may not detect. A 2021 *PLOS One* study failed to find a statistically significant association with voting to recommend drug approval and disclosed COIs among Gastrointestinal Drug Advisory Committee (GIDAC) members across 34 meetings from 1998 to 2018.[98] Yet, studies of all meetings in aggregate can mask the impact of COIs in consequential or particular types of votes. The evidence shows the potential of select cases with significant consequences, as were the cases of Yaz and Yasmin along with Vioxx and Bextra.

Moreover, a 2016 *JAMA Internal Medicine* article examined twenty-eight of the forty-nine Oncologic Drugs Advisory Committee (ODAC) meetings from 2009 to 2014 that had public hearings discussing cancer drugs.[99] There were 103 public speakers, of which 31 (30.1 percent) had direct financial ties to the company seeking marketing approval or were there representing an organization that had received funding from the company. Fifty-eight speakers (56.3 percent) reported connections with organizations relevant to the drug or the treated cancer. Similarly, a 2018 *JAMA Internal Medicine* piece examined Anesthetic and Analgesic Drug Products Advisory Committee (AADPAC) meetings from September 2009 to April 2017 relating to drug approval.[100] There were fifteen meetings involving ninety-one individuals who made 112 speaking appearances. Such speaking appearances are standard, as advisory committee meetings usually include public speakers who provide statements about the subject matter at hand.[101]

For the 112 speaking appearances, 28 (25.0 percent) had disclosed or undisclosed financial ties to the company seeking approval, which the authors verified existed prior to the meeting. Support for approval among all speakers was 68 percent, and this jumped to 86 percent for those with known prior COIs. When counting the additional 15 speakers with COIs—in which the authors could not determine when they occurred—conflicted speakers were more than eight times as likely to support approval compared to speakers without financial ties.[102] Accordingly, a previous 2014 analysis from *The Milbank Quarterly* examined the reported financial interests of 1,379 members of the FDA's CDER advisory committees along with their voting behavior from 1997 to 2011.[103] Individuals with financial interests exclusively in the sponsoring company and those who were on the advisory board solely for the sponsor were around one and a half and five times more likely, respectively, to vote in favor of the sponsor.

In 2018, *Science* revealed the weakness of just examining disclosed COIs.[104] The investigation scrutinized compensation records for the physicians who advised the FDA on whether to approve twenty-eight psychopharmacologic, arthritis, and cardiac or renal drugs between 2008 and 2014. Out of the 107 physician advisers, 66 (61.7 percent) received financial compensation from the drugmakers whose product they voted on or their competitors for travel/consulting or via research subsidies. The degree of compensation varied, as 26 got between $1,000 and $10,000, 14 received between $10,000 and $100,000, 20 received between $100,000 and $1,000,000, and 6 got more than $1,000,000. Therefore, nearly 4 in 10 (37.4 percent) and a quarter (24.3 percent) of the physicians received more than $10,000 and $100,000 in compensation, respectively. Critically, *Science* found that the FDA's COI review process was "primarily an honor system and seems to miss obvious conflicts." Eleven of the seventeen top earners acknowledged to *Science* financial ties to relevant drugmakers, yet the FDA disclosed none and issued no waivers.

In another example of COIs at play in a consequential committee meeting, the FDA's Circulatory System Devices Panel of the Medical Devices Advisory Committee voted 13–1 that the benefits of TriClip—a cardiac device from device manufacturer Abbott—outweighed the risks in February 2024.[105] By April 2024, the FDA approved TriClip for the purpose of treating leakage from the heart's tricuspid valve.[106] Yet, the FDA had not publicly disclosed that the vast majority of the committee, ten members (71.4 percent), had either previously received payments from Abbott or had their research funded by the manufacturer. From 2016 to 2022, these ten members received $650,000 from Abbott, and every one of them voted in favor of TriClip. One of these committee members, Dr. Craig Selzman, benefitted from $181,000 in associated research funding from Abbott to the University of Utah Hospitals & Clinics. Questioned on whether the public could question his and other members' impartiality based on the payments, he said, "people from the outside looking in would probably say yes."

Ultimately, significant numbers of individuals on FDA advisory committees have had ties to not just industry but the very companies for which their decisions are relevant. To sway votes, a few members with financial COIs may be all that is required to swing an outcome. The public speakers who directly pressure committee meetings also often have ties to industry. While laws are in place to limit such conflicts, they are very weak in practice and provide significant discretion to the FDA on which conflicts are significant enough to matter and, if so, when it is permissible to grant waivers. These conflicts add onto the fact that nonvoting industry representatives serve on advisory committees, although new FDA policy in April 2025 bars industry representatives from serving as official members except where required under law.[107] Thus, the FDA has relied on advisory committee votes cast and influenced by individuals with significant financial ties to regulated companies, corrupting their commitment to the public interest and signaling regulatory capture.

## Funding and Priorities

As there is a revolving door between the FDA and industry, and advisory committees have many financially conflicted members, the agency also relies on the companies it regulates for funding. The 1992 PDUFA and its multiple reauthorizations fundamentally shifted the FDA from a standard executive agency reliant on congressional appropriations to a regulatory institution that not only relies on funding from the very companies it regulates, but one that negotiates with industry regarding the conditions accompanying such funding for every five-year reauthorization. As increases in user fee funding have outpaced increases in funding from congressional appropriations, the share of industry funding has significantly increased and, thus, the importance of good industry relations.

Nearly half of the FDA's entire budget came from user fees in FY 2024; however, the areas of the agency that approve industry products receive the largest shares of industry funding (except for tobacco regulatory activities that are 100 percent funded by user fees).[108] The FDA's human drugs, biologics, and devices/radiological health programs received 69.2 percent, 53.1 percent, and 43.7 percent of their funding from user fees, respectively. This funding has not come without consequence for the FDA's focus and priorities. Higher levels of funding accompanied the agency abiding by performance goals from each PDUFA iteration. These performance goals largely focus on the agency implementing faster review times for both standard and priority review applications. At the same time, Congress has created new expedited pathways for medical products to get approved faster and with less evidentiary requirements. This transition has significantly shifted the burden to prove efficacy and safety toward the period after regulatory approval rather than beforehand.

While Congress has ultimately passed the laws instituting the aforementioned changes to the priorities of the FDA, the pharmaceutical and other regulated industries have had significant influence and input. When Congress contemplates what to include in PDUFA reauthorizations, it considers recommendations put forth by the FDA. Since PDUFA III in 2002, the agency has been mandated to directly consult with the industry it regulates.[109] Compared with members of the public, medical professionals, and other interested parties, industry has significantly more resources and a greater financial interest in pushing its priorities on the FDA. Reflecting this situation, the FDA holds significantly more meetings with industry compared to other groups to the extent that PDUFA IV forced the FDA to hold at least one meeting a month with patient and consumer advocacy groups during the periods in which it interacted with industry.[110]

FDA negotiations with industry do not take place on equal footing. Dr. Joseph Ross—a Yale University professor of medicine—described agency reliance on user fees as a "devil's bargain," where every five years, consultations with industry result in "the F.D.A. essentially asking industry, 'What can we do to secure this money?' "[111] Additionally, the pharmaceutical, biotechnology, and medical device industries have spent billions of dollars on lobbying agency officials and legislators in Congress. According to the Union of Concerned Scientists, from 2009 to 2011—the years preceding the PDUFA V reauthorization—the aforementioned industries spent over $700 million on lobbying federal officials.[112] This spending is not unique. According to OpenSecrets, the pharmaceutical/health products industry—which includes drugmakers, medical product dealers, and dietary supplement companies—spent approximately $6.4 billion on federal lobbying from January 1998 to April 2025.[113] For just the full years from 2021 to 2024, the industry spent over $1.5 billion on federal lobbying.

While pouring in immense resources to present their information and priorities to FDA officials and legislators, industry also spends large sums of money to fund the campaigns of the members of Congress who ultimately pass legislation, approve funding, and instruct the FDA. Congress has prohibited corporations from directly making campaign contributions since the 1907 Tillman Act.[114] However, companies are allowed to form political action committees (PACs) to make contributions to candidates, political party committees, and other PACs. Additionally, individuals within corporations—like executives—can contribute funds to the aforementioned recipients. These contributions are subject to federal limits. For example, individuals and PACs can make contributions up to $3,500 and $3,500–$5,000 (depending on the PAC type) to a candidate committee per election in the 2025–26 cycle.[115] Yet, individual donors can give almost $1.1 million to committees for political parties each year in 2025–26 ($360,000 for most PACs).[116] From 1990 to 2024, individuals and corporate PACs within the pharmaceutical/health products industry spent $522.4 million on campaign contributions.[117] Most of this funding—$306.2 million (58.6 percent)—came from individuals while $216.2 million (41.4 percent) came from PACs.

Corporations can directly spend money on elections through independent expenditures—spending in support or opposition to clearly identifiable federal candidates that are made independently, meaning there is no coordination between the spender and recipient. The Supreme Court legalized such infinite spending in its 2010 *Citizens United v. Federal Election Commission* decision.[118] From 2010 to 2024, the pharmaceutical/health products industry spent $93.6 million via this outside spending.[119] Therefore, FDA negotiations with industry take place in the context of (A) considerable industry spending to dominate the information that agency officials and legislators are exposed to via lobbying and (B) industry funding of the campaigns of members of Congress who the FDA must appeal to every five years to pass their recommendations.

Further representing the accuracy of Dr. Ross's conclusion that the FDA essentially asks industry what it can do to secure its funding, each PDUFA reauthorization involves negotiations over performance measures. The reauthorizations outline performance goals for the FDA to prove that they are properly using the increased funding to meet various measures, such as expedited review times. For example, the 2023 PDUFA performance report that the FDA submitted to Congress lauds how the agency "is currently meeting or exceeding the 90-percent performance level for nine performance goals," meaning that the agency has acted on at least 90 percent of submitted applications and supplements within certain time frames.[120] The focus of these performance goals is not patient-focused through measures of better efficacy and safety review. The performance goals largely reflect the interests of industry: faster review times, more approvals based on less evidence, an enhanced transition to postmarketing surveillance, and greater collaboration between the FDA and industry during product development and review.

FDA negotiations with industry result in commitment letters that outline the performance goals the agency works to meet for each PDUFA reauthorization. In the most recent commitment letter, the FDA described its mission to put more drugs on the market to increase the availability of medications to Americans.[121] To fulfill this mission, the agency will enhance communications between the FDA and industry sponsors, use more and newer surrogate endpoints, and further explore basing approvals on real world evidence like observational studies rather than high-quality randomized trials.

Lack of FDA acquiescence to industry demands can have severe consequences as user fee funding sunsets every five years. The FDA accepted PDUFA II's weakening of evidentiary standards compared to a clean reauthorization of the original legislation due to fear of budget cuts.[122] Reliance on user fee funding has only exponentially increased since. Dr. David Wheadon—the senior vice president of scientific and regulatory affairs at PhRMA—recognized in 2012 congressional testimony relating to PDUFA V that "failure to reauthorize PDUFA in a timely fashion would have catastrophic effects" on the FDA's ability to function.[123] Such leverage grants great power to industry to impose its priorities. In 2022, negotiations for MDUFA V stalled between the agency and the medical device industry due to disagreements where medical device companies opposed how the FDA wanted to use increased user fee funding.[124] For example, the FDA proposed funding for the total product lifecycle program (TAP) with the primary goal of expediting patient access to new medical devices.[125] The device industry did not like that the agency had not cleared the idea with them.

Industry not only maintains significant influence during the PDUFA reauthorization process, but the FDA engages regularly with industry during the development and review process for its products. In the case of Aduhelm, Biogen worked with FDA officials so extensively that their work was hard to distinguish in their joint report to the PCNS Advisory Committee, and the agency overrode the committee and switched the drug to the accelerated approval pathway to get it to market.[126] Although the 2022 report by the Committees on Oversight & Reform and Energy & Commerce declared this case to be atypical and improper, it represents an exaggeration of the standard dynamic between the regulator and regulated. The FDA actively communicates and advises product sponsors during the drug development process, and industry representatives present their pointed cases for approval in front of the agency's advisory committees. These cases rely upon clinical trials that industry both designs and runs, and these studies also result in more pro-industry conclusions compared to nonindustry sponsored trials.

Rather than combat industry influence on the regulatory process, top FDA officials have embraced and shared many of the same priorities while seeking to further entrench collaboration between both sides of the regulatory fence. In her 2011 congressional testimony to the House regarding PDUFA V, future acting FDA commissioner Janet Woodcock bemoaned the "patent-cliff" that faced the pharmaceutical industry "where many of the most profitable brand-name products" were set to face generic competition.[127] While acknowledging the benefit to consumers by not having to pay monopoly prices, she made note that drug manufacturers "will lose large sources of profit." Such industry sympathies are not unique to Woodcock, as former FDA commissioner Andrew von Eschenbach lamented in 2012:

> Consumer groups distrustful of industry have led Congress to erect ever greater barriers between regulators and those they regulate. The FDA can convene advisory committees of outside experts, but these experts weigh in only at the end of the regulatory process. Worse, congressionally mandated conflict-of-interest rules keep many of the most knowledgeable academic and industry scientists off advisory committees out of fear that industry ties might bias their judgment.[128]

In his view, there should be even greater collaboration between the FDA and the industry that it regulates. Eschenbach also proclaimed that the US biomedical industry is "one of the crown jewels of the American economy," and he argued that the FDA must approve products faster while leaving "efficacy to be proven in later trials."[129] Eschenbach's view reflects editor-in-chief of *The Lancet* Dr. Richard Horton's 2004 critique: "Too often, the FDA saw and continues to see the pharmaceutical industry as its customer—a vital source of funding for its activities—and not as a sector of society in need of strong regulation."[130]

The view also exists that expediting times for drug development and review is an answer to the issue of high costs for consumers. In May 2024, then-CBER director Dr. Peter Marks claimed that every time the FDA approved a new gene therapy and the manufacturer announced the price of the treatment, he received a short email from FDA commissioner Dr. Robert Califf.[131] When Orchard Therapeutics announced that its product, Lenmeldy, had a price tag of $4.25 million, Marks received an email from Califf with just the price followed by an exclamation point. While Marks noted that the FDA does not factor cost into its approval decisions, he made a point that regulatory steps raise costs for companies. Thus, he believes the FDA can reduce costs "by shortening the time to development."

In his aforementioned *New York Times* op-ed following the FDA's approval of Aduhelm, Dr. Kesselheim and his coauthor Dr. Jerry Avorn—both medical professors at Harvard University—concluded their piece with a clear admonishing of the FDA's ties to industry.[132] Writing that pressure from drugmakers and their lobbyists have compelled FDA administrators to weaken their standards, they called for the creation of an HTA organization similar to other countries that is entrusted with reviewing drug approvals and making evidence-based analyses of their clinical impact. In their view, this additional oversight is necessitated by "the continuing failure of the F.D.A. to listen to its advisers, stand up to industry and consumer-group pressure and draw clear distinctions between drugs that work and drugs that only cause changes in lab tests of uncertain relevance."

The FDA has not only prioritized industry interests; it has clamped down on internal dissent. *The Washington Post* reported in 2012 that the FDA secretly spied on its own scientists who had expressed concerns about poor review standards for medical devices that put Americans at risk.[133] In 2007, six FDA employees working at the Office of Device Evaluation began making complaints internally about the approval of around a dozen radiological devices that had not proven their effectiveness and that they thought could lead to safety risks. For example, the doctors feared that several colon cancer screening devices used enough radiation to actually risk causing cancer in healthy individuals. However, the FDA had not acted upon their concerns, approving at least some of the devices they raised concerns about. Thus, the employees began reaching out to members of Congress and the press. In January 2009, the FDA started monitoring the communications of these scientists, identifying twenty-one congressional officials, agency employees, outside medical researchers, and journalists as collaborators who were helping to bring negative publicity to the agency.[134] Of the six scientists, four were fired by 2011.

Ultimately, the institution that the public has entrusted to ensure the efficacy and safety of medical treatments is filled with future employees of the industry that it regulates, is directly and indirectly influenced by former officials now working for industry, relies on industry for the funding to conduct its operations, views industry as its collaborative partner, and shares the same priorities of faster and increased levels of approvals. This situation fits the definition of regulatory capture. The FDA not only identifies with and protects the interests of the industry that the public has charged it with regulating—contrary to the public interest of guaranteeing safety and effectiveness—but it actively strives to meet performance goals it negotiates with industry. As director of the Bioethics Program at Penn State University Jonathan H. Marks describes:

> [Industry relationships with policymakers] form webs of influence that undermine the integrity of public health agencies; distort public health research and policy; and lead to the framing of public health problems and their solutions in ways that are least threatening to the commercial interests of powerful industry actors.[135]

8

# Why Do Doctors Accept This?

This book has investigated significant problems among key institutional actors—industry, medical journals, clinical guidelines, and government—that collectively undermine medical knowledge. However, these actors do not actually provide care to patients. Clinicians work one-on-one with patients, determining how to best diagnose and treat them. Patients entrust them with absorbing the relevant medical knowledge and best utilizing it to improve their health. Thus, why do many doctors deal with this system of industry dominance, the inability to vet clinical trial results, and weakening standards of evidence?

The answer is quite simple: doctors are people, not magicians. Their job is to provide the best care possible for their patients, and they rely on designated authorities to tell them how. Throughout their careers, doctors rely on sources of power to not just educate them on what is correct but what sources themselves are trustworthy. Questioning such authorities is not only another job in and of itself, but it leaves the question: if they are not trusted sources, who is? This reality is not limited to doctors, as educated professionals generally rely on institutions for their expertise. As Dr. Abigail Zuger explained in *The New York Times* about the widespread prescribing of opioids, doctors were "mostly ... just well-intentioned schlubs with prescription pads, dutifully following then-current practice guidelines."[1]

Along with education, nearly every phase of doctors' careers is influenced by industry, as the institutions and sources of authority they rely upon are intertwined with commercial interests. Many doctors are personally involved in such entanglements, forging not just conflicts of interest but reliance on skewed information that benefits companies' bottom lines. It is very difficult for an individual doctor to tackle these issues considering their long working hours caring for their patients.

## How Doctors Are Taught

In 1962, the University of Chicago published one of the most cited philosophical books on science of all time: *The Structure of Scientific Revolutions* by Dr. Thomas Kuhn.[2] Kuhn argued against the idea that science progresses through gradual building up of knowledge in a linear process. Rather, there were periods of "normal science" with a certain accepted paradigm in a scientific field, and significant change occurred through revolutions that tore down and created new paradigms and new types of normal science.[3] Thus, science progressed in spurts, where lengthy periods of stasis and limited progress within the consensus viewpoint were followed by dramatic shifts that laid the groundwork for new accepted science. Furthermore, Kuhn wrote:

> Normal science … is predicated on the assumption that the scientific community knows what the world is like. Much of the success of the enterprise derives from the community's willingness to defend that assumption, if necessary at considerable cost. Normal science, for example, often suppresses fundamental novelties because they are necessarily subversive of its basic commitments.[4]

Medical school serves as among the first primary experiences where students are taught what is normal, acceptable science. Scientific education is rigorous and rigid, producing answers that "exert a deep hold on the scientific mind."[5] According to Kuhn, this education perfectly equips scientists to conduct work within what is normal; outside of this, they are often not prepared. Kuhn is just one individual, and his work was published over a half century ago. However, the structure of medical education supports his description.

To become a doctor, prospective students undergo extensive education. Before medical school, undergraduate students usually go to college as part of a four-year premed program. The premed track is not a degree in and of itself, but the majority of medical school applicants get a degree in the biological sciences—such as biochemistry, chemistry, or biology—as part of their premed program.[6] But, other medical school applicants have gotten degrees in specialized health sciences, social sciences, physical sciences, and math and statistics. These four-year degree programs vary, but—like undergraduate degrees generally—they offer basic education in the relevant fields along with laboratory and research work. Ultimately, premed students prepare to take the standardized Medical College Admission Test (MCAT) to prove their proficiency to medical schools. The MCAT tests the level of foundational knowledge in scientific fields such as biochemistry, along with individuals' abilities to read, comprehend, and analyze passages of text.[7]

After applying and getting accepted into medical school based on such standardized testing and relevant research experiences, prospective doctors undergo another four years of rigid education. The first two years of traditional medical school predominantly focus on the mass absorption of scientific knowledge in fields like biochemistry, microbiology, pharmacology, and anatomy.[8] According to Med School Insiders, a private organization that offers tutoring and other services to premed and medical school students, "the sheer volume of material will take some time to adjust to … studying in medical school is often described as drinking out of a fire hydrant."[9] These years lead to the taking of another standardized test: the United States Medical Licensing Examination (USMLE). The USMLE has three parts, the first of which usually follows the second year of medical school and is a multiple-choice test largely on the foundational knowledge of basic sciences.

In the third and fourth years of medical school, students work in clinical settings via clinical rotations/clerkships in various fields, such as internal medicine, family medicine, and pediatrics.[10] Rather than simply absorbing mass amounts of information, success in these years heavily depends on getting good evaluations from attending physicians.[11] Thus, students learn how to provide care by following the direction and example of their superiors. During these two years, often the beginning of the fourth year, students take another standardized exam for the second part of the USMLE. This exam is also multiple-choice and tests foundational clinical knowledge along with applying knowledge to clinical scenarios.

While graduating medical school grants students a degree—traditionally a Doctor of Medicine (MD)—doctors still have several more years of training and additional tests to take before becoming a practicing physician. Toward the end of medical school, individuals apply to residency programs. If accepted (which nearly all medical students are), they go through three to seven years of supervised clinical training depending on the chosen specialty, involving sixty to eighty hours of work per week.[12] Residents follow the supervision and direction of their attending physicians while directly providing care to patients. Throughout the length of their program, supervising doctors evaluate residents, highly influencing the standards of care and information residents use.

Often in their first year, resident physicians take the third and final part of the USMLE, which is a two-day test involving multiple-choice questions and computer-simulated testing of clinical decision-making. Doctors ultimately can only become practicing physicians if they get licensed in the state or territory in which they want to practice. The USMLE testing throughout the medical education process comes from the Federation of State Medical Boards (FSMB) and the National Board of Medical Examiners (NBME), and it is a prerequisite to getting an initial license. Doctors who went to osteopathic school and have a Doctor of Osteopathic Medicine (DO) degree rather than an MD often take their equivalent of these tests called COMLEX-USA.[13]

Following residency, doctors can choose to apply to a fellowship program that provides further specialized training and usually lasts between one and three years.[14] Fellowships allow doctors to train in subspecialties, such as cardiology, endocrinology, geriatrics, and so on.[15] Like residency, fellows receive guidance and follow the direction of attending physicians.

Overall, individuals can take as long as eighteen years to fully complete their medical training through premed, medical school, residency, and a fellowship depending on their field of practice. Throughout many years of rigorous study, doctors' ability to listen to designated authorities determines their success. In *Overdosed America*, Dr. John Abramson describes this dynamic:

> We have been taught in medical school and during our residencies to accept information that modifies our practice only after it has been "blessed" by doctors farther up the chain of command. In training, these authority figures are the residents, fellows, and attending physicians, depending on where you are in the hierarchy. Practicing physicians in turn look to recognized experts, usually with prestigious academic affiliations.[16]

Predominantly, this education does not focus on teaching doctors to be critical of the reigning medical consensus or paradigm. In the words of Kuhn, scientists in the same field "have undergone similar educations and professional initiations; in the process they have absorbed the same technical literature and drawn many of the same lessons from it."[17] Thus, medical education is meticulous and thorough in having doctors absorb and believe in the tenets of accepted, normal science.

However, for all the years of training, relatively little education is spent on teaching doctors to conduct critical appraisals of the evidence. They are taught that peer-reviewed medical journals are the premier source of knowledge, and their education ensures widespread understanding of the terminology and concepts necessary to understand what published articles say. There is little instruction on evaluating the quality and trustworthiness of the evidence itself even if it comes from a mainstream, respected source like *JAMA* or *NEJM*.[18]

Dr. Abramson initially developed the required skills to become an expert in critically evaluating the medical literature through a two-year fellowship from the Robert Wood Johnson Foundation (RWJF) following his residency in family medicine. This fellowship included instruction on "research design, statistics, epidemiology, and health policy," and it was critical for Dr. Abramson's recognition of severe problems in the medical literature, including during the Vioxx crisis.[19] Through reading the August 2001 published results of Merck's VIGOR trial for Vioxx in *NEJM*, he knew that the trial population differed significantly from the likely patient population because the former took more steroids.[20] Scrutinizing the data, he figured out that the article's published conclusion that Vioxx resulted in significantly less gastrointestinal side effects than the comparable treatment (naproxen) was false for the nonsteroid-taking segment of the trial population that better reflected the actual patient population.

However, far more meticulous examination uncovered the significant threat that Vioxx posed and why it killed an estimated 30–60 thousand Americans.[21] While an initial November 2000 *NEJM* article noted that the VIGOR trial assessed the differences in cardiovascular events following treatment with Vioxx and naproxen, it did not report that Vioxx caused more dangerous cardiovascular events.[22] Rather, while noting that Vioxx led to more heart attacks than naproxen, the authors chalked this result up to only the patients who should have been taking aspirin. Eleven of the twelve named authors had financial ties to Merck and other pharmaceutical companies, and two were Merck employees.

In the subsequent August 2001 *NEJM* article, the authors did report that people who took Vioxx had twice as many heart attacks, strokes, and cardiovascular deaths.[23] However, they downplayed that result as possibly reflecting "the play of chance" because there were only seventy cardiovascular events even though the difference was statistically significant. Yet, they did not posit that the misleadingly claimed gastrointestinal benefit was due to chance when there were only fifty-three of such serious complications. Abramson's training helped him understand not just the hypocrisy of the article's authors, but that the dismissal of a statistically significant result revealed significant bias and ultimately "made no sense."[24] Both authors had received grant funding and served as consultants for Merck along with other drug companies.[25]

Through finding publicly available FDA review documents and searching through their contents, Dr. Abramson found that Vioxx not only caused significantly more serious cardiovascular complications, but that the twenty-seven excess cardiovascular events were more than the twenty-one fewer gastrointestinal complications.[26] These numbers were not only not reported in either *NEJM* article, but the published results omitted three heart attacks reported to the FDA. If the heart attacks had been correctly reported in the November 2000 *NEJM* article, the results would have shown that Vioxx caused a statistically significant increase in heart attacks alone compared to naproxen regardless of recommended aspirin usage.[27] For all cardiovascular events, the risk more than doubled for those taking Vioxx.

Additionally, the FDA documents revealed that Vioxx caused 21 percent more serious adverse events generally leading to hospitalization or death compared to naproxen.[28] For every 200 people treated with Vioxx, there were five more hospitalizations or deaths each year. Neither *NEJM* article reported this. In fact, the *NEJM* editors admitted in 2005 that they did not have access to the relevant data.[29] For patients with a history of cardiovascular disease specifically, seven to eleven more people would experience serious cardiovascular events for every 100 treated with Vioxx.[30] One FDA reviewer had stated that naproxen was likely the preferred treatment compared to Vioxx.

Dr. Abramson was among few medical professionals like Dr. Jennifer Hrachovec who critically analyzed the *NEJM* articles, examined the FDA review documents, and called out the danger of Vioxx.[31] His efforts resulted from significant initiative and adequate training. In contrast, the vast majority of doctors not only did not know about the issues with Vioxx until it was too late, but they had not been trained to. Not only do not all doctors pursue fellowships, but all fellowships do not specifically train doctors to appraise evidence like the RWJF program Dr. Abramson took part in. By the end of 2001, Vioxx was among the top ten selling drugs in the United States, constituting over a quarter of total US spending on prescription arthritis medication and bringing in over $2 billion.[32] Between the FDA's approval of Vioxx in May 1999 and Merck's withdrawal in September 2004, almost 107 million prescriptions of the drug were dispensed in the United States.[33]

While the Vioxx case study may be extreme due to its death toll, it undercounts the problems facing doctors. Dr. Abramson was able to find crucial information not included in the published *NEJM* articles because they happened to be included in publicly available FDA review documents. However, while the FDA has access to the underlying clinical trial data, it does not publicly release all of it. Thus, Abramson was fortunate that the relevant data was revealed at all. For the preponderance of industry-sponsored trials where the companies keep the underlying data hidden from journals and the public, most doctors are not just ill-equipped to critically appraise the evidence before them, but they wouldn't be able to examine the real, full data if they were.

Even if doctors were widely trained to scrutinize published trial results, they are taught to trust designated sources of authority. According to the University of California San Francisco (UCSF)—a widely acclaimed medical school ranked among the top schools in the nation by US News & World Report—information provided by medical institutions and government health agencies are the most credible.[34] As

Chapter 3 discusses, medical professionals revere peer-reviewed journals as the gold standard of medical knowledge, and the EBM movement further pushed clinicians to rely on peer-reviewed articles and clinical guidelines for their decision-making. Clinicians currently receive alerts from information services for when new information is published in the medical literature, and there are specific filters that prioritize clinical guidelines and systematic reviews.[35]

Additionally, regulatory capture at the FDA can make relying on the agency untenable. The estimate of 30–60 thousand deaths from Vioxx comes from research done by Dr. David Graham, who served as associate director for science and medicine in the FDA's Office of Drug Safety.[36] His supervisor and acting director of the Center for Drug Evaluation and Research (CDER) Dr. Steven Galson personally contacted *The Lancet* editor-in-chief Richard Horton to block publication of Graham's research, delaying the release until a week before Merck pulled Vioxx from the market.[37] After leaving the FDA, Galson worked for pharmaceutical company Amgen for over a decade, self-describing his work as representing "Amgen to the FDA and other regulatory bodies on matters involving development, manufacturing, testing and distribution of investigational and marketed products."[38] He sits on the board of BioCryst Pharmaceuticals.

Following Vioxx's withdrawal, FDA management attempted to discredit Graham, who testified before Congress.[39] Prior to the Government Accountability Project legally supporting Graham, an agency management official filed an anonymous complaint to the group accusing Graham of bullying.[40] Congressionally obtained emails also revealed that deputy director of the Office of Drug Safety Dr. Anne Trontell (1) asserted that the FDA agreed to inform Merck prior to any agency publication about their drug products and (2) criticized Graham's research, arguing Merck "needs to know before it becomes public so they can be prepared for extensive media attention that this will likely provoke."[41]

In light of publicly reported debacles involving severe errors by journals, guidelines, and government institutions—such as Vioxx, Tamiflu, and OxyContin—doctors still rely upon these sources of authority. In March 2023, the de Beaumont Foundation published a national survey of 806 physicians.[42] The poll asked about trusted sources, and 89 percent of physicians reported using medical or scientific journals somewhat or very often. Eighty-one percent reported relying on their colleagues and 60 percent used medical conferences as sources. In 2021, the *International Journal of Medicine* published survey results from 404 physicians at the University of Florida Gainesville.[43] Among these respondents, 68.8 percent reported adhering to clinical guidelines highly or very highly. Over 85 percent of physicians deemed current guidelines to be evidence-based.

During the COVID-19 pandemic, many physicians rallied around the government health agencies. The American Medical Association (AMA)—the professional lobbying group on behalf of physicians, residents, and medical students—put out a strongly worded piece in September 2020 entitled "Words and Actions That Erode Trust in the CDC Hurt Us All."[44] The statement derided any risk to "the credibility of institutions such as the Centers for Disease Control and Prevention (CDC) or the Department of Health and Human Services for partisan political purposes."

In 2021, the National Opinion Research Center (NORC) at the University of Chicago and the American Board of Internal Medicine (ABIM) Foundation surveyed 600 US physicians, finding that 78 percent somewhat or completely trusted government health agencies like the CDC or FDA compared to just 14 percent who slightly or completely distrusted them.[45] Physician trust in government far surpassed trust in other institutions including the health care system as a whole (63 percent), hospitals and health systems (61 percent), health care leaders and executives (54 percent), pharmaceutical companies (47 percent), and health insurance companies (20 percent). These figures may understate physician's relative trust in government, as not more than 8 percent of physicians reported completely trusting the other entities, while 23 percent had complete trust in public health agencies. Additionally, trust in government may have been previously higher. A plurality (43 percent) of physicians reported that the pandemic decreased their trust in health agencies while only 21 percent reported increased trust: a 22 percent net decrease.

These results do not prove that doctors have not recognized individual cases of poor government behavior. In light of the Aduhelm situation, the private firm Spherix Global Insights surveyed 252 specialists in dermatology, gastroenterology, nephrology, neurology, and rheumatology in July 2021.[46] Only 36 percent of respondents reported a high level of assurance in the FDA with almost 50 percent saying that their confidence eroded over the past year. These negative findings were most due to perceived bias/politicization, the speed of FDA reviews, and lack of transparency with the medical community. According to one respondent:

> The erosion [of my confidence] is based on the disastrously bad decision to approve aducanumab [Aduhelm], which seems like a poorly developed and even possibly corrupt decision. I cannot remember a similar situation in which there was so much dismay and disbelief created by an FDA decision. We do not plan to use aducanumab at this time and we no longer know what to think about and how much to trust any future FDA decisions.

However, the Aduhelm example is unique in that it received significant public coverage. The House Committees on Oversight & Reform and Energy & Commerce conducted an eighteen-month investigation culminating in a report that lambasted the agency's decision-making and close collaboration with industry.[47] Yet, as Chapters 5, 6, and 7 discuss, such a fusion between regulators and the companies they oversee is not just widespread but actively encouraged. Thus, how would doctors respond if there were many more reports like the House committees' on Aduhelm?

## Industry Influence

On top of the weaknesses of medical education's general structure, industry has significantly intertwined itself early in doctors' education and directly influenced medical students. A 2011 *PLOS Medicine* systematic review examined thirty-two peer-reviewed research articles published on and before May 2010, including twenty-five articles published in the 2000s.[48] These studies encompassed 9,850 medical students attending seventy-six medical schools or hospitals. Between 89 percent and 98 percent of medical students during the clinical years of their education reported having accepted food from the pharmaceutical industry. As many as 90 percent of surveyed students reported getting textbooks, journal reprints, or other educational materials from industry. While the studies were not isolated to the United States, the United States had the most industry exposure. Greater exposure to industry was associated with more positive attitudes about pharmaceutical marketing.

One of the studies, a 2005 *JAMA* article, reported 826 responses to a 2003 survey of third-year students at eight US medical schools.[49] It found that 93.2 percent were asked or required by a physician to attend an industry-sponsored lunch and 80.3 percent thought they were entitled to gifts. Among the minority of students who thought accepting a gift from industry worth less than $50 was inappropriate, 86.3 percent reported having accepted such a gift. On average, students interacted with industry at least once per week.

Research shows that even relatively small industry payments and gifts can affect doctors' behavior. A 2016 *JAMA* investigation examined industry payments to and the prescribing patterns of 279,669 physicians in 2013 relating to four classes of drugs: (1) statins, (2) beta blockers, (3) angiotensin-converting-enzyme (ACE) inhibitors and angiotensin-receptor blockers (ARBs), and (4) selective serotonin and serotonin-norepinephrine reuptake inhibitors (SSRIs and SNRIs).[50] They found that doctors who received a single industry-sponsored meal with an average value under $20 were significantly more likely to prescribe the brand-name products promoted by the meal sponsors compared to competitors. More expensive meals produced an even higher likelihood of prescribing a sponsoring company's drug.

Similarly, a 2019 *JAMA Internal Medicine* letter analyzed CMS prescribing data from 2014 to 2016 alongside industry payments reported via the Open Payments Program.[51] The manufacturers of three brand-name gabapentinoids made nearly 510,000 payments to physicians totaling almost $11.5 million, meaning the average payment was around $22.46. Doctors receiving such payments were almost twice as likely to prescribe the three brand-name drugs compared to generic alternatives.

Gifts need not serve as blatantly direct quid pro quo (this for that) bribes; rather, they are mechanisms to make physicians feel more favorable to industry. In 2008 testimony to the Senate Aging Committee, former Eli Lilly sales representative Shahram Ahari explained that the purpose of "these gifts is to draw attention to the pharmaceutical products and to serve as reminders of the company's generosity. These reminders generate a conscious or subconscious desire to return the 'favor.'"[52]

A 2020 *Annals of Internal Medicine* systematic review included thirty-six studies on the influence of financial payments from industry to physicians, of which thirty-five were from 2016 to 2020.[53] Thirty studies (83.3 percent) identified that industry money was associated with higher levels of physician prescribing while six (16.7 percent) had a combination of similar and null findings. Eighty-nine (88.1 percent) out of 101 total individual analyses found a positive association between industry payments and prescriptions of the paying company's drug, higher prescription costs, and more prescriptions of branded drugs.

One of the studies, a 2019 *JAMA* study, employed a unique design that examined how pharmaceutical company payments to physicians in 2,208 US counties from August 2013 to December 2015 were associated with opioid prescribing and overdose mortality.[54] Adjusting for potential confounding factors, counties with higher numbers of payments to physicians and larger numbers of physicians receiving such payments had significantly more opioid prescriptions and overdose deaths.

Given the corrupting influence of industry money, the American Medical Students Association (AMSA) established its national PharmFree campaign in 2002 to educate students on the pharmaceutical industry's impact on medical training.[55] Its website stated, "we must advocate for better professionalism training and in particular resist the penetration of medical education by the pharmaceutical industry."[56] The campaign presented questions to students such as "does that one slice of pizza matter?" where the organization noted how providing food "influence[s] physician prescribing patterns in ways that do not optimize patient care."[57] This campaign involved a PharmFree pledge, where medical students would promise not to accept money, gifts, or hospitality from the industry, agree to pursue unbiased information not coming from drug companies, and avoid COIs in their medical education and practice.[58] In December 2004, the AMSA marched on Pfizer headquarters in New York City, where students demonstrated in front of the building and returned paraphernalia they had received from drug representatives, including more than 500 pens.[59]

In 2007, the AMSA began producing scorecards for medical schools to assess their COI policies.[60] Assigning schools letter grades, the initiative drew national attention. In March 2009, *The New York Times* highlighted Harvard Medical School, which had received an F, as it had no effective COI policy for all scorecard measures like gifts/meals, consulting relationships, and school curriculum.[61] In 2008, pharmaceutical companies gave the university $11.6 million for basic research and continuing education classes, although the school said it could not track the total amount of industry support it had received. Additionally, Merck had built a corporate research center directly across from Harvard's own research and class building in 2004.

The day after the *Times* story was published—which mentioned a Pfizer employee taking cellphone photos of Harvard students protesting against drug company influence—Senator Chuck Grassley (R-IA) sent Pfizer a letter raising "concerns that Pfizer is attempting to intimidate young scholars."[62] He requested a detailed account of Pfizer payments and/or benefits given to all Harvard doctors, including the 149 faculty members the *Times* reported having received payments from Pfizer.

Following the AMSA's success in bringing public scrutiny to industry's influence on medical education, many schools began adopting stricter COI policies. In June 2008, the Association of American Medical Colleges (AAMC) published a report on industry funding of medical education.[63] The report recommended institutions adopt stricter regulations, such as banning industry-provided food in academic medical centers, prohibiting travel funds from industry (not including "legitimate reimbursement or contractual services"), and discouraging faculty participation in industry-sponsored programs. In 2008, only

4.7 percent of medical schools received an A grade from the AMSA, increasing to a quarter (25.9 percent) by 2013.[64] Nearly three quarters of schools had As and Bs in 2013.[65]

The AMSA revised its methodology in 2014 to be more rigorous and strict. In 2016, *BMC Medical Education* analyzed the effect of the new policy on school scores in 2014.[66] The researchers found that fewer schools scored As (16.1 percent) and Bs (50.6 percent), but the significant majority still had these higher grades. Importantly, more COI policies did not mean that actual industry influence in medical schools went away.

While levels of providing direct gifts like pens and meals decreased, they were still significant following reforms. In 2013, a *Journal of General Internal Medicine* national survey received responses from 1,610 first-year and fourth-year medical students along with 739 third-year residents.[67] A third (33.0 percent) of first-year medical students reported receiving a gift from the pharmaceutical industry, and this significantly increased to a majority for fourth-year students (56.8 percent) and third-year residents (54.0 percent). Similarly, while only 17.2 percent and 16.7 percent of first-year students spoke with a pharmaceutical representative or attended a company-sponsored lecture, respectively, these percentages rose to 44.4 percent and 40.0 percent by the fourth year of medical school and remained similar for residents (49.1 percent and 35.9 percent). Thus, as these students entered clinical care settings, their interactions with industry substantially rose. Importantly, the researchers also found that the strength of a medical institution's COI policies as measured by the AMSA was not associated with lower probabilities of medical students reporting accepting industry gifts even though students at such institutions perceived greater faculty-industry separation.

Many students and residents also reported favorable attitudes toward industry involvements. Significant majorities of first-year students (64.1 percent), fourth-year students (67.5 percent), and residents (79.8 percent) agreed that physicians got "useful education about new treatments" from drug representatives. At the same time, all groups recognized that such physicians may become biased toward the company's product (78.9–86.4 percent). Yet, around two-thirds of respondents did not believe that receiving gifts or food from industry would affect their own prescribing behavior, and 30.1–45.5 percent viewed company materials as useful ways to learn about new drugs.

The study's corresponding author, Dr. Aaron Kesselheim, highlighted how putting "the policy on the books is one thing … [ensuring] that it's implemented and isn't being skirted around" is another.[68] Indeed, a 2010 ProPublic investigation found that while Stanford University barred its physicians from giving paid promotional talks for industry, over a dozen of its doctors violated the policy with two earning six figures in 2009.[69] Fourth-year medical student and coauthor of the 2013 study Kirsten Austad urged medical schools to invest in educating students on "how to interpret clinical trials and ways to approach evidence-based prescribing so trainees can learn to critically evaluate industry promotion."[70]

Moreover, prospective doctors have still reported significant industry exposures before even entering medical school. In 2019, the journal *Family Medicine* published 2017 survey results of 911 students who had accepted admission but not yet matriculated into fourteen US medical schools.[71] Most students (70.9 percent) reported having received or observed someone else receiving marketing gifts, food, articles, or samples from the pharmaceutical industry. Additionally, the most frequent environment where students reported encountering direct pharmaceutical marketing was when shadowing doctors and during previous employment (53.6 percent and 50.0 percent, respectively).

Severely limited research has suggested that industry influence through direct payments may not be as widespread with resident physicians in training. An October 2023 *JAMA* article examined 65,376 residents in the three largest primary-care specialties and three largest surgical disciplines.[72] From 2020 to 2021, 13.4 percent had accepted payments from industry, as reported in the Open Payments database, totaling nearly $4.0 million with a median payment of $64.40. In comparison, 39.6 percent of residency program directors received industry money, totaling over $5.2 million. Among all 124,715 residents in training programs during 2020–21, around 11.9 percent took industry payments, totaling $6.4 million with a median payment of $119.55. However, a significant caveat to these reported figures is that federal regulations do not require the reporting of industry payments to residents; thus, these numbers are almost certainly an underestimation.

Indeed, a 2022 *JAMA* article investigated industry payments made between 2015 and 2021 to 45,745 newly independent physicians from residency or fellowship programs within three specialties: orthopedic surgery, neurosurgery, and internal medicine.[73] The OPP showed that 77.2 percent of these physicians received general industry payments, including three quarters of those in internal medicine and around 98 percent for both the other specialties. Per year, physicians got $229.43 on average, but this varied by specialty as orthopedic surgeons got $1,183.95 compared to just $187.92 for those in internal medicine. Among those who got industry money, most received it by one year since becoming an independent physician. By two years, 94.7 percent, 91.8 percent, and 58.8 percent of orthopedic surgery, neurosurgery, and internal medicine physicians got industry money, respectively.

Additionally, the OPP requires disclosure of industry payments to fellows, and a 2021 *Journal of General Internal Medicine* study examined OPP data from July 2016 to July 2018 on general payments to all fellows who matriculated in the 2016 academic year.[74] The study found that 54.2 percent of fellows received industry payments within their first two years, totaling over $1 million. Payments were especially prevalent in cardiology (75.1 percent) and gastroenterology (74.0 percent) and less likely for infectious diseases (27.4 percent). The vast majority (86.6 percent) of program directors received industry payments from 2013 to 2018, totaling over $14.4 million. The median payment per fellow and program director was $136.33 and $1,989.66, respectively.

Even though industry influence on medical students remained prevalent, the AMSA discontinued its grading of medical schools following the 2016 scorecard.[75] The organization chose to transition to focusing on developing a scorecard for Congress because of "the changing landscape of conflicts of interest ... [like] the overreaching pharmaceutical influence in important sectors such as health policy." Now, people can only access the AMSA's scorecards through the Internet Archive's Wayback Machine.

Years later in June 2024, the AMSA announced that it would start taking industry funding.[76] The organization amended its policy of not accepting any industry cash to allow up to 25 percent of their operating budget to come from the pharmaceutical, medical device, and health insurance industries.[77] The AMSA removed its ban on direct industry advertising and explicitly endorsed accepting journal advertising and exhibit hall fees from industry as long as they advance AMSA priorities. Additionally, these amended rules allow funding from industry-backed nonprofit organizations.

Further highlighting the limited success of the AMSA's short-lived scorecards, medical schools still rely on significant funding from pharmaceutical companies. The June 2008 AAMC report found that "medical schools and teaching hospitals have become increasingly dependent on industry support of their core educational missions" over the last several decades.[78] After this report and the introduction of the AMSA scorecards, Stanford University accepted a $3 million grant from Pfizer in 2010 to finance a new continuing education curriculum for its physicians and other health care professionals.[79] However, this deal pales in comparison to the Yale School of Medicine's $100 million research contract covering the decade from 2011 to 2021 with the biopharmaceutical company Gilead Sciences.[80] According to the chair of Yale's pharmacology department, Dr. Joseph Schlessinger, "Yale and Gilead have established strong links, productive collaboration, and common goals, and function as a harmonious couple."

In April 2024, Harvard's student newspaper, *The Harvard Crimson*, highlighted the medical school's "Deal with the Devil."[81] In 2021, the university signed a five-year $30 million research deal with drugmaker National Resilience, and the medical school dean, Dr. George Daley, said that they were trying to diversify their funding sources.[82] Correspondingly, Harvard Medical School reported increases in revenue and sponsored research from commercial sources in FY 2022.[83] In 2024, Daley said that because NIH funding did not sufficiently increase with inflation, Harvard was more motivated to get funding from private sources like biopharma, which had become increasingly interested in working with institutions like Harvard Medical School.[84] The school's executive director of therapeutics translation, Mark Namchuk, celebrated industry funding and collaboration, as many students' careers would be in industry. Thus, greater exposure would boost their careers.

Jonathan Kagan, a professor of pediatrics at Harvard, warned that it is "one of those classic 'you signed a deal with the devil' mindsets, where you could say you're getting a lot of money, but it comes with this massive string attached." Several professors explained that such strings include companies' not wanting academics to publish research findings and industry directing researchers away from desired scientific pursuits that are not deemed profitable. Overall, Harvard Medical School's ready acceptance of industry funding generally is not unique. According to the UCSF website, the university maintains "unique and close relationships with many large pharmaceutical and biotech companies that are excited to fund early research at UCSF within their strategic areas of interest."[85] Johns Hopkins lists nineteen pharmaceutical company funders of its drug discovery program, including Pfizer, Bayer, and J&J's subsidiary Janssen Research & Development.[86]

## Continued Education

While doctors go through many years of rigorous study to become independently licensed physicians, their education never actually stops while they are licensed. Most states require physicians to go through continuing medical education (CME) to maintain their state licenses.[87] There are some exceptions like Indiana which does not require a particular number of CME credit hours for license renewal.[88] To meet CME requirements, physicians must obtain credits from educational activities including but not limited to lectures, seminars, conferences, and coursework.[89] Additionally, credit-eligible activities are certified or sponsored by providers accredited by the Accreditation Council for Continuing Medical Education (ACCME) or a medical society recognized by the ACCME.

In 2007, the US Senate Finance Committee bipartisanly released a report on pharmaceutical industry involvement in CME.[90] The report revealed that ACCME records showed several cases from 2004 to 2007 where drug companies "had too much influence over the content of supposedly independent educational programs."[91] These companies used educational grants to "increase the market for their products."[92] In 2004, the twenty-three pharmaceutical companies surveyed in the report had budgets for educational grants ranging from under $2 million to $117 million, which predominantly went to fund accredited educational programs. Total CME-supporting expenditures exceeded $1 billion. The report concluded:

> Continuing medical education has developed into a multi-billion dollar a year industry, much of which is funded by pharmaceutical manufacturers. It seems unlikely that this sophisticated industry would spend such large sums on an enterprise but for the expectation that the expenditures will be recouped by increased sales.[93]

In 2010, the University of Michigan became the first major medical school to announce that it would stop accepting any industry funding for its medical education programs.[94] The head of the university medical school's Clinical and Educational Conflict of Interest Committee, Dr. Paul Lichter, reasoned, "industry does not give money without a profit purpose."[95] Thus, the only rational explanation for industry funding of educational courses is "that they will be able to tell their shareholders that the money was given to support and increase profit."

While industry support to ACCME-accredited providers has lessened over the years, it is still significant. In 2006, almost $1.2 billion (50.3 percent) of their income came from commercial funding.[96] This figure may undercount industry support, as providers also got significant funding—$244.9 million (10.3 percent)—from advertising and exhibits that industry uses to educate medical professionals.[97] Comparatively in 2023, commercial interests provided $858.0 million (24.3 percent) of ACCME-accredited providers' income.[98] An additional $668.3 million (18.9 percent) came from advertisement and exhibit income. Most advertising money (64.8 percent) came from nonprofit physician membership organizations, which are often greatly funded by industry.[99] From 2015 to 2023, CME providers got over $7.0 billion (27.5 percent) of their income in commercial funding.[100]

Moreover, industry-funded CME often results in educational material favorable to the sponsors' medical products.[101] According to the 2009 IOM report on COIs in medicine, recipients of industry funding "may have an implicit understanding that additional industry funds will not be offered in the future if the course does not present topics of interest to the company and use speakers who are favorable to the company's products."[102] In a brazen reflection of such bias, Concepts in Professional Education and Communications—a company that helped drug companies with marketing and education—wrote on its website in 2000:

> Medical education is a powerful tool that can deliver your message to key audiences, and get those audiences to take action that benefits your product ... Whatever combination of [health care professional or consumer] audiences you need to motivate in order to exert maximum leverage on the marketplace, we can help you identify them, reach them, and influence their behavior.[103]

The company, now CPE Communications, currently adopts a less blatant messaging strategy, describing its leadership as a "diverse and seasoned group of pharmaceutical industry professionals."[104] It works to keep "clinician behavior and patient outcomes at the heart of all we do."[105]

Contemporary, widespread research on the extent of bias is lacking; however, individual case studies demonstrate the findings of the Senate Finance Committee report and the IOM. A 2015 *Journal of Medical Ethics* study examined fourteen industry-funded, online, and free CME courses on hypoactive sexual desire disorder (HSDD) in women before the FDA approved the drug flibanserin in 2015, which it had rejected twice before.[106] Persistent themes were that HSDD was underdiagnosed, clinicians can screen for HSDD—with tools made by companies backing drugs to treat HSDD—and there was an unfortunate lack of treatment options for HSDD. A 2020 *Journal of the American Board of Family Medicine* article examined twenty-seven CME activities on binge-eating disorder (BED) in 2015.[107] All these CME activities were sponsored by Shire: the drug manufacturer that received the first FDA approval in 2015 for a treatment, lisdexamfetamine, targeting BED. Common themes across the various CME programs were the prevalence and severity of BED along with the message that lisdexamfetamine was a highly effective treatment while other treatment options were inferior.

Another documented tactic for industry to influence the information doctors encounter is developing financial relationships with key opinion leaders (KOLs) in specific medical disciplines who often give presentations at CME events.[108] Various consulting companies exist where the service they provide to medical manufacturers is identifying KOLs.[109] For example, the consulting company H1 says on its website that its Medical Science Liaisons (MSLs) "act as the point of contact between the pharmaceutical company developing a new drug or therapy and the healthcare professional (HCP), or key opinion leader (KOL) treating patients and influencing the world of science and research."[110] The company even offers artificial intelligence–powered KOL mapping and engagement platforms.

Many KOLs are thoroughly paid by industry. A 2020 *BMJ* article identified the top ten deadliest disease areas in the United States from 2015 AHRQ data, 328 leaders of ten professional medical associations relevant to these areas, and industry payments to those individuals from 2017 to 2019 recorded in the OPP.[111] Two hundred and thirty-five leaders (71.6 percent) had financial ties to industry, totaling nearly $130 million. For eight of the ten associations, over 80 percent of their US-based medical leaders had financial ties. Payment amounts varied, as the median payment to leaders of the American Psychiatric Association was $212, while it was $518,000 for leaders of the American Society of Clinical Oncology. The overall median amount was $31,000.

A 2022 *JCO Oncology Practice* article examined oncologists who received the highest industry payments—over $100,000—in 2018 according to the OPP.[112] Overall, 139 medical oncologists received over $100,000, representing just 1.3 percent of all US oncologists but 36.8 percent of industry payments. These individuals disproportionately represented key leadership positions, as 71.9 percent held faculty appointments, 60.4 percent served in hospital leadership, 23.7 percent served on journal editorial boards, 20.9 percent led specialty associations, and 10.1 percent were clinical guideline authors.

Companies employ KOLs to increase the credibility of information that promotes the need for, efficacy, and safety of their products.[113] A 2008 *BMJ* article entitled "Key Opinion Leaders: Independent Experts or Drug Representatives in Disguise?" investigated this dynamic and interviewed a former drug sales representative, Kimberly Elliott.[114] She worked for eighteen years for large companies like GSK and Novartis, where her job was to cultivate relationships with local and national opinion or thought leaders. According to Elliott, KOLs "were salespeople for us, and we would routinely measure the return on our investment, by tracking prescriptions before and after their presentations … If that speaker didn't make the impact the company was looking for, then you wouldn't invite them back." Thus, she would pay these doctors who were respected by other physicians $2,500 per lecture and provide them company-supplied presentation slides.

Elliott's descriptions are not unique, as others who have worked in the industry have made similar statements. The medical director for the Association of the British Pharmaceutical Industry revealed, "companies will employ consultants to help advise on marketing strategies … and present and speak at conferences." In a November 2019 *Washington Post* piece, former Eli Lilly sales representative Shahram Ahari divulged that he recruited speakers among his "high-volume prescribers" who had Ivy League educations, demonstrated they could speak well in their local lectures, and spoke favorable of Eli Lilly products.[115] Company-backed speakers could make hundreds of thousands of dollars a year, and the company benefited from producing a supposed "established scientific consensus" that was "key to establishing a drug's legitimacy." Regarding the promotion of OxyContin, Purdue Pharma hired 3,000 doctors to serve on its speakers bureau to do the same thing.[116]

On November 16, 2020, the HHS OIG sent out a "Special Fraud Alert" about industry speaker programs where companies pay physicians and other medical professionals to speak or make a presentation to their colleagues about their products.[117] The alert documented that the OIG and DOJ had found multiple cases of fraud where drug and device companies rewarded doctors who highly prescribed their products with "lucrative speaker deals" and even conditioned payments on sales targets. For example, the DOJ got Novartis to pay a $678 million settlement for illegal conduct like hosting "tens of thousands of speaker programs and related events under the guise of providing educational content, when in fact the events served as nothing more than a means to provide bribes to doctors."[118] Relatedly, the alert called out how speaker programs often took place at entertainment venues and recreational events like expensive restaurants, "wineries, sports stadiums, fishing trips, golf clubs, and adult entertainment facilities."[119] The central reason HHS warned about illegal behavior was due to the explicit kickbacks identified in its investigation. However, generally giving large payments and luxury accommodations are not inherently illegal and are a known industry practice.

Industry not only rewards scientists, it targets its critics. In October 2001, senior Merck employees discussed scientists calling out the cardiovascular risks of Vioxx, with one writing, "we may need to seek them out and destroy them where they live."[120] The company maintained a list of doctors to neutralize and discredit.[121] Merck seemingly neutralized individuals through payments to purchase favor; when unsuccessful, the company moved to discredit them.[122]

### Direct Contact

Drug representatives' direct lobbying of doctors is another major industry influence strategy. Sales representatives engage in a practice called detailing, where they present brochures, journal article reprints, and other educational material to convince doctors to prescribe their products.[123] These efforts are not restricted to doctors, as they also affect pharmacists and other health care providers.[124]

Sales representatives' jobs are to selectively present information favorable to their employer. Indeed, their income depends on earning commissions through building relationships with medical professionals and increasing prescriptions and sales.[125] Additionally, representatives can earn more money through performance-based raises from exceeding sales targets.[126] According to Ahari, his experience selling the drugs Prozac and Zyprexa revealed "how easy it is to cherry-pick studies and present them as straightforward, neutral information."[127] Testifying under oath before the Senate Committee on Aging, Ahari described the intent of sales representatives: "To provide a skewed perspective; one where our product is presented in the best possible light" while disparaging competing products and persuading doctors to use their company's product "when a non-medication therapy would be a better alternative."[128]

From 1996 to 2001, the number of pharmaceutical sales representatives doubled to around 90,000 people.[129] In 2001, the KFF ran a national survey of 2,608 physicians, finding that nearly three quarters found information from drug industry representatives about diseases or treatments to be very or somewhat useful.[130] More than four in five physicians described information from these salespeople to be very or somewhat accurate. Over the past quarter century, the number of pharmaceutical representatives has only increased, with there being over 156,000 in 2021.[131] In 2016, pharmaceutical companies spent $5.6 billion on prescriber detailing, meaning sales visits to providers.[132] A 2020 *JAMA Internal Medicine* study found that among 2,333 outpatient physicians' practices from a national survey, around half (49.7 percent) experienced weekly detailing from the pharmaceutical industry between June 2017 and August 2018.[133]

In recent years, industry has complained about declining willingness of doctors to see sales representatives, but this has been largely due to physicians' time constraints. In 2019, the consulting company Decision Resources Group published a report finding that among 1,285 surveyed physicians, only 54 percent met with a drug representative within the last six months compared to 67 percent the previous year.[134] However, the market struggles of sales representatives do not reflect diminishing industry impact, as 46 percent of physicians viewed pharmaceutical websites as credible sources of information, up from 27 percent in 2017. Additionally, a May 2020 survey found that 61 percent of physicians reported interacting more with drug representatives during the COVID-19 pandemic compared to beforehand.[135] Since the pandemic, physician-sales representative interactions have shifted toward virtual calls; yet, 66 percent of surveyed physicians in 2021 reported that in-person visits from drug representatives had impacted their clinical decision-making.[136]

These figures do not count medical device sales representatives whom the industry uses for the same reason as pharmaceutical companies: to sell their products.[137] Although device representatives may be even more involved than their drug counterparts, as they are often in the room when doctors use their products. In 2016, *PLOS One* published a qualitative study where researchers held two focus groups with a total of fourteen surgeons at two academic medical centers.[138] They found that surgeons frequently relied upon device representatives to help guide them in using their products. One orthopedic surgeon stated, "nowadays, a [device] rep is in the OR [operating room] for every case that you're using his or her stuff." These findings were not unique. In a separate survey of ninety neurosurgeons, 100 percent stated that they worked with device sales representatives in the operating room.[139] Additionally, 92.1 percent revealed that the majority of the education they received about using the new equipment came from the sales representatives. Ultimately, cultivating relationships with doctors is very lucrative for device representatives, as they can earn a commission between 10 percent and 50 percent for any used equipment.

Sales representatives and their industry employers also directly influence doctors through providing gifts and payments. In the 2002 KFF survey, 92 percent of physicians reported having ever accepted free drug samples from sales representatives along with 61 percent having received meals, tickets to entertainment events, or free travel.[140] According to a 2003–04 national survey of 1,662 physicians published in *NEJM*, 93.5 percent of physicians reported some time of relationship with the pharmaceutical industry.[141] The most frequent types of relationships were receiving food and drinks (83.4 percent) in the workplace and drug samples (75.5 percent). In the two decades since, such industry initiatives are not lacking. In 2016, the pharmaceutical industry spent $13.5 billion on free drug samples to physicians along with $979 million on direct physician payments relating to specific drugs, such as speaking fees and meals.[142]

In 2023, the OPP reported that drug, device, biological, and medical supply manufacturers spent $12.69 billion in payments and ownership/investment interests to physicians, nonphysician practitioners, and teaching hospitals.[143] There were over 15.6 million payment records, meaning that the average payment was roughly $811.38. Overall, over 630 thousand physicians received such payments, meaning around 62.4 percent of all active physicians got industry money.[144] Physicians received more in general payments like meals and consulting fees ($2.3 billion) compared to research payments ($71.1 million). The average general payment to physicians was $3,617.37, albeit the median was likely noticeably lower due to a minority of very-high-paid doctors.

These figures are not unique to 2021, as physicians received over $12.1 billion in direct payments from 2013 to 2022, including consulting services, speaker fees, food and beverages, travel and lodging, education, grants, gifts, entertainment, honoraria, and charitable contributions.[145] A majority (57.1 percent) of eligible physicians received a payment; the median value was $48. Yet, this amount varied greatly among specialties, with the highest median payment of $2,339 for gastrointestinal surgery. Almost all payments were associated (93.8 percent) with at least one marketed medical product.

As this chapter describes earlier, payments both small and large can affect doctors' decision-making. A 2020 *JAMA* study found that among 4,435 physicians who implanted cardioverter-defibrillators (ICDs) or cardiac resynchronization therapy-defibrillators (CRT-Ds) to 145,900 patients from 2016 to 2018, 93.6 percent were paid either before or after by at least one of four device manufacturers.[146] Payments ranged from $2 to $323,559 with a median of $1,211. Physicians were between two and seventeen times more likely to implant patients with the device from the manufacturer that they received the most money from, depending on the manufacturer, while patients with higher-paid doctors were more likely to receive a device from the paying manufacturer.

## The Odds Are Not in Doctor's Favor

From the outset, many doctors are not properly equipped to challenge the current regime of industry control of medical research, lack of transparency and effective peer review, and the overall weakening standards of evidence—all of which question the reliability of medical knowledge. Years of rigorous medical education focus on absorbing large amounts of information along with listening to and following the lead of superiors. However, there is not significant focus on learning how to become critical appraisers of the evidence and the authorities that doctors rely upon like medical journals and clinical guidelines. Even if doctors were thoroughly educated on appraising the evidence, they are taught that sources like journals, guidelines, and public health agencies are very trustworthy and legitimate.

At the same time, the medical industry—predominantly pharmaceutical companies—entangles itself in almost every stage of doctors' education and careers.

Before even entering medical school, premed students are exposed to gifts, food, samples, and educational material from drug companies. When in medical school, students similarly receive gifts, attend events, and get at least part of their education from industry. The medical schools themselves have embraced industry through signing deals worth millions of dollars for research. Many residents, fellows, and newly independent physicians receive direct payments from medical product companies.

Following years of education necessary to become a licensed physician, most doctors must earn CME credits throughout their career to maintain their state licenses. CME providers have received billions of dollars from the pharmaceutical industry as part of a publicly recognized strategy to increase their sales. Drug and device companies also cultivate relationships with KOLs, often paying them thousands of dollars to give speeches, lectures, and presentations to their colleagues, using their respected, influential statuses to push industry products. While such behavior is not inherently illegal, the DOJ has gotten companies to pay hundreds of millions of dollars for alleged illegal kickbacks from the most brazen *quid pro quo* relationships with such leaders. Additionally, industry hires thousands of sales representatives to directly lobby doctors, presenting skewed information in favor of their products and providing gifts like free meals. Drug and device companies have spent billions on direct payments to physicians, where even small individual payments less than $20 can influence prescribing behavior.

One case study that highlights the pharmaceutical industry's own account of its influence on doctors is that of gabapentin—otherwise known by the brand name Neurontin. In 2006, the *Annals of Internal Medicine* published an analysis of around 8,000 internal documents from Pfizer and Parke-Davis resulting from federal litigation.[147] One Parke-Davis document titled a section on strategy as "MEDICAL EDUCATION DRIVES THIS MARKET!"[148] Another document revealed the strategy of influencing "physicians from the bottom up," such as solidifying the company's "role in the resident's mind as he/she evolves into a practicing physician" (see Figure 10).[149] The company would also strategically and selectively place research and educational grants to buttress their marketing. From 1996 to 1998, between one half and two-thirds of the promotional budget for gabapentin went toward professional education, such as developing a speaker bureau and holding dinner meetings.[150] The Parke-Davis 1998 strategic plan stated that the company should "continue to develop and leverage thought leader support throughout the community" to increase their "business potential."[151] Outlining its strategies to penetrate influential hospitals, the company named specific doctors who served as key influencers within each hospital.[152] Sales representatives would track physicians' prescribing behaviors before and after advisory board and counseling meetings with physician participants, and these doctors would receive honoraria, paid travel, lodging, and amenities at luxury hotels and resorts where the events took place.[153]

Given all these obstacles, doctors also face the reality that their time is significantly constrained. In 2024, Doximity, an online networking service for medical professionals, published findings from several surveys, drawing data from a total of 33,000 physicians in 2023.[154] One 2023 survey of 2,600 physicians found that 81 percent reported

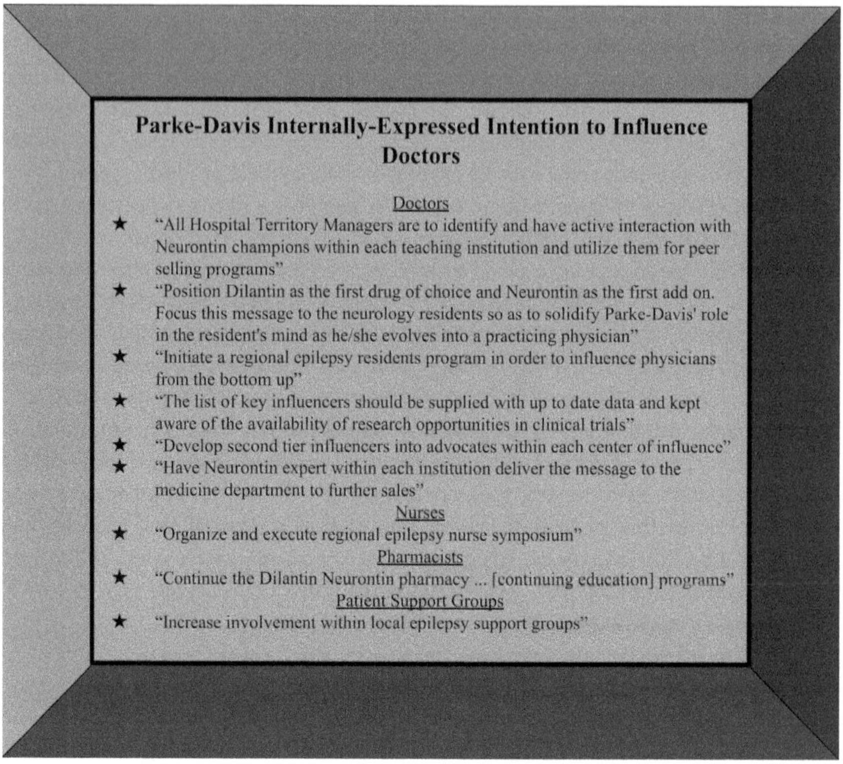


**Figure 10** Quotes from an internal Parke-Davis document marketing strategy of influencing "physicians from the bottom up" along with patient support groups and key actors throughout medicine. *Source*: Natasha Giordano et al., "Business Strategies to Penetrate the Hospital Segment of the Northeast Customer Business Unit," Parke-Davis, accessed June 27, 2024, https://www.industrydocuments.ucsf.edu/drug/docs/#id=nsyd0217.

being overworked; the same was true for 86 percent in 2022. A 2024 survey of 1,100 physicians found that 88 percent reported being impacted by a shortage of physicians, including 74 percent who said such impact was moderate or severe. According to the 2023 Medscape Compensation Report, physicians worked fifty hours a week on average, which was over fifteen hours more than the average hours worked weekly for all private-sector employees.[155] Therefore, on top of their fifty-hour average workweek, doctors would have to conduct arguably another job to review and scrutinize the medical literature and trusted sources they rely upon.

However, improving the accuracy and quality of such sources could positively impact doctors' clinical decision-making. A 2021 *JAMA* analysis observed the opioid prescription behavior of 10,246 physicians from 2009 to 2017 for Medicare fee-for-service patients based on their performance on the ABIM's Maintenance of Certification (MOC) examinations.[156] From the mid-2010s onward, the authors noted that numerous medical societies and organizations changed their guidelines to limit opioid prescriptions due to revelations of their addictive consequences. Correspondingly, in 2015–17, physicians with the highest scores on their MOC tests issued statistically significantly less opioid prescriptions compared to those with the lowest scores, representing a 4.6 percent absolute and 20 percent relative decrease in prescribing rates. There was no significant difference in the previous periods. While the magnitude of this change is not incredibly high, it suggests the ability for better sources of knowledge to change physician behavior.

Ultimately, American doctors face a stacked deck if they desire to challenge the established authorities and institutions that they were taught and conditioned to trust. However, the numerous issues underlying medical knowledge outlined in this book, including industry influence on doctors, stems from root, systemic incentives. The next chapter delves into these incentives and outlines potential alternatives.

# 9

# The Root Incentive: Patents

The current system to incentivize medical research and innovation in the United States and globally is based on intellectual property (IP) protections through patents. While patents allow discoverers of new treatments to overcome research and development (R&D) costs and, thus, profit, they come at the expense of high costs borne by patients, employers, and governments. At the same time, this system has not primarily incentivized innovation to improve health outcomes; rather, it has encouraged exploitation of monopoly protections to charge high prices with minimal added clinical benefits from new products.

By tying financial rewards to patent protections and successful marketing rather than health outcomes, the patent system explains industry behaviors against public health: pushing shorter FDA reviews and lower standards of evidence, designing biased studies to favor their product, keeping data from clinical trials hidden, and corrupting the organizations and researchers who evaluate evidence. If a product is not better than alternative treatments, companies need not worry about their bottom line as long as their product stays on the market, physicians prescribe it, and advertising successfully reaches patients and their physicians. However, the patent system is not the only avenue to incentivize innovation. Other proposals such as publicly funded research via contracts and prize funds aim to reward researchers and innovators while also tying financial rewards to better health outcomes.

## The Current System

The market for medical products—drugs, biologics, devices, and so forth—is inherently not free. In a genuinely free market, private actors would have little financial incentive to conduct research into new, innovative treatments. Pharmaceutical companies and other medical manufacturers often spend billions of dollars on R&D to bring their products to market. In 2019, pharmaceutical companies spent $83 billion on R&D, which is ten times greater than R&D spending in the 1980s adjusted for inflation.[1] A 2021 analysis in *INQUIRY: The Journal of Health Care Organization, Provision, and Financing* reviewed previous studies attempting to identify the cost of R&D for drug companies.[2] In 2025 dollars, the estimated cost to bring a drug to market ranged from roughly $144.4 million to $7.7 billion.[3]

In a completely free market, spending $1 billion to bring a drug to market would put a company at a significant competitive disadvantage. Without IP protections, competing companies would wait for the original manufacturer to incur all the R&D costs and then simply produce the drug themselves. Thus, the original manufacturer would have to immediately compete with other companies while being the only company having spent $1 billion. This situation inherently disincentivizes innovation, as it is more profitable to be the competitor free riding off the work of others than the original creator of new treatments.

This market failure produces a purpose for the government to intervene to incentivize innovation and improve public health. The contemporary policy of the United States and the rest of the world is to grant monopoly control over medical innovations to the original creator for a designated period. With competitors barred from producing and selling novel drugs, pharmaceutical companies can recoup their R&D losses and earn a profit. In turn, the public benefits from access to new treatments that ideally improve the standards of care available to them and, thus, their health outcomes.

This situation is not unique to pharmaceutical companies and other medical producers. Patents protect the makers of computers, special purpose machinery, cars, machine tools, semiconductors, and much more.[4] Without copyright laws, book authors and movie developers would not have exclusive rights over their creations. Profitability would sink, as others could legally and freely share their works, destroying the possibility for people to have careers as innovators—whether by revolutionizing computers or writing inspirational novels. Thus, patents are widespread in the US economy. A 2012 report from the Economics and Statistics Administration (ESA) and United States Patent and Trademark Office (USPTO) identified seventy-five IP-intensive US industries, meaning the industries that use the most patents, trademarks, and copyright protections.[5] These industries accounted for 18.8 percent of all employment in 2010, adding roughly $5.1 trillion (34.8 percent) to the US gross domestic product (GDP).

While these industries similarly benefit from government-granted monopoly protections, the health industry is unique regarding the structure of the market and the stakes for consumers. Unlike most product markets, individuals predominantly do not shop among competing products. Rather, patients visit their doctors who diagnose and prescribe treatments like pharmaceutical drugs. For most Americans, individuals do not pay the entire cost of treatments up front as their health insurer at least partially covers the cost.[6] Additionally, if the price of a new computer is too high for someone's budget, they can choose not to buy the product. However, if an individual has a significant medical condition requiring treatment, and their doctor prescribes a potentially lifesaving drug, there is not much choice for the patient due to the high stakes. The demand for medical products is much more inelastic than other types of goods, meaning that it is less subject to change with higher prices.[7] Thus, drug and device companies can afford to charge increasingly high prices without losing enough patients to hurt their profits.

Asymmetry of information exacerbates these dynamics.[8] In a market transaction involving the sale of a computer, the customer can generally research the components and quality of the computer, and they can see if the product works (e.g., Does it turn on? Do the buttons work? Does it run smoothly?). However, the clinical trial data revealing the traits of drugs and devices can be extremely complex requiring expert review. Outside of the FDA approval process, medical experts and doctors predominantly do not have access to the data from clinical trials. Thus, patients rely on their doctors on what treatments to use, and the clinicians don't have access to the required information to make truly informed recommendations.

## Medical Patent Law: A Brief History and Overview

Patents are firmly rooted in American law, as the US Constitution itself grants Congress the right to protect innovative technologies and creations. Article I Section 8 Clause 8 of the Constitution states: "Congress shall have power … to promote the progress of science and useful arts by securing for limited times to authors and inventors the exclusive right to their respective writings and discoveries."[9] The Intellectual Property Clause serves as the foundation for US copyright and patent laws, granting two distinct authorities.[10] First, the Constitution gives Congress the right to grant authors exclusive rights over their writings—including a wider variety of works besides literal writings like movies and software. Second, it allows Congress to protect inventors' exclusive rights over their discoveries. For both patents and copyrights, the purpose of Congress's authority is "to promote the progress of science and useful arts."[11] For medical innovation, patents should promote the progress of science through the development of technologies and treatments better than existing methods of care.

Through passing the Patent Act of 1793, Congress allowed US citizens to patent "any new and useful art, machine, manufacture or composition of matter or any new and useful improvement on any art, machine, manufacture or composition of matter, not known or used before the application."[12] While the original Patent Act of 1790 created a Patent Board to issue patents, a patent office was not formally created until 1802.[13] The Patent Act of 1836 formally established the Patent Office. Since 2000, the United States Patent and Trademark Office (USPTO) is in charge of accepting, reviewing, and making decisions on patent applications, and it is led by the under-secretary of Commerce for Intellectual Property and director of the USPTO.[14]

While US patent law began as early as the Constitution, the 1800s were not a period with frequent patenting of medicines.[15] The Patent Act of 1836 especially dampened medicine patenting, as it introduced a mandatory examination of novelty for something to be patented. In 1875 and 1880, the Patent Office issued fourteen and twenty-five patents for explicitly identified medical compounds or cures out of nearly 15,000 and over 13,000 issued patents, respectively.[16] While the term "patent medicines" was common, it did not refer to legally patented drugs.[17] Rather, patent medicines predominantly meant those sold by a single manufacturer containing "a secret combination of ingredients." At the time, patients and physicians alike largely did not know what constituted the medicines they took. However, medical patents particularly took off by the mid-twentieth century, as scientific progress made it much more difficult to keep the ingredients of medicines secret, and patents were the primary means of protecting inventions.

American physicians largely opposed medical patents throughout the nineteenth and early twentieth centuries, viewing them as unethical and a hindrance to scientific progress. They believed advances in medical knowledge should be shared freely and benefit patients more so than commercial interests.[18] The American Medical Association led efforts to get Congress to appoint a commission that studied excluding medicines from patent and trademark laws in 1898; but, this did not happen.[19] In 1896, the association barred a doctor from becoming a member due to applying for a patent. The AMA's 1903 *Principles of Medical Ethics* held that holding patents "for any surgical instruments or medicines" was "derogatory to professional character for physicians."[20] In 1921, the then major pharmaceutical company H. K. Mulford refused to patent its products.[21]

Industry reliance on and medical professionals' acceptance of patents emerged after the First World War and really took off after the Second World War.[22] In 1938, *JAMA* editor Morris Fishbein wrote an article entitled "Are Patents on Medicinal Discoveries and on Foods in the Public Interest?"[23] He recognized the considerable cost associated with R&D and viewed patents as an ethical and necessary tool; however, he argued for nonprofit control of patents rather than control by for-profit corporations. Over the first half of the twentieth century, the medical industry gradually began patenting their products and winning over acceptance from physicians and medical professionals. By the 1950s, medical industry had wholly embraced patents to commercialize their discoveries or those that they purchased.[24]

The Patent Act of 1952 significantly changed the landscape for medical patents by changing the definition of patentable matter from the 1793 Patent Act.[25] It exchanged the word *art* with *process*: "Any new and useful process, machine, manufacture, or composition of matter, or any new and useful improvement thereof, may obtain a patent."[26] This change of words, however small, is significant in the case of biomedical research. In *Halliburton Oil Well Cementing Co. v. Walker* (1946), the US Supreme Court ruled that patent claims formed based on what "the most crucial element" in a new combination will do rather than a specific description of its "physical characteristics or its arrangement in the new combination" were legally invalid.[27] The 1952 law explicitly overruled *Halliburton* through the aforementioned change along with the following clause:

> An element in a claim for a combination may be expressed as a means or step for performing a specified function without the recital of structure, material, or acts in support thereof, and such claim shall be construed to cover the corresponding structure, material, or acts described in the specification and equivalents thereof.[28]

Thus, contrary to *Halliburton*, Congress allowed patent filings based on what the function of an element is rather than its specific material or structure. For a new pharmaceutical, a drug company could file this type of claim—otherwise known as a means-plus-function (MPF) claim—and prevent a generic competitor from replacing an element in the formulation of the pharmaceutical that is patent protected by its function.[29] Thus, the protection of process and function further entrenches the monopoly authority of pharmaceutical companies and other relevant actors over their patented products.

In the 1980 Bayh-Dole Act, Congress expanded the patentability of medical innovations.[30] Beforehand, patents generally were only retained for commercial interests in the private sector, meaning that private researchers and companies paid for and conducted research behind patented products. However, facing global competition in innovation—particularly from the Japanese automobile industry—Congress passed the Bayh-Dole Act to spur American innovation, allowing researchers receiving federal funds to retain patent rights over their discoveries and commercialize their findings, including selling them off to industry.[31] Thus, universities, research institutions, private companies, and other contractors receiving federal funding could then patent medical innovations for financial gain. Yet, the law also grants the federal government march-in rights, meaning the ability to force a patent holder to license the federally funded patent to third parties under four specific situations.[32] One of these situations allows the government to march in after determining "action is necessary to alleviate health or safety needs which are not reasonably satisfied by the contractor, assignee, or their licensees." However, the federal government has yet to ever use march-in rights.

Throughout US history, Congress has changed how long patents grant exclusivity and monopoly pricing power over products.[33] The original 1790 Patent Act provided fourteen years of patent exclusivity without extensions following issuance. The 1836 Patent Act kept the original exclusivity at fourteen years, but it created the possibility of a seven-year extension for a total possible exclusivity period of twenty-one years. In 1861, while Congress removed the seven-year extension, it increased the baseline exclusivity period to seventeen years. However, in 1994, Congress passed the 1994 Uruguay Round Agreements Act to comply with the international Uruguay Round Agreements (URA), further extending the patent exclusivity length to twenty years starting in 1995 with exclusivity starting after the date of filing rather than patent issuance.[34] Importantly, the twenty-year patent term begins upon the date of filing the patent, which—due to lengthy pharmaceutical R&D periods—means often just seven to ten of these years protect a drug once it is actually on the market.[35] The URA represented a significant advancement in the globalization of IP rights and patent law. The URA established the World Trade Organization (WTO), comprising 123 global members in 1995, increasing to 166 in 2024.[36]

Along with establishing the twenty-year baseline, the creation of the WTO included provisions known as Trade Related Aspects of Intellectual Property Rights (TRIPS). These provisions required member countries to adopt a uniform set of IP protections, although there has been a phase-in period for developing countries that has been repeatedly extended.[37] For example, India only adopted patent law protections in line with TRIPS in 2005—a decade after the WTO's creation—even though it was an original member.[38] TRIPS provisions are meant to prevent the foreign pirating of technologies. However, TRIPS can also prevent poorer, developing nations from producing affordable generic versions of drugs and other medical products that are produced in developed nations at higher prices than developing countries and their citizens can afford.

The primary US law governing the introduction of generic competition is the 1984 Drug Price Competition and Patent Term Restoration Act, otherwise known as the Hatch-Waxman Act.[39] Prior to Hatch-Waxman, bringing a generic drug to market was especially costly and long. Generic manufacturers had to file the same application—the FDA's NDA—as originally approved drugs, forcing many companies to pay for independent trials and studies proving the safety and efficacy of their products that had the same chemical makeup as what was already approved. Additionally, they could not start developing generics before the expiration of the original patent.[40] Therefore, Hatch-Waxman created a new type of application—the Abbreviated New Drug Application (ANDA)—that generic manufacturers would file to receive FDA approval. If a generic drug has an active ingredient bioequivalent to the approved drug, then the manufacturer can file an ANDA based on the safety and efficacy data from the original manufacturer's clinical trials. Generic companies can also use data that is available in the published literature; however, this practice predated Hatch-Waxman. Additionally, the legislation allows generic manufacturers to begin development and work on generic versions of approved, patented drugs during the lifetime of a patent.

Congressional debates behind the legislation essentially amounted to a negotiation between brand-name and generic drug companies; thus, the law also granted several favors to brand-name manufacturers.[41] Hatch-Waxman allows drug patent holders to apply with USPTO for an extension that is no more than five years to cover a portion of the period during clinical testing and FDA review, and no more than fourteen years can remain on the patent following FDA approval.[42] Additionally, the legislation grants five-year regulatory exclusivity for new chemical entities (NCEs), meaning that competitors cannot file an application for approval of a drug with the same active core molecule for five years. The legislation also grants a three-year marketing exclusivity for an already approved drug when a new NDA or supplemental NDA contains new clinical studies essential to regulatory approval. Thus, if the FDA approves changes to a drug's active ingredients, strength, dosage form, or means of administration, then the FDA cannot approve an application for any generic version of the new version of the drug for three years.[43]

Since 1984, Congress has passed several laws following the framework of Hatch-Waxman. For example, as part of the Affordable Care Act, Congress passed the Biologics Price Competition and Innovation Act (BPCIA), which included the creation of an expedited pathway for the approval of biosimilars, the biologic-specific version of generic drugs.[44] At the same time, this legislation granted a twelve-year reference product exclusivity, which is much longer compared to the five-year exclusivity granted to NCEs for pharmaceutical drugs.[45] Under this exclusivity, branded biologics are protected from competition for twelve years even if no patents exist.[46]

Ultimately, congressional policy over the last half century has both lengthened the possible monopoly protections for medical products while also promoting the increased development and marketing of generics. The current era represents an embrace of a patent-based system not always welcomed by medical professionals and manufacturers throughout US history. Rather, the patent system—permitted by the

Constitution—was the chosen avenue by private actors and policymakers alike to spur and incentivize medical innovation.

## Consequences of the Patent System

While the patent system addresses the failure of the theoretical free market of medical products by successfully incentivizing innovation, it ultimately has resulted in the pursuit of monopoly pricing power and legal protections over actual benefits to public health. This incentive structure places the profit-motive of the medical industry in opposition to public health, leading to industry control over key aspects of medical research that is similarly against the public interest.

### Exorbitant Patent-Based Profits

Patents allow pharmaceutical companies and other medical manufacturers to recoup their R&D losses; however, they also provide extraordinary profits far exceeding R&D costs. Prices are much higher than what it takes to actually produce treatments.[47] For example, a single shot of the Moderna vaccine cost $2.85 to produce, yet Moderna marked up the price by over 4,000 percent to between $110 and $130 in 2023.[48] While the costs of branded and generic drugs are both higher than production costs—as necessary to make a profit—branded drug prices are considerably higher. Compared to brand-name drugs, generics typically cost 80–85 percent less according to the FDA.[49] Yet, price decreases with generic competition can take years and several generic entrants. A 2021 FDA report found that for all 321 drug products that received a generic approval in 2021, 60.9 percent experienced a price decrease of 10–40 percent while 24.7 percent and 3.6 percent had price declines of 40–70 percent and over 70 percent, respectively, after the first twelve months following generic approval.[50]

Government-granted market exclusivity and monopoly pricing power has led to significant drug price increases far outpacing inflation. A 2019 *JAMA Network Open* analysis looked at the forty-nine top-selling branded drugs in 2017 with available net pricing data, finding that the median cost increase from 2012 to 2017 was 76 percent, while inflation over the period was just 6.8 percent.[51] A similar 2020 *JAMA* analysis examined the list and net prices of 602 branded drugs between 2007 and 2018. List prices rose by 159 percent while net prices—prices after accounting for trade discounts—rose by 60 percent. Inflation from 2007 to 2018 was nearly 21.2 percent.[52]

R&D costs do not explain these prices. While inflation-adjusted R&D costs increased nearly tenfold from the 1980s to 2019, drug companies have taken in considerably more revenue overall and earned higher profits.[53] Among the top 27 largest pharmaceutical companies from 2000 to 2018, net revenues grew over 241 percent from around $300 billion to nearly $725 billion while R&D spending as a percentage of net sales grew 12–17 percent.[54] In contrast, investor payouts and stock buybacks doubled from 10 percent to 20 percent of net sales, rising from $30 billion to $146 billion. A 2023 *BMJ* analysis examined the financial records of the fifteen largest pharmaceutical companies globally from 1999 to 2018.[55] While the companies spent $1.4 trillion on R&D over the period, they spent $2.2 trillion on selling, general, and administrative activities. These activities encompass nearly all business costs not directly related to production or performing services, including marketing and advertising.

Moreover, other analyses have shown that large pharmaceutical companies spend more on stock buybacks—a practice where a company buys its own shares to raise its stock price and increase shareholder profits—and dividends—direct corporate payouts to shareholders—than R&D. A 2021 report from the Democratic majority staff on the US House Committee on Oversight & Reform investigated pharmaceutical industry drug pricing.[56] From 2016 to 2020, the 14 largest drug companies spent $577 billion on stock buybacks and dividends, which is $56 billion more than the $521 billion spent on R&D. A 2017 Institute for New Economic Thinking paper examined the 18 drug companies within the S&P 500 Index in January 2016 which were publicly listed from 2006 to 2015.[57] While spending $516 billion on buybacks and dividends, these companies spent just $465 billion on R&D. Ninety-nine percent of their total profits went directly to shareholders through stock buybacks (50 percent) and dividends (49 percent). A similar analysis of the top 14 drug companies from 2013 to 2022 found that they distributed 105 percent of their net income to shareholders, meaning they spent more than they took in.[58] Just $701 billion went toward R&D compared to $773 billion on buybacks and dividends.

In 2022, Congress passed the Inflation Reduction Act (IRA), allowing Medicare to directly negotiate drug prices with manufacturers for limited numbers of drugs starting in 2026.[59] In 2023, the government announced the ten drugs Medicare planned to negotiate prices for. A 2024 Public Citizen report examined the 2022 finances of the manufacturers of the ten drugs, finding that, in 2022, they spent over $107.6 billion on stock buybacks, dividends to shareholders, and executive compensation compared to $97.3 billion on R&D.[60] Roughly 56.6 percent of executive compensation came from equity-based rewards that are directly tied to share prices, demonstrating a key trait of stock buybacks: executive enrichment.

High spending on stock buybacks and dividends strongly demonstrates extreme profit-making, as these costs are not for necessary expenditures, reinvestments to expand business operations, or even advertising. They are central methods to maximize profits for shareholders. Companies that can spend billions more on stock buybacks and dividends than on R&D are not approaching financial trouble, but they are making exorbitant profits from patent monopolies.

Overall, pharmaceutical companies bring in considerably more profits compared to other industries. A 2020 *JAMA* study examined the profits of 35 large pharmaceutical companies compared to 357 large companies from other industries within the S&P 500 Index from 2000 to 2018.[61] Pharmaceutical annual profit margins were significantly greater than other industries, and the net income as a percentage of revenue was nearly double (13.8 percent compared to 7.7 percent). A 2017 GAO report found that the largest 25 drug companies had annual profit margins between 15 percent and 20 percent from 2006 to 2015 compared to just 4–9 percent among the 500 largest nondrug companies.[62] Examining top pharmaceutical companies is important, as the GAO estimated that the top 25 companies controlled 73.4 percent of industry revenues in 2015. Rough estimates for more recent years vary, with the top 25 drug companies controlling between 53 percent and 78 percent of global prescription drug sales annually from 2022 to 24.[63]

The costs to bring a drug to market are also not associated with prices. A September 2022 *JAMA* investigation examined sixty-three new drugs that the FDA approved from 2009 to 2018.[64] No correlation existed between both estimated R&D costs and list prices at launch along with net prices one year after launch and R&D costs. The authors reasoned that if R&D "costs justified drug prices, an association between the 2 variables would be found."

Furthermore, monopoly pricing power is especially profitable in the United States due to the lack of direct government negotiation of drug prices. In 2022, the United States spent 2.78 times more for all drugs compared to Organisation for Economic Co-operation and Development (OECD) countries, and this inflated to 3.22 times more for branded drugs even when accounting for rebates.[65] A large cause of this disparity is that other developed countries—like France, Canada, and Germany—negotiate prices with drug manufacturers.[66]

Through the 2003 Medicare Modernization Act, Congress barred the US government from negotiating drug prices as part of Medicare's prescription drug benefit. A report by Common Cause revealed that a top priority for PhRMA's lobbying campaign during negotiations over the bill was "industry protection," as pharmaceutical companies feared the power of the federal government to reduce their profits through significantly lowering prices for Medicare beneficiaries.[67] PhRMA spent at least $72.6 million lobbying Congress in 2003. A key indication of how the lack of price negotiation inflates the pricing power of drugs overall and especially patented drugs is the US Departments of Veterans Affairs (VA) and Defense (DoD). Both the VA and DoD can negotiate drug prices, and they have historically paid around half the price for prescription drugs compared to the rest of Americans.[68]

## Disincentivized to Promote Public Health

The patent system's extremely high profits have incentivized industry to prioritize maintaining monopoly power over innovating new technologies with significant added health benefits. The 2021 House Committee on Oversight & Reform report obtained internal industry documents, finding that the investigated pharmaceutical companies devoted a "significant portion of their R&D" spending on research tailored "to extend market monopolies, support the companies' marketing strategies, and otherwise suppress competition."[69] For example, Abbott and AbbVie—the pharmaceutical companies behind one of the best-selling drugs in the world (Humira)—specifically focused R&D spending to create "enhancements" to Humira to "raise barriers to competitor ability to replicate" (see Figure 11).[70]

Accordingly, there were 247 filed patents on Humira by 2021, delaying competition and aiming to obtain thirty-nine years of patent protection.[71] AbbVie filed 122 (49.4 percent) of these patents from 2014 onward even though the FDA approved

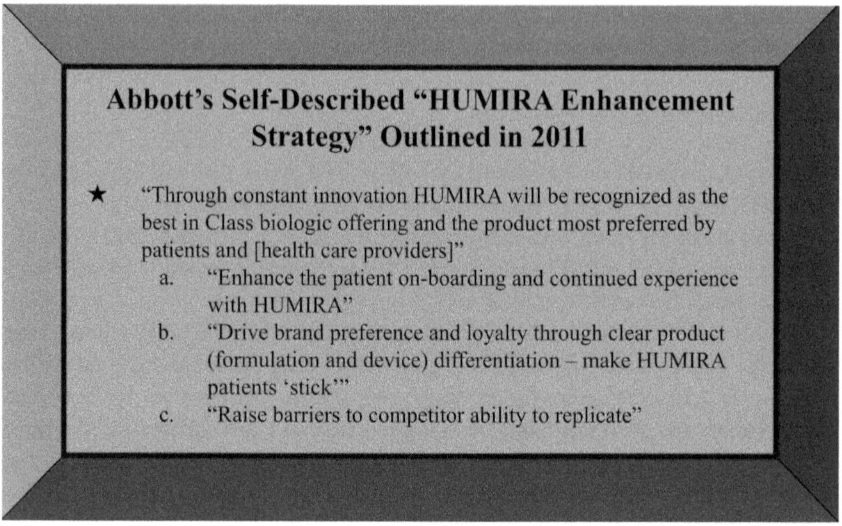

**Abbott's Self-Described "HUMIRA Enhancement Strategy" Outlined in 2011**

★ "Through constant innovation HUMIRA will be recognized as the best in Class biologic offering and the product most preferred by patients and [health care providers]"

a. "Enhance the patient on-boarding and continued experience with HUMIRA"
b. "Drive brand preference and loyalty through clear product (formulation and device) differentiation – make HUMIRA patients 'stick'"
c. "Raise barriers to competitor ability to replicate"

**Figure 11** Quotes from an internal Abbott document revealing the company's strategy to create "enhancements" to Humira to "raise barriers" to competition. *Source*: Committee on Oversight and Reform, "Drug Pricing Investigation: Majority Staff Report," 173, US House of Representatives, December 2021, https://oversightdemocrats.house.gov/sites/evo-subsites/democrats-oversight.house.gov/files/DRUG%20PRICING%20REPORT%20WITH%20APPENDIX%20v3.pdf.

Humira in 2002. These patents were part of efforts to slightly change aspects of Humira just to maintain patent-granted monopoly control. For example, AbbVie executives informed their board of directors in 2015 that getting approval for a new high-concentration Humira formulation was part of its "defense strategy" against biosimilars.[72] Approval and patent protection allowed AbbVie to maintain monopoly pricing power through directing patients toward this new formulation before generic competition began for the original formulation. Humira lost patent exclusivity in 2023, representing a successful delay of six years from when it was previously meant to face biosimilar competition.[73]

AbbVie's strategy is not unique. According to the Initiative for Medicines, Access, and Knowledge (IMAK), companies behind the ten best-selling drugs in 2021 filed nearly 143 patent applications, obtaining over 74 (51.9 percent) and reflecting 40.5 years of patent protection on average from the date of filing each patent, over double the twenty years intended by Congress.[74] Additionally, 63 percent and 66 percent of these filed patents in 2019 and 2021, respectively, were filed after FDA approval, demonstrating the companies' focus on extending market exclusivity.

Evergreening—extending patent protections through slight, functionally insignificant modifications of old products—is also prevalent. From 2005 to 2015, 78 percent of drugs tied to new patents were not actually novel.[75] Manufacturers recycled and repurposed old drugs through methods like patenting a drug in tablet form because the patent on the capsule formulation was expiring. Among the top 106 best-selling drugs, 71.7 percent extended their patent past their original monopoly protection periods at least once, and 50.9 percent did so multiple times.

Many treatments involve both drug and device components, such as inhalers. A 2022 *Health Affairs* study examined all patents and exclusivities on inhalers for asthma and chronic obstructive pulmonary disease (COPD) between 1986 and 2020.[76] Most patents (55.1 percent) at the time of FDA approval were for the devices rather than medications, and only one inhaler had an active ingredient with a new method of action for treatment. Yet, 73.6 percent of patents after approval were for devices, some including small adjustments like adding a dose counter. Numerous device types were not uniquely necessary for medicine usage, as manufacturers put active ingredients into other devices—"device hopping"—for 26.4 percent of brand-name inhalers, lengthening total patent protection to a median of 28.1 years.

In 2022, Brookings looked at all FDA approvals of branded products and combination products containing new molecular entities from 2011 to 2021.[77] Just 36 percent of brand-name product launches pertained to new molecular entities, increasing to 46 percent when including new combination products. The remaining 54 percent included approvals for new indications, formulations, dosage levels, and combinations of existing drugs.

Ultimately, as the patent system rewards companies with the ability to earn exorbitant profits as long as they keep monopoly power, they are incentivized to focus their resources on maintaining patent protections. They are not directly rewarded for producing new treatments that provide added clinical benefit to existing therapies. As Chapter 3 describes, studies using information from French and German HTA organizations show that 57.9–77.6 percent of new medicines entering the market did not provide any added clinical benefit over standard therapies.[78] A 2023 *JAMA* study investigated the added clinical benefit of forty-nine of the top fifty best-selling drugs in Medicare in 2020.[79] Twenty-seven (55.1 percent) of these top-selling drugs had a low-added therapeutic rating, meaning that there was "limited or no evidence that these drugs offer benefits to patients over existing treatments."

As the patent system does not primarily reward drugs with added clinical benefits, companies often target their resources on treatment areas with known high profitability and an already existing base of treatments to get a share of the high profits.[80] A 2014 National Bureau of Economic Research paper examined the impact of the 2003 creation of Medicare Part D—which expanded pharmaceutical drug coverage for Medicare beneficiaries, thus, growing the market—on the development of new drugs and biologics.[81] While the number of treatments brought to market increased, they found that new products were "concentrated among products aimed at diseases that already have multiple existing treatments." More specifically, they found that the program yielded a spike in development of new biotechnologies where there were already five or more existing treatments.

Moreover, the patent system incentivizes industry sponsors of clinical trials to hide the underlying clinical trial data from the public and any entity outside of what is legally required to obtain FDA approval. Clinical trials are tools to get approval and marketing material; thus, outside scrutiny from independent researchers and others—which may reveal limitations or harms of their product—threaten product profitability. With Tamiflu, Roche earned $18 billion globally from a drug that offered minimal benefits due to hiding the underlying clinical trial data from the public and Cochrane reviewers.[82]

The patent system's incentives to keep information secret and proprietary can harm the advancement of medical knowledge. As argued by the physicians and medical professionals opposed to patents up until the early-mid-twentieth century, patents harmed science by stopping the sharing of knowledge. Instead of building upon each other's research, researchers must work around barriers of information secrecy resulting from patent protections.[83] In a 2013 *Journal of Political Economy* article, researcher Heidi Williams estimated that IP protections for DNA sequences held by the firm Celera resulted in 20–30 percent reductions in subsequent scientific research and product development.[84]

Furthermore, the patent system significantly distorts the research agenda for industry, as the ultimate goal to maximize profits is to maintain monopoly power. Profits are not directly tied to developing and pushing drugs with higher added clinical benefit, as demonstrated by the 2023 *JAMA* analysis of the 150 top-selling drugs in the United States in 2020 that showed drug companies spent more money advertising less clinically beneficial drugs and those with higher sales.[85] Therefore, companies conduct trials to meet FDA regulatory standards, get published in medical journals, and produce marketing material for physicians and medical professionals regardless of a new product's actual clinical benefit. As Chapter 1 explains, industry-sponsored research is significantly more likely to produce results favorable to industry. A patent-based system rewards companies for biasing their trial design and selectively publishing favorable trials, as this increases the chance of getting FDA approval. These biased results also populate the medical journals and CPGs that doctors and other medical professionals rely upon.

The biasing of the research agenda prevents important studies for public health from being conducted unless otherwise funded by government or nonprofit entities. The social determinants of health show that medical care only determines up to 20 percent of population health, while the remaining 80 percent is determined by health behaviors (30 percent) like diet and exercise, social and economic factors (40 percent), and one's physical environment (10 percent).[86] Yet the vast majority of medical research focuses on the 20 percent. Around $116 billion (95.9 percent) of US medical and health services research in 2011 went toward new drugs and devices compared to only around $5 billion (4.1 percent) for better delivery of health services.[87]

Largely, the clinical trials underlying FDA approval at best use active comparators to prove efficacy; however, they often use placebos and sometimes no comparator at all. This reality grew as FDA standards of evidence weakened over the last several decades as Chapter 5 describes. Yet, even using other treatments as active comparators is not sufficient to identify the best methods of treatment. For example, a 2019 systematic review and meta-analysis of twenty-nine prospective cohort studies studied the effect of a Mediterranean diet on the most important clinical outcome: all-cause mortality.[88] The HHS and US Department of Agriculture guidelines along with those of the

American Heart Association and European Society of Cardiology have recommended this diet to improve health and prevent diseases, such as heart disease.[89] Each two-point increase in adherence to the diet yielded a 10 percent decrease in all-cause mortality. However, the authors rated the quality of the included studies as low because they were observational, highlighting the importance of randomized trials.

The public would benefit from RCTs that not only study the effect of a Mediterranean diet on all-cause mortality but also compare it to drug treatments. For example, trials could test the efficacy of statin therapy compared to Mediterranean diet, both, and placebo. Yet, conducting studies that test products alongside unprofitable substitutes like lifestyle modifications is not in statin makers' or other drug companies' interests. The Diabetes Prevention Program Research Group study comparing lifestyle modification through diet and exercise with taking metformin to reduce the risk of type 2 diabetes demonstrates this dynamic.[90] Diet and exercise were significantly more effective in lowering the incidence of type 2 diabetes compared to the drug. As Dr. John Abramson noted, the trial results showed that lifestyle modification delayed the incidence of type 2 diabetes while costing just around $1,100 a year, which is significantly less than the cost of earning an additional year of healthy living with other medical interventions that can cost up to $150,000 a year.[91]

Ultimately, one of the patent system's most apparent effects is high costs. Exorbitant profits for producers of branded products come from the ability to charge monopoly prices. Between 2011 and 2021, prescription drug spending rose from $366 billion annually to $603 billion adjusted for inflation, representing a 64 percent increase in real prices.[92] In 2018, a Democratic Senate Homeland Security & Government Affairs Committee report showed that the prices for the twenty most-prescribed brand-name drugs increased at an annual rate ten times higher than inflation from 2012 to 2017.[93] In March 2024, the Kaiser Family Foundation found that 28 percent of surveyed Americans responded that it was somewhat or very difficult to pay for their prescription drugs.[94] Historically, relief in drug prices has come from generic competition. A 2022 report from the Association for Accessible Medicines found that from 2012 to 2021, the availability of generic drugs and biosimilars saved the US health care system $2.6 trillion.[95]

When addressing the free-market problem for medical innovation, there are several potential issues to consider such as incentivizing investment, developing the most clinically beneficial treatments, and lowering costs for patients so that they have access to the best care. Ultimately, the patent system primarily targets the need to incentivize investment into research and development. It fails to promote the advancement of medical knowledge centrally in service of public health, and it keeps prices high for patients.

## Alternatives

### Contract-Based Public Funding of Research

One alternative to a patent-based system for medical products is the public funding of research through federal contracts. As patents' purpose is to reward private actors for significant investments in R&D, this alternative model would have taxpayers directly foot the bill. In exchange for financing medical R&D, the public would gain access to cheaper products that immediately face competition after launch, and the government can regulate the conduct of research.

In his 2016 book *Rigged: How Globalization and the Rules of the Modern Economy Were Structured to Make the Rich Richer*, economist Dean Baker outlines such a public financing model based on government-awarded contracts in similar fashion to how the DoD contracts with weapons and military technology companies.[96] The federal government would primarily finance R&D to private firms under contracts with clear rules and guidelines for the research and its results. These regulations would aim to ensure that public financing does not have the same primary ills of the current patent system.

The results of all publicly financed research—including product information and underlying clinical data—would become publicly available. Therefore, generic competition could immediately enter the market, and manufacturers could use the public information to relatively quickly get FDA approval. Any tools, procedures, and other forms of relevant information that could augment and improve future research would also become publicly available. Through "copyleft" regulations, such information disclosure requirements would also apply to products derived from the information disclosed from publicly funded research.

Medical journal peer reviewers, guideline authors, medical researchers, doctors, and anyone else would have access to clinical trial results, including CSRs, anonymized individual participant data, and the metadata. Therefore, patients and doctors would not have to rely on unvetted partial releases of data from industry sponsors as the sources of medical knowledge. Additionally, information would enter the public domain as it is created, meaning that preclinical research results would be available to the public. Secrecy would not be necessary for companies conducting research due to already receiving awarded funding from their contracts. Delays in making information public would constitute "grounds for revoking the contract."[97]

Baker's model also seeks to minimize the extent to which the government directly sets the research agenda. Funding would take the form of long-term contracts—he suggests ten to fifteen years—where private firms would decide where to use funds and what topics to prioritize investigating. The government would maintain an oversight role to ensure there is no waste, fraud, and abuse with the taxpayer funds. The terms of the contracts would include broad, "less well-defined outcomes" that would point contractors in a general direction while not micromanaging exactly what research they do.[98] Contractors would also be allowed to subcontract as they deem necessary for efficiency in similar fashion to defense contractors.

Simultaneously, through government input into the funding of research, trial designs can incorporate elements otherwise not included in industry trials within a patent system. More studies like that of the Diabetes Prevention Program Research Group could take place, where new products would be tested alongside forms of lifestyle modification rather than just a placebo or other medicines. Overall, the research agenda could better reflect the social determinants of health so that 95.9 percent of medical research is not focused on medical care that only reflects 20 percent of population health.[99]

Furthermore, the public would not have to rely on industry to conduct high-quality preapproval or postmarketing studies in a timely manner. Contracts can mandate that trial designs meet high standards of participant size, endpoint usage, randomization, double blinding, and more. They can also ensure that multiple studies are conducted to analyze different target populations. For treatments that may get FDA approval based on weaker standards of evidence due to the lack of existing treatments and the serious nature of a disease or condition, contracts could include strict requirements for postmarketing research that include robust designs and the usage of relevant clinical endpoints rather than weak surrogate endpoints.

In 2004, Representative Dennis Kucinich (D-OH) proposed a similar publicly financed system in his Free Market Drug Act (FMDA).[100] The bill would have established a National Institute for Biomedical Research and Development (NIBRD) to oversee the R&D for drugs, biological products, and devices conducted both within federal laboratories and via third parties, such as universities and private companies.[101] The NIBRD director would create ten new laboratories within NIH with each one subjected to a ten-year performance review with the possibility of termination for poor performance. The NIBRD would also make information publicly available online relating to discoveries from the taxpayer-financed research, including the identification of each discovery along with "all raw data developed … in carrying out research and development activities" and the findings from such R&D.[102] Kucinich's proposal would have the government hold or "reasonably be expected to obtain" the patent for any discoveries made with federal research; but, the NIBRD would issue nonexclusive licenses to private manufacturers to create competition and lower drug prices. Additionally, the FMDA would have barred the government from transferring patent ownership to any nonfederal entities.

Furthermore, Kucinich's proposal would have appropriated over $19.9 billion to the NIBRD for FY 2004 with increasing amounts listed up until 2008. For context, total medical R&D spending in 2004 exceeded $59.1 billion, including $38.8 billion from the pharmaceutical industry.[103] Therefore, the FMDA would have represented roughly one-third of total medical R&D in 2004 and not have supplanted the patent system. Rather, it would have provided a significantly funded alternative. Additionally, the FMDA would have appropriated $50 million in prize funds for individuals or organizations who may not have produced a product but whom the NIBRD director found to have made "significant advances in knowledge regarding a disease, disorder, or other health condition, including new treatments or diagnostic techniques."[104]

Such a program of public financing would build off billions of dollars in existing funding for medical research from the federal government. For 2024, Congress appropriated $47.1 billion in funding for the NIH—the primary agency with the mandate to both support and perform biomedical and behavioral research—and the agency reports spending roughly 83 percent of its budget ($39.1 billion) funding medical research through competitive grants.[105] Additionally, around 11 percent of the NIH budget (nearly $5.2 billion) goes toward funding research in its own laboratories. Thus, the NIH spent approximately $44.3 billion (94.1 percent) toward financing medical research in 2024. While total NIH funding is less than total industry R&D spending, the time value of such research is substantial by supporting the foundation for successful medical products, including 99.4 percent of FDA-approved drugs from 2010 to 2019.[106]

Total spending on medical and health R&D in 2020 was $245.1 billion.[107] Of this spending, industry contributed $161.8 billion (66.0 percent) compared to $61.5 billion (25.1 percent) from the federal government, $16.8 billion (6.9 percent) from academic and research institutions, $3.0 billion (1.2 percent) from voluntary health associations and professional societies, and $2.1 billion (0.9 percent) from state governments. For the federal government to have fully replaced the patent system with public financing in 2020, it would have needed to increase spending by roughly $183.6 billion. This represented less than 0.9 percent of the US GDP in 2020 along with roughly 2.8 percent of federal spending and 5.4 percent of federal revenues.[108]

There are several limitations and potential drawbacks to a system of public funding through government contracts. First, as Baker notes, the United States is involved in international agreements—such as TRIPS through being a WTO member—and any changes to intellectual property systems would need to consider such agreements and international relations.[109] Thus, in his model, companies can still choose the route of the current patent-based system; however, they would be competing against companies with almost guaranteed funding from government contracts. However, the United States may be able to abolish patent monopolies in medicine without violating TRIPS (further discussed in the next section).

Second, a publicly financed system based on government-granted contracts inherently places the power of directing medical research in the hands of government officials. Even with the usage of broadly defined outcomes that allow researcher flexibility, there is still baseline government control of where the funding goes. Conversely, this system replaces a patent model, where private actors without democratic accountability to the public direct research funding primarily to maintain monopoly control rather than improve public health. Additionally, such a system could involve the government regularly receiving advice and input from outside experts, medical professionals, and other relevant stakeholders as to what general areas to award research contracts toward. Yet, public officials would hold power over the selection of such experts.

Third, political corruption could harm a contract-based system. Medical research contractors could spend hundreds of millions of dollars on lobbying government officials, including executive agency employees and members of Congress, to receive larger shares of the government funding pie. According to OpenSecrets, defense contractors spent $149.4 million on federal lobbying in 2024 alone, and they have spent over $3.2 billion since 1998, including nearly $2.1 billion since 2010.[110] Such spending occurs due to the fact that the size of all defense contracts is worth hundreds of billions of dollars annually. In FY 2024, the federal government granted $455.7 billion in defense contracts.[111] Contracts for medical R&D would also be worth hundreds of billions of dollars overall. Importantly, both lobbying expenditures and the number of employed revolving door lobbyists are significantly correlated with the size of awarded contracts.[112] While the patent system ties financial rewards to maintaining monopoly power, a publicly financed system would tie rewards not necessarily just to health outcomes but also the ability to convince government officials and/or selected experts to award contracts.

Fourth, public contracts compensate companies for R&D prior to the actual carrying out of research. Therefore, the funding is not directly tied to the quality of what is produced. In a system where lobbying has significant influence on who wins contracts, there is a real possibility of wasting public funds. However, such waste would likely differ from what occurs with defense contractors, as the government uses defense companies to directly purchase products that lack competition due to consolidation and required secrecy for information on military technology. This has led to situations with immense prices, such as how the RTX Corporation—formerly known as Raytheon—increased the price of its Stinger missiles by around 700 percent from 1991 to 2024, far outpacing the period's roughly 130.2 percent total inflation.[113] Additionally, medical research contracts do not involve the government directly purchasing products. Rather, the government would pay for advances in medical knowledge that would be publicly available, and resulting products would quickly face competition.

The third and fourth limitations could be addressed by following the recommendations of Dr. Peter Gøtzsche. Gøtzsche has advocated for public funding of medical R&D solely through "nonprofit public health-focused institutions" rather than for-profit companies.[114] Through nonprofits, he argued clinical trials could become "a public enterprise, done for the public good, and performed by independent academic institutions." Nonprofits would face difficulty lobbying their way to success like defense contractors have, due to their grant-based system of funding. Unless Congress directly authorizes such spending, the Congressional Research Service (CRS) has noted that "federal contract or grant money may not be used for any lobbying."[115] Theoretically, nonprofits could obtain funding from private sources for lobbying; however, the extent to which this would occur is unknown. Generally, funding nonprofits would significantly reduce the possibility of political corruption as the tax code requires them to mostly spend on the mission-driven activities that afforded them their nonprofit status.[116] For example, tax-exempt 501(c)(3) nonprofits include scientific research organizations that can only engage in very minimal amounts of lobbying that cannot exceed $1 million annually.[117] With less opportunity for lobbying and potential corruption, the government would face less pressure to fund wasteful research.

Furthermore, usage of nonprofit institutions and academic researchers would additionally benefit from them not needing to seek industry funding. Since the 1980s, many academic researchers have had to seek out industry funding and make concessions, such as giving industry control over trial data, to carry out research and find career success.[118] Public financing would remove corrosive influences of industry over the integrity of medical research, better allowing the topics of research, designs of trials, and sharing of data to reflect the advancement of science rather than the profit-seeking motives of industry.

Overall, acknowledging the limitations to a publicly financed system of medical research based on competitively awarded contracts, this alternative model would address the key issues with the current patent system. Medical product manufacturers would no longer be incentivized to maintain monopoly power at the expense of improving health outcomes. All taxpayer-financed research would become publicly available, allowing for free advancement of medical knowledge and vetting of clinical trial data. Contracts could ensure that trial designs are of high quality and the resulting evidence pertains to the most relevant clinical outcomes. All products resulting from such research would be subject to competition immediately following FDA approval, lowering prices for patients and insurers.

## Publicly Funded Prize Fund System

Another alternative to the patent system similarly involves the public funding of medical research. However, awards are tied to research outcomes in the form of prizes rather than granted beforehand via contracts. Rather than rewarding companies with patent monopolies, prize funds would reward innovators based on identified improvements to public health that their discoveries produce.

Representing the most prominent, official effort to present an alternative to the patent system thus far in the United States, Senator Bernie Sanders has introduced several iterations of the Medical Innovation Prize Fund Act (MIPFA) during both his time in the US House of Representatives and the Senate.[119] The March 2017 bill presents his latest model for a prize-funded system. The bill would prohibit any individual or entity from having "the right to exclusively manufacture, distribute, sell, or use a drug, a biological product, or a manufacturing process for a drug or biological product in interstate commerce."[120] This restriction would only apply to products developed following enactment of the bill. Products already on the market at the time of enactment would be eligible for prize payments for at most ten fiscal years. Notably, the bill does not mention medical devices; however, similar legislation could do so.

Importantly, the MIPFA includes a "notwithstanding clause" regarding the current patent laws that provide exclusivity rights, meaning that the bill's medical patent prohibition would supersede those laws.[121] As the Supreme Court held in *Cisneros v. Alpine Ridge Group* (1993), "the use of such a 'notwithstanding' clause clearly signals the drafter's intention that the provisions of the 'notwithstanding' section override conflicting provisions of any other section."[122] Ultimately, the Sanders model eliminates the patent system for future drugs and biologics rather than creating a competing system.

The proposal would create a Medical Innovation Prize Fund (MIPF) that rewards whoever is first in getting FDA approval/market clearance for a drug or biologic based on how their discoveries improve public health.[123] The same reward system would apply for the holder of a patent for a manufacturing process. The MIPF board would determine recipients of prizes based on criteria that consider how many patients would benefit from the discovery and the added therapeutic benefit relative to existing treatments and processes. The board could also reward products created at the same time and compare them with previous treatments rather than each other. Additionally, prize allocation would consider the extent to which a discovery addresses "priority health care needs" like global, severe, and neglected diseases along with if it improves manufacturing process efficiency. Regarding products that may become less effective over time like antibiotics, the board would also account for the discovery's "expected life cycle benefits." For potential threats to public health, such as a pandemic, the board would consider the risk-adjusted benefits of stockpiling a product.

One critique of a prize-based system, especially in comparison to a contract-based model, is that it incentivizes secrecy like the current patent system, since a company only receives a reward if they are the first to get credit and approval for a discovery. Therefore, the MIPFA also includes open-source dividend prizes to "induce greater access and the open sharing of knowledge, data, materials and technology." Individuals, groups, or other entities who "openly shared knowledge, data, materials, and technology on a royalty-free and nondiscriminatory basis" relating to the development of drugs, biologics, and manufacturing processes that received prize rewards would be eligible for open-source dividend prizes. Nominations for open-source dividend recipients and the evidence supporting such nominations would be publicly available and open for comments.

The Board of Trustees for the MIPF would ultimately make the decisions about how to allocate prize funds within the bill's directives. The board would have thirteen members including the administrator of CMS, the FDA commissioner, the NIH director, the CDC director, and nine presidentially appointed and Senate-confirmed persons. These nine members must include two representatives of employers that provide health insurance, two health insurance industry representatives from entities that help fund the MIPF (explained later), two medical R&D representatives—including at least one from the nonprofit medical R&D sector—and three consumer and patient interest representatives, including at least one representing patients suffering from orphan diseases. Each of these nine members would serve four-year terms, and the members would elect a chair with a term length of two years.

The thirteen members would make determinations by majority vote, and they could hold hearings, collect testimony, and gather evidence to support their decisions. All proceedings and determinations of the board would be "transparent" and "supported by a description of the methods, data sources, assumptions, outcomes, and related information" that would allow the public to know how the board made its decisions. Additionally, the board would be supported by six independent advisory committees for the following topics: (1) economic evaluation of therapeutic benefits, (2) business models and incentives structures for innovation, (3) R&D priorities, (4) orphan diseases, (5) financial control and auditing, and (6) open-source biomedical science. Every five years, the GAO would audit the board and determine its effectiveness in bringing products to market in a cost-effective manner along with "addressing society's medical needs."

To fund the prize fund program, the bill would mandate the US Treasury to appropriate funds equal to 0.55 percent of the US GDP in the preceding fiscal year. Additionally, any leftover funds from a given year would be usable by the fund for three years and then returned to the Treasury. Thus, the bill would have allocated nearly $150.5 billion for 2024.[124] This level of funding would roughly cover current

R&D spending by industry for the bill's limited targeting of drugs, biologics, and the manufacturing processes behind drugs and biologics. Of the $161.8 billion that industry spent on medical and health R&D in 2020, about $122.2 billion went to biopharmaceuticals.[125] In comparison, the MIPFA's funding mechanism would have allocated nearly $118.4 billion to the prize fund or almost 96.9 percent of industry spending on biopharmaceutical R&D.[126]

The MIPFA also specifies specific percentages of the prize fund that can go toward various discoveries and research.[127] The bill prohibits the board from awarding any single drug, biologic, or manufacturing process with more than 5 percent of the appropriated funding for the MIPF, representing a ceiling of $7.5 billion in 2024. Additionally, at least 4 percent of funding ($6.0 billion in 2024) would have to go toward global neglected diseases, 10 percent ($15.0 billion) toward orphan diseases, and 4 percent for global infectious diseases and other worldwide public health priorities such as AIDS research. Another minimum threshold of 5 percent of funds must go toward open-source dividends to reward sharing of medical knowledge.

While most funding for the prize fund would come from the US Treasury, the bill also includes funding from an annual fee on all nongovernmental health insurance providers that earn more than $25 million annually in net premiums. The fee increases with higher levels of net premiums and is based on other factors such as the sum of all health insurers' net premiums along with all federal spending on health insurance and reimbursements not counting long-term care. Furthermore, the fund's board could authorize multiple nonprofit intermediary organizations funded by the health insurers that co-fund the MIPF to manage and allocate prize payments.[128] These payments would go toward open-source dividend prizes and projects conducting interim R&D that fall short of producing a final product but that are deemed of value to the development of products.[129] All recipients of prizes would have to "provide open, nondiscriminatory and royalty free licenses to relevant intellectual property rights."

A primary benefit of a publicly financed prize system compared to a contract model is that government officials in a concentrated body do not directly decide where R&D spending goes toward. The larger, more diversified field of all medical researchers and research companies/institutions would choose what to research based on areas they deem to help the most people and/or fit unmet medical needs. Additionally, the prize system encourages competition based on measured outcomes rather than competition based on convincing government officials to award a contract before any research outcomes are known.

Prize funds can incentivize high-quality trial designs and the usage of the most clinically relevant endpoints due to how rewards are tied to public health benefits. Thus, if a pharmaceutical company develops a drug with minimal added benefit that gets FDA approval, they would not receive a significant reward from the prize fund. However, the prize fund system does not inherently guarantee high-quality study designs in the same direct manner as publicly financed contracts could.

A significant weakness of Sanders's proposal in comparison to Baker's contract model is that the prize fund does not require that all the research and information behind products' receiving prizes are made publicly available. However, there is no barrier for another proposal for a prize-based system to have such a requirement once a product receives FDA approval, as whoever is first in getting market clearance is eligible for prize funds. In this case, not only would a prize system immediately allow for generic competition due to the elimination of patent monopolies, but the information behind such products would boost the time to regulatory approval for generics. However, transparency would occur at a slower pace than under the contract model, as information would not be publicly available prior to approval.

Mandatory disclosure of research information, including the underlying data from clinical trials, is essential for a prize system to allow proper vetting of results. Most importantly, the group deciding allocation of the prize fund—the MIPF board in Sanders's bill—and all relevant advisory committees and groups need to be able to vet the highest quality evidence. Otherwise, industry would still be incentivized to bias trials to receive more funding. Additionally, public disclosure would allow other key dispersers of medical knowledge, namely medical journals and clinical practice guidelines, to also have access to the necessary data to understand the results and limitations of clinical research.

There are several limitations to a publicly financed prize fund system for medical R&D. First, the benefits of a prize fund regarding the quality of medical research highly depend on the ability of those determining prize rewards to measure public benefits. The prize fund would need to function as an HTA organization. While Sanders's bill provides a set of criteria for the prize fund's board to consider, it is ultimately up to the board to accurately measure and weigh each criterion. For example, one metric to measure benefits to patients is quality-adjusted life years (QALYs) that, according to the independent HTA organization ICER, "is the academic standard for measuring how well all different kinds of medical treatments lengthen and/or improve patients' lives."[130] However, while researchers and medical experts have spent years developing sophisticated ways to measure quality of life, there are inherent limitations to being able to accurately and fully do so.[131] Additionally, QALYs do not account for benefits not directly tied to health outcomes, such as faster return to and enhanced performance in school or work. While the MIPFA's criteria seek to be expansive enough to cover a variety of concerns—such as considering if a product addresses a severe illness affecting a small patient population—there is inherent difficulty in capturing and predicting all factors that determine the quality of a discovery. Even if the criteria is of the highest possibility standard, there is the limitation of the board's subjective ability to make prize allocation decisions.

Second, while prize funds have a very similar benefit as contracts in that the government can require companies to meet specific rules and standards to qualify for prizes, they inherently incentivize some secrecy before FDA approval. Prize funds encourage competition between researchers, research institutions, and companies to receive FDA approval to qualify for financial rewards. The government could not realistically require the sharing of data prior to regulatory approval, as then the wrong people could get credit and receive prizes for others' discoveries. Thus, the sharing of information to advance scientific knowledge would be delayed in comparison to a contract system.

While the MIPFA includes a provision that at least 5 percent of prize payments go toward "the open sharing of knowledge, data, materials and technology," that still leaves up to 95 percent of the fund going toward the first individual or entity to bring their product to market.[132] Considering the prize fund's budget from the US Treasury for 2024 based on the proposed MIPFA, open-source dividends would be worth at least more than $7.5 billion compared to up to $143.0 billion for the rest of the fund.[133] Five percent is the minimum for open-source dividends; however, such payments would likely be significantly smaller than rewards for first getting market clearance. Future proposals for a prize fund could allocate larger rewards for the open sharing of research to further incentivize collaboration.

Third, a prize fund system must guard against the potential for political corruption. Although the board must follow a set of criteria when making decisions, industry could spend significant sums of money on lobbying to bias what areas of research members of the board favor. As Chapter 7 explains, federal laws surrounding the revolving door between industry and government are weak. Thus, stronger rules—such as barring board members outside of the two medical R&D representatives from having worked or going to work for entities receiving prize funds indefinitely or for long periods of time (e.g., ten to fifteen years)—are key to separate the interests of those providing and receiving research awards. Additionally, no board member should have any financial conflict of interest with industry or others receiving prize funds. These rules may require a different board composition than outlined in the MIPFA, which has specific individuals guaranteed a spot like the heads of the CDC and FDA regardless of their industry ties. The two medical R&D representatives must not make decisions on whether to reward research from entities they are connected to. Such strong rules must also apply to the six independent advisory committees; otherwise, members of these committees might have the same prevalent COIs that the FDA advisory committees do.

Much like the system of public contracts, a prize fund system would better guard against issues of corruption if prize funds are limited to only nonprofit institutions. Nonprofit competition for prize funds would similarly base medical research more on the mission to advance medical knowledge rather than maximize profits. However, within a system that includes for-profit research institutions under the premise that it further spurs innovation, a prize fund proposal could ensure that a minimum proportion of payments goes toward nonprofits.

Fourth, the United States would need to successfully demonstrate that using prize funds rather than patent monopolies would not violate TRIPS if policymakers want to comply with international agreements. Advocates for Sanders's proposed MIPFA have argued that eliminating patent monopolies need not violate TRIPS due to various flexibilities and exceptions.[134] For example, paragraph four of the 2001 Doha Declaration on TRIPS and Public Health states, "the TRIPS Agreement does not and should not prevent members from taking measures to protect public health … and promote access to medicine for all."[135] The declaration thus affirms the right of WTO members to use TRIPS flexibilities to protect public health. For example, Article 30 of TRIPS allows exceptions to patents given that they "do not unreasonably conflict with a normal exploitation of the patent and do not unreasonably prejudice the legitimate interests of the patent owner."[136] The United States could argue that the numerous aforementioned benefits of replacing the patent system to "protect public health" and "promote access to medicine for all" are reasonable. Additionally, the billions of dollars in prize funds would sufficiently award patent owners and not unreasonably prejudice their interests to recoup losses and profit off innovations.

Moreover, the United States also boasts the largest economy and military budget.[137] Even if a prize system violated TRIPS, the United States has the power to implement its own domestic agenda and potentially create new international standards for medical patents. Implementation of an alternative to patents could garner significant support from developing countries that struggle to afford patented medical products, and the United States could also use its significant influence to get support from wealthy allied nations. The WTO's own Working Group on Public Health, Innovation and Intellectual Property has suggested alternatives to the patent system, including prize funds.[138] In 2006, Bangladesh directly called for prize funds to replace patents: "We note with great interest a shift in the global policy discussion, away from the status quo of TRIPS compliant patent regimes for medicines and toward new models for rewarding innovation, such as prize funds."[139]

Ultimately, the limitations of a publicly financed prize fund system do not negate its improvements upon the weaknesses of the patent system. R&D incentives would be delinked from monopoly prices and attached to public health benefits. Thus, the model disincentivizes biasing trial designs and weakening evidence, as that would hurt one's chances of winning prize payments. Eligibility criteria for prize payments can include mandatory sharing of research and trial data with the public after regulatory approval, allowing for the advancement of medical knowledge and vetting of trial results. Prize payments for open sharing can further incentivize the free flow of research before regulatory approval. Medical product prices would be significantly lower due to the removal of patent monopolies and the immediate allowance of generic competition following approval.

The weaknesses of the patent system in addition to many of the issues this book discusses—such as lack of trial data transparency and weak standards of evidence—do not just reflect the whole US system. These issues have manifested and significantly affected the most substantial matters of public health in many Americans' lifetimes. In the next chapter, I delve into the case study of COVID-19 and the research, development, and policy rollout of the vaccines. This story positively shows how even within a system with significant weaknesses and limitations, US medical research and development can create products that save many lives relatively quickly. However, it also serves as a cautionary tale that industry is not the only source that can use lack of transparency, weakening standards of evidence, and dishonesty to mislead the public.

# 10

# The COVID-19 Case Study

The COVID-19 pandemic became a lightning rod for public scrutiny of the integrity of medical knowledge and public health institutions. While the numerous areas of concern described in previous chapters preceded COVID-19, the pandemic did demonstrate an exacerbation of several key issues. The US government's collaboration with industry—Operation Warp Speed (OWS)—successfully developed effective vaccines given the emergency. However, vaccine distribution efforts suffered from a legally unnecessary subservience to patent exclusivity rights and lack of data transparency.

These issues did not stop the development of effective, lifesaving vaccines. However, federal policymakers and public health institutions pursued a simplified, one-size-fits-all approach for the vaccine rollout that neglected differences between demographic groups, separating their decisions from the available evidence. Reflecting the weakening of evidence standards, the FDA and other public health officials also pushed a universal vaccine booster program that continuously relied on less evidence at the same time as the danger of COVID-19 decreased. Thus, the pandemic revealed how federal officials—not just industry—can perpetuate unreliability in medical knowledge, thereby fueling public mistrust.

## Public Funding and Private Profit

The COVID-19 vaccines were developed very quickly following the 2019 outbreak of SARS-CoV-2 in China due to both the Trump administration's OWS and decades of prior publicly funded research. On January 31, 2020, HHS secretary Alex Azar declared that the coronavirus outbreak was a public health emergency, and the World Health Organization declared COVID-19 to be a pandemic on March 11, 2020.[1] A few months afterward on May 15, 2020, HHS and DoD launched an interagency partnership to quickly develop, acquire, and distribute medical countermeasures against COVID-19.[2] These efforts largely focused on vaccines.

The federal government had already provided hundreds of millions of dollars to support vaccine development prior to the announcement of OWS. On March 30, 2020, HHS provided $456 million to Johnson & Johnson for development of a COVID-19 vaccine.[3] On April 10, 2020, HHS gave $483 million to support Moderna's own vaccine development program.

OWS significantly expanded upon the federal funding granted to pharmaceutical companies for vaccine development. By March 1, 2021, seven companies had received more than $18.2 billion in federal funding for vaccine development, manufacturing, and distribution.[4] The original goal of such spending was to produce 300 million doses of vaccines and have initial doses available by January 2021.[5]

While vaccine development traditionally takes between five and ten years, OWS successfully propelled development so that Americans began getting vaccinated in under one year.[6] Chinese scientists published the genetic sequence of COVID-19 online on January 11, 2020, and Moderna sent the initial doses of its vaccine to the NIH for testing only a month afterward on February 24.[7] By July 22, DoD and HHS agreed to purchase 100 million doses of Pfizer-BioNTech's vaccine candidate given that it received FDA authorization for being reasonably safe and effective.[8] The government similarly promised to purchase 100 million doses of Moderna's vaccine candidate on August 11, 2020. On December 11 and 18, 2020, the FDA granted emergency use authorizations for the Pfizer and Moderna vaccines. By December 24, over 1 million Americans had received vaccine doses.

However, the swift period that it took to develop COVID-19 vaccines can obscure the decades of publicly/taxpayer-funded research that provided the foundation for industry development of the vaccines. Prior to thc COVID-19 outbreak, the US government provided $336.8 million to fund R&D into the mRNA technologies underlying the main COVID-19 vaccines.[9] Of this money, $148.4 million (44.1 percent) came from the Biomedical Advanced Research and Development Authority (BARDA), $116.4 million (34.6 percent) came from NIH, and $72.0 million (21.4 percent) came from DoD. While BARDA provided a plurality of the funds, NIH provided all the $89.2 million in funding for the basic and translational science behind the mRNA technology. In other words, NIH funded research of the basic processes along with taking those processes and applying them so that they could be turned into treatments. The remaining $247.6 million went toward mRNA vaccine development and trials predating the COVID-19 pandemic.

As recently as 2016, NIH scientists working with academic researchers discovered the exact spike protein technology utilized by the main COVID-19 vaccine makers in the United States, namely Moderna and Pfizer-BioNTech but also J&J and Novavax.[10] Government involvement in vaccine development was especially true for the Moderna vaccine, where NIH scientists helped design and test Moderna's vaccine, and the government accordingly filed two patent applications covering integral vaccine components.[11] Yet, Moderna's patent application for the vaccine only named its own employees as inventors, and the company disputed the role of federal scientists for years.[12] In December 2022, Moderna eventually agreed to compensate NIAID—an institution within NIH—with $400 million in a "catch-up payment" along with promising to pay "low single-digit royalties" to the government for vaccine sales.[13] This payment represented just over 1 percent of the roughly $36 billion in COVID-19 vaccine sales Moderna brought in during 2021 and 2022 alone. In comparison, seven other vaccine makers, such as BioNTech, had already paid NIH to license the government's patented spike protein technology by the end of 2021.[14]

Overall, decades of publicly funded research made the fast development of the COVID-19 vaccines possible. mRNA vaccines work by having the body make proteins that trigger an immune response that protects the body from specific viruses.[15] The COVID-19 mRNA vaccines cause the body to produce a specific protein called a spike protein, which triggers an immune response, trains the body to combat the virus, and ideally prevents severe illness from a future COVID-19 infection. An advantage of the mRNA technology for quickly emerging threats to public health like the COVID-19 pandemic is that vaccines are developed and manufactured faster relative to other types of vaccines.[16]

While the government spent hundreds of millions of dollars on the R&D behind COVID-19 vaccines and billions more to fund their rapid development, manufacturing, and distribution, federal policymakers allowed the pharmaceutical manufacturers to maintain patent monopolies. There was no firm legal barrier stopping OWS from reflecting a version of Baker's contract-based medical R&D system, where the billions in public money would result in vaccines without patent exclusivities that would be immediately subject to competition and be sold at low prices.

Instead, the government agreed to purchase vaccine doses in bulk from the pharmaceutical companies, delivering them billions in profits from products that taxpayers and federal scientists were instrumental in developing. According to former HHS deputy chief of Staff for Policy Paul Mango, "our role was to enable the private sector to be successful."[17] As of March 1, 2021, Pfizer-BioNTech received $5.97 billion to deliver 300 million doses of vaccine, Moderna received $4.94 billion for another 300 million doses along with $954 million for vaccine development, AstraZeneca/Oxford University received $1.2 billion for 300 million doses, J&J received $1 billion for 100 million doses and $456 million for vaccine development, Novavax received $1.6 billion for 100 million doses, and Sanofi/GSK received $2.04 billion for 100 million doses and $30.8 million for vaccine development.[18]

The vast majority of Americans received either the Pfizer-BioNTech or Moderna vaccines. As of April 26, 2023, 96.8 percent of administered COVID-19 vaccine doses in the United States were from these two companies, not counting additional booster doses.[19] Pfizer-BioNTech and Moderna's original vaccines received over $12.1 billion and $9.6 billion in federal funding through 2021, respectively.[20] While it cost Pfizer and Moderna roughly $1.20 and $2.85 to produce a vaccine dose, the government purchased them at around $19.50–$24.60 and $15.25–$16.52 per dose, respectively.[21] The 2022 federal booster shot purchases gave another $3.2 billion to Pfizer ($30.48 per dose) and over $1.7 billion to Moderna ($26.36 per dose).[22] In 2021 and 2022, Pfizer-BioNTech generated $75 billion in sales for its COVID-19 vaccine compared to $36 billion for Moderna.[23]

With immense purchasing power and decades of research funding, the federal government also gave away intellectual property rights. As noted by *The New York Times*, "the government used unusual contracts that omitted its right to take over intellectual property or influence the price and availability of vaccines."[24] Pfizer had the most restrictive contract based on the unredacted portions of the released contracts. Pfizer's OWS contract explicitly provides the company with total ownership of intellectual property for its vaccine, and it explicitly bars the government from using any march-in rights granted under the Bayh-Dole Act.[25] In justification, the contract repeatedly states that the government did not provide funding for the R&D for the vaccine, even though the technology behind the vaccine relied on knowledge discovered through federally funded research. Consequently, after the government supplies of Pfizer and Moderna's vaccines ran out, the companies significantly raised the prices of their shots to between $110 and $130 per dose in 2023—four to nine times greater than the prices for government purchases.[26] Due to the IP protections the federal government granted in contracts, these price hikes were perfectly legal while also preventable.

Along with receiving billions of dollars from taxpayers and then charging significantly higher prices by 2023, companies have further tried to benefit from patent monopolies by suing each other. In 2022, Moderna sued Pfizer and BioNTech for patent infringement, alleging that the two companies had illegally copied its IP, such as Moderna's mRNA chemical modification.[27] Within the same year, Pfizer and BioNTech countersued Moderna.[28] While the USPTO ruled against Moderna in March 2025, the European Patent Office (EPO) upheld the validity of one of the two disputed patents in May 2024.[29] Ultimately, Moderna is seeking to gain a share of the vaccine profits from Pfizer and BioNTech.

While the COVID-19 pandemic represented a global health crisis, the US government did not mandate that the contracted companies provide low-cost access to their products in developing and poorer nations. Until June 2022, developing nations lacked access to COVID-19 vaccines, such as those produced by Pfizer and Moderna, and they were barred from producing their own generic versions under international law.[30] On June 17, the WTO decided to provide a five-year TRIPS waiver, temporarily removing patent exclusivities for inventions necessary to produce COVID-19 vaccines.

Along with IP protections for the vaccine products themselves, the federal government granted Pfizer, Moderna, and other vaccine makers control and ownership over the data from their clinical trials. Thus, while the FDA had access to the underlying data when deciding whether to authorize their use, most independent researchers, doctors, and members of the public could not conduct their own analyses. Such independent access to trial data can be extremely important. In 2020, the NIH appointed an eleven-member Data and Safety Monitoring Board (DSMB) that consisted of independent experts to monitor the then-ongoing clinical trials testing the efficacy and safety of COVID-19 vaccine candidates.[31] The DSMB determined that AstraZeneca cherry-picked and used "outdated information" from their clinical trial when releasing a press release touting their vaccine's efficacy.[32] The company claimed that their vaccine had 79 percent efficacy against symptomatic infection and 100 percent efficacy against severe disease and hospitalization.[33] Despite their claims, the FDA has never authorized the usage of AstraZeneca's vaccine to protect against COVID-19 due to a myriad of issues regarding delays in its US clinical trial and lack of transparency.[34]

In this case, the NIH-appointed body of experts caught misbehavior by AstraZeneca. However, for vaccines meant for usage by hundreds of millions of

Americans and billions of people worldwide, maximizing the number of experts to analyze all the clinical trial data would more fully fit the public interest of transparency. As this book has discussed systemically and with individual cases like Vioxx, independent analyses outside of government can yield previously unknown observations like benefits, trial design limitations, and adverse events—especially in unique populations. Yet, the US government made the active policy choice not to require such data disclosure.

In 2021, researchers in a *BMJ Evidence-Based Medicine* article made the case for data transparency:

> Critical appraisal of clinical trials is vital to inform decision making at the personal, professional and governmental level, but cannot be credibly performed on journal publications alone. Access to clinical trial data and related trial documents … allows for independent and informed assessment of trials. By understanding details of how studies were designed and how data were collected, one can understand if endpoints were reliably operationalised and measured … [it] allows for independent verification of results, assessment of heterogeneity of treatment effects for specific subgroups, and facilitates the formation of new research questions.[35]

These benefits are especially relevant during a period of quick decisions made by government officials because of a serious public health emergency. Independent examination of trial data could catch missed data from expedited product development and regulatory review.

The researchers asserted why the COVID-19 trials specifically should have shared data. For example, because the vaccines are reactogenic—meaning that they cause short-term adverse events—and the placebo groups received a saline solution, they argued that "a thorough analysis of the underlying individual participant data [IPD]" is necessary to ascertain if unofficial unblinding biased results because participants knew they got the vaccine.

Furthermore, federal contracts with the vaccine manufacturers absolve them of almost any liability for potential COVID-19 vaccine injuries barring proof of willful misconduct.[36] In March 2020, HHS secretary Alex Azar protected the pharmaceutical companies from lawsuits by invoking the 2005 Public Readiness and Emergency Preparedness (PREP) Act.[37] While the granted immunity is temporary, the government has amended the PREP Act declaration twelve times; the latest amendment on December 11, 2024, extended the liability shield through December 31, 2029.[38]

This immunity expanded upon the existing protections afforded by the National Childhood Vaccine Injury Act of 1986 that protects vaccine makers from civil lawsuits from vaccine-related injuries or deaths caused by unavoidable side effects or the manufacturers' failure to directly warn patients.[39] At the same time, the federal government granted pharmaceutical companies both guaranteed billions of dollars in public funding via bulk vaccine purchases and patent monopolies. Liability shields, guaranteed profits, and patent monopolies can incentivize companies to hide or downplay negative trial results. Full access to CSRs and de-identified individual participant data would allow independent researchers to identify signals of adverse events caused by each respective vaccine product.

As of June 27, 2021, the *BMJ* researchers found that none of the clinical trials conducted by Pfizer-BioNTech, Moderna, AstraZeneca/Oxford, J&J, Novavax, and others had publicly released their IPD.[40] They listed Pfizer as the only company with publicly available documents from its clinical study report, albeit not the full CSR. Additionally, pre-study data for twelve (50 percent) of the twenty-four examined clinical trials—including trial protocol, statistical analysis plans, and so on—was unavailable. Of the twelve trials with such data available, six only made the protocol available without the statistical analysis plan. By this date, over 179 million people in the United States had received at least one COVID-19 vaccine dose and over 153 million were fully vaccinated.[41]

Additionally, the FDA actively worked in the interest of Pfizer to block the release of underlying data from their clinical trials. On August 23, 2021, the FDA granted full approval to Pfizer-BioNTech's COVID-19 vaccine for those aged sixteen years and older.[42] As the FDA has copies of the clinical trial data for approved vaccines, the nonprofit organization Public Health and Medical Professionals for Transparency (PHMPT) filed a FOIA request for all the roughly 455,000 pages of trial information in response.[43] PHMPT requested expedited processing to start receiving access in a timely manner, but the FDA refused. The agency claimed that it would take seventy-five years to fulfill their request, so the group sued. A federal judge from the US District Court for the Northern District of Texas ruled in 2022 that the FDA had to start releasing documents at a far faster pace: 55,000 pages a month.[44] By the time of the judge's ruling on January 6, 2022, almost 246 million Americans had received at least one COVID-19 vaccine dose, over 207 million were fully vaccinated, and nearly 73 million had received a booster shot.[45]

Another significant dimension to the lack of data transparency for the COVID-19 vaccine clinical trials specifically is the impact on public trust. No official survey has specifically asked Americans a question about clinical trial data transparency, yet polls have shown that the pandemic has shaken trust in public health officials and vaccines. A 2023 American Enterprise Institute (AEI) survey of US adults found that the percentage of respondents expressing trust in scientists and medical scientists fell from 87 percent and 89 percent in 2019 to 69 percent and 75 percent in 2023, respectively.[46] However, the numbers are far worse for government officials. A 2024 Edelman survey found that while 83 percent of Americans trusted their own doctor to tell the truth about health issues, only 39 percent trusted government leaders.[47]

A January 2025 KFF poll found a still significant, but less extreme, disparity with 85 percent of Americans trusting their own doctor compared to trust levels of 66 percent for NIH scientists, 61 percent for the CDC, 55 percent for HHS, 54 percent for CMS, 54 percent for state and local public health officials, and 53 percent for the FDA.[48] Trust in prominent health leaders was low, with 43 percent for the now HHS secretary Robert F. Kennedy Jr. and 53 percent for Anthony Fauci—the NIAID director from 1984 to 2022 and chief medical advisor to the president from 2021 to 2022 (in an earlier 2022

KFF poll).[49] In the 2025 survey, distrust was especially prevalent among Republicans, who had trust levels of 84 percent for their own doctors but just 39 percent for the CDC and FDA. In the AEI poll, 47 percent of adults expressed concern about "adverse health effects of vaccines."[50] This view was especially prevalent among Republicans (67 percent) and Americans with less educational attainment—57 percent and 52 percent for those with at most a high school diploma or some college, respectively.

A 2022 *JAMA Network Open* survey showed American support for general FDA transparency by asking 1,035 adults if they supported ten transparency measures regarding medical trials and products.[51] None of the measures included releasing clinical trial information, but they included disclosing when and under what scientific basis the FDA speeds up a review and how "special safety measures" for certain medications are working. The significant majority of respondents supported all measures with support ranging from nearly two-thirds (65.0 percent) to nine in ten (90.7 percent). Disclosure of the strength of FDA review and safety of medications received 80.5 percent and 83.2 percent support, respectively, showing consistent support for transparency about product safety and effectiveness.

Declining levels of trust and public desire for transparency support that failing to share the underlying data from COVID-19 vaccine trials likely only further fuels distrust. Indeed, in the Texas ruling mandating that the FDA expeditiously release documents from Pfizer's vaccine trial, Judge Mark Pittman wrote that "there may not be a 'more important issue at the Food and Drug Administration … [than] getting every American vaccinated, [and] making sure that the American public is assured that this was not … rush[ed] on behalf of the United States.' "[52]

## The Effective COVID-19 Vaccines

While the first reported American death from COVID-19 took place on February 6, 2020, weekly deaths involving COVID-19 reached as high as 17,201 by April according to death certificate data posted by the CDC's National Center for Health Statistics.[53] The first 100,000 Americans to reportedly die with COVID-19 occurred as early as May, crossing the 200,000 threshold in September. On December 12, the day after the FDA authorized the distribution of Pfizer's vaccine, the CDC reported that 321,531 Americans had died due to COVID-19. Through the winter of 2020–21 when Americans began getting vaccinated but the vast majority of people had not received their first dose, CDC-reported COVID-19 deaths spiked to 487,729 at the end of January and 544,754 around the beginning of March.

Debate exists over the exact accuracy of this death certificate data where some reported deaths due to COVID-19 may rather have been deaths not due to but alongside COVID-19.[54] Others point to potentially substantial undercounting from a failure to track and record all COVID-19-caused deaths.[55] Nonetheless, the death toll was significant.

Given the significant number of deaths, the development of COVID-19 vaccines was expedited, including the clinical trials meant to prove their efficacy and safety along with the FDA review process. The emergency use authorization mechanism allows the FDA to make "medical countermeasures" like vaccines available faster during public health emergencies.[56] The central difference between clinical trials for traditionally approved treatments and those for EUAs is that the former collects more data over a longer period. Johns Hopkins University School of Medicine finds that typical vaccine development that includes phase I, II, and III clinical trials can take five to ten years with two to four years for phase III trials.[57]

Despite a shorter overall process, the clinical trials for COVID-19 vaccines were randomized, placebo-controlled, and officially blinded in addition to including tens of thousands of participants. For example, the *NEJM* published results from Pfizer's phase III clinical trial including around 43,500 participants along with Moderna's phase III trial that had over 30,400 participants.[58]

While there are costs with expedited trials, the pandemic's death toll was significant. Both Pfizer and Moderna's trials only tracked participants for a median period of two months following their last dose, meaning that they could not observe vaccine efficacy and safety for long periods of time. Theoretically, participants injected with either vaccine could suffer long-term adverse events that the trials would not detect. Yet, given hundreds of thousands of reported American deaths, public health officials determined that the benefits of reducing COVID-19 deaths and serious illness outweighed potentially undetected vaccination risks.

Both clinical trial results strongly suggested that the major COVID-19 vaccines had efficacy in fulfilling the primary purpose of vaccination: curbing death and severe illness from the virus. In the *NEJM*'s published accounting of Pfizer's phase III trial results, two doses of the vaccine caused a 95.0 percent relative risk reduction (RRR) of getting any form of symptomatic COVID-19 infection—meaning being infected with the virus and displaying symptoms—for those aged sixteen years or older.[59] While the absolute risk reduction was just 0.84 percent, the total number of people getting infected was low in both groups: 162 people who got placebo and 8 people who got the vaccine. Similarly, Moderna's phase III trial published results showed two vaccine doses led to a 94.1 percent relative risk reduction in symptomatic infection (1.24 percent ARR) compared to placebo for those aged eighteen years or older.[60] The only individuals to get severely infected were in the placebo group. While the ARRs appear low, they estimated that 119 and 81 people needed to receive two doses of Pfizer and Moderna, respectively, to avoid a symptomatic COVID-19 infection over a few months. Thus, if 100 million people got the Pfizer and Moderna shots, the trials predicted around 840,000 and 1.24 million people would avoid symptomatic COVID-19 infection for that period in the pandemic.

Dr. Paul Offit—the director of the Vaccine Education Center at the Children's Hospital of Philadelphia who also coinvented the rotavirus vaccine—was a voting member on the FDA's Vaccines and Related Biological Products Advisory Committee (VRBPAC) in December 2020, which voted to recommend authorization of both the Pfizer and Moderna vaccines.[61] According to Dr. Offit, all committee members "were informed" they could "reasonably recommend" authorization if the vaccines were just 50 percent effective (RRR), and Dr. Fauci predicted that they may be as high as

70 percent effective.[62] Thus, the results far exceeded the expectations of key public health officials.

While the trials' primary endpoint was symptomatic COVID-19 infection, the key takeaway from the results was that the vaccines would likely reduce severe disease and death. In his 2024 book, *Tell Me When It's Over*, Dr. Offit explains that the spread of viruses with long incubation periods—meaning there are at least several weeks between infection and symptom manifestation—can be eliminated by vaccination.[63] In contrast, respiratory viruses such as COVID-19 have relatively short incubation periods—the CDC states two to fourteen days for COVID-19—resulting in the extremely low possibility of stopping mild infection over time.[64] Vaccine- or infection-induced antibodies—which are virus-specific and can protect against mild illness—are short-lasting and may only prevent mild infection for up to around six months. In the aforementioned phase III clinical trials, researchers tracked participants for a median of two months following their second dose to catch any serious safety concerns. During this period, they likely benefited from antibody protection. In comparison, severe illness and death are more so prevented by memory B and T cells that can last for decades. T cells especially remain effective against viral variants that contain similar components of the original strain for which a vaccine was designed to protect against or with which someone was previously infected.[65] Both COVID-19 vaccine trials indeed found fewer cases of severe illness among vaccinated participants, but the total number of cases was small (ten with a 9:1 split in Pfizer-BioNTech's trial and thirty with a 30:0 split in Moderna's trial).[66]

While the phase III RCTs were not designed to directly measure vaccine impact on COVID-19 deaths, observational analyses buttressed their findings on symptomatic infection and demonstrated that unvaccinated individuals were much more likely to be hospitalized or die from COVID-19. In August 2023, *Cureus: Journal of Medical Science* published a meta-analysis of seven studies published from 2020 up to July 2022, including data on over 21.6 million COVID-19 patients.[67] Unvaccinated patients were almost 2.5 times more likely to die from a COVID-19 infection compared to infected patients who had received at least one dose of any COVID-19 vaccine. A September 2022 investigation published in *JAMA Internal Medicine* examined data from January 2021 through April 2022 and similarly found that unvaccinated individuals were several times more likely to be hospitalized compared to vaccinated people.[68]

The vaccines were especially effective in preventing severe disease and death for populations at highest risk of the worst outcomes: the elderly, the immunocompromised, and those with various underlying health conditions.[69] For example, on October 9, 2021, Americans aged sixty-five to seventy-nine who were unvaccinated had a weekly death rate of 52.50 per 100,000 compared to 2.05 of those who were vaccinated.[70] The discrepancy between the unvaccinated and vaccinated death rates shrank to 12.61 compared to 0.54 for those aged fifty to sixty-four, 2.94 to 0.08 for those aged thirty to forty-nine, 0.25 to 0.0 for those aged eighteen to twenty-nine, 0.08 to 0.0 for those aged twelve to seventeen, and 0.1 to 0.0 for those aged five months to four years. While the exact numbers change over time, the smaller difference in death rates between the vaccinated and unvaccinated for younger populations remains. The CDC reported that 80.7 percent of COVID-19 deaths in 2020 occurred in people aged sixty-five and older, and this dynamic has stayed roughly true throughout the pandemic.[71] Regarding severe disease, the discrepancy in COVID-19 hospitalization rates based on vaccination status also decreased with younger age groups.[72]

The immunocompromised—people living with weakened immune systems—had especially high risk of poor COVID-19-related outcomes, making vaccine-reduced risk particularly beneficial. A 2022 CDC report showed that among 22,345 US adults hospitalized for laboratory-confirmed COVID-19 from March 1, 2020, through February 28, 2022, 2,209 (9.9 percent) were immunocompromised, which is over three times greater than their share of the total US population.[73] These immunocompromised patients were significantly more likely to get admitted to the intensive-care unit (ICU) or die from COVID-19 compared to the other studied patients. In 2023, *The Lancet* published a retrospective cohort study of individuals twelve years and older in England over the entirety of 2022.[74] While immunocompromised people only comprised 3.9 percent of the study population, they accounted for 21.9 percent of hospitalizations, 28.4 percent of ICU admissions, and 23.8 percent of COVID-19-related deaths. Around 84 percent of the sampled immunocompromised population had at least three COVID-19 vaccine doses. Thus, the authors concluded that "while vaccines may be sufficient to safeguard most immunocompetent individuals against severe COVID-19," the population still has an enhanced risk from COVID-19.

Another group at enhanced risk of severe disease was overweight and obese individuals. In March 2021, the CDC released a report with data from March to December 2020.[75] Among the 148,494 adults who had received a COVID-19 diagnosis from an emergency department or inpatient hospital visit, nearly four in five (79.1 percent) were obese or overweight with a majority (50.8 percent) being obese. Of the 71,491 people hospitalized (48.1 percent), a similar 78.0 percent were obese or overweight with a majority (50.2 percent) being obese. Among the 8,348 deaths (5.6 percent), 73.3 percent were obese or overweight with almost half (46.0 percent) being obese. These numbers are based on BMI values that do not account for body fat percentage. Thus, the percentages may understate the role of excess fat in increasing severe COVID-19 risk as higher BMIs would also include individuals with more muscle mass.

Correspondingly, a 2022 *Frontiers in Endocrinology* study looked at data for over 450,000 individuals of European ancestry from the UK Biobank and found that body fat mass was significantly associated with severe COVID-19 illness and hospitalization while fat-free mass was not.[76] More specifically, every 9.6 kg (21.2 lb) increase in body fat mass nearly tripled (2.91 times) the risk of severe COVID-19 and more than doubled (2.38 times) the risk of COVID-19-induced hospitalization. The CDC has stated that "obesity may triple the risk of hospitalization due to a COVID-19 infection."[77] As a significant number of Americans are overweight or obese, the COVID-19 vaccines were especially protective for millions of Americans due to their increased risk. The CDC's pre-pandemic survey from 2017 to 2020 found that 41.9 percent of US adults aged twenty years and older and 19.7 percent of children aged two to nineteen were obese.[78] CDC data from 2017 to 2018 found that the age-adjusted percentage of obese and overweight adults (twenty years old and older) was 73.1 percent.[79]

Further underscoring the impact of individual health on COVID-19 risk, the CDC notes physical inactivity also increases the risk of severe COVID-19.[80] This corresponds with a 2021 *British Journal of Sports Medicine* study that examined 48,400 adult patients diagnosed with COVID-19 from January 1, 2020, through October 21, 2020.[81] The researchers found that self-reported consistent physical inactivity more than doubled the risk of hospitalization (2.26 times) and death (2.49 times) compared to those meeting physical activity guidelines. Given that the CDC in 2022 found that a quarter of US adults were "not active enough to protect their health," the vaccines may have been especially important for tens of millions of inactive Americans.

A widely covered instance of breakthrough infections—infections among vaccinated individuals—in the summer of 2021 highlighted both the effectiveness of COVID-19 vaccines against severe disease and their predictable inability to stop infections and transmission.[82] In July 2021, several public gatherings of thousands of people—mostly men—occurred in Provincetown, Massachusetts. During this time, the Delta variant of COVID-19 was extremely prevalent, and 469 people caught COVID-19 from July 3 to 17 in Barnstable County, which contains Provincetown.[83] Of these cases, 346 (73.8 percent) happened in fully vaccinated people, meaning they had received two doses of the Pfizer or Moderna vaccines or one dose of the J&J vaccine. Most infections (274 or 79.1 percent) among vaccinated individuals were symptomatic. While nobody died, five people were hospitalized, four of whom were fully vaccinated. Therefore, while COVID-19 vaccination did not stop symptomatic COVID-19 infection like a literal reading of the clinical trials may have predicted, only 4 (0.1 percent) out of 346 vaccinated people who got COVID-19 were hospitalized. One unvaccinated person (0.8 percent) out of the 123 people with COVID-19 who were unvaccinated, partially vaccinated, or had an unknown vaccinated status were hospitalized. Predictably for a virus with a short incubation period, vaccine-generated memory B and T cells likely protected against severe illness and death while antibodies did not stop infection or transmission.

Overall, the available data strongly supports that the COVID-19 vaccines were effective in preventing severe illness or death for likely millions of Americans.[84] The RCTs backing vaccine approvals were not designed to measure impact on death and much of the aforementioned evidence comes from lower certainty observational studies. However, the randomized trials showed the vaccines conferred protection by temporarily reducing symptomatic infection, the real-world death rate among the unvaccinated was many times greater than for the vaccinated (over sixteen times greater the week of October 9, 2021), and most Americans had a high-risk condition for COVID-19.[85] Accordingly, the vaccines were especially important for the elderly and the significant majority of Americans who were overweight or obese along with the roughly 3 percent of immunocompromised Americans, the quarter of inactive US adults, and others with underlying health conditions.[86]

## The Mandate and Child Vaccination

The benefit of vaccines is that they can train the body to protect itself from infection without the cost of an actual infection. When someone is infected by a virus, their body similarly learns how to protect itself from future infections. This natural immunity, or infection-induced immunity, provides individuals who have had COVID-19 with significant protection from severe illness.[87] For example, a CDC published study examined COVID-19 cases and hospitalizations in California and New York from May through November 2021, although hospitalization data was only available for California.[88] While 11.5 per 1000 unvaccinated people without a previous COVID-19 diagnosis were hospitalized with the virus, the rate was only 0.3 per 1000 for unvaccinated individuals who previously had COVID-19. This was the same rate as previously infected people who had been vaccinated and lower than vaccinated people who had not gotten COVID-19 (0.7 per 1000).

In a March 2023 systematic review and meta-analysis published in *The Lancet*, researchers examined sixty-five observational studies from nineteen countries published up through September 2022 that studied the effect of infection-induced immunity.[89] Their results broadly mirrored the evidence for vaccines, finding that infection-induced immunity gave protection against symptomatic infection that waned after forty weeks (around nine months). This protective effect was weaker and waned faster against newer variants, such as the Omicron variant that spread throughout the United States in early 2022.

At the same time, natural immunity conferred very strong protection against severe disease—defined as hospitalization and death—against all variants including Omicron. The authors concluded that the protective effect of natural immunity "against re-infection, symptomatic disease, and severe disease appears to be at least as durable, if not more so, than that provided by two-dose vaccination with the mRNA vaccines for ancestral, Alpha, Delta, and Omicron BA.1 variants." These results buttressed a 2021 Israeli study that found that natural immunity incurred greater protection against the Delta variant compared to those who got two doses of the Pfizer-BioNTech vaccine.[90] At the same time, the lead author of *The Lancet* study, Dr. Stephen Lim, made clear that vaccination was "the safest way to acquire immunity," as it did not involve the risks of actually getting infected.[91]

On August 23, 2021, the FDA approved the first COVID-19 vaccine, the Pfizer-BioNTech mRNA shot, for everyone aged sixteen years and older.[92] Congressional testimony on June 26, 2024, from Dr. Philip Krause—who served as deputy director of the FDA's Office of Vaccines Research and Review from December 2010 through September 2021—revealed that this approval was allegedly accelerated for political reasons outside of the FDA's official role.[93] Pfizer completed its application for approval on May 16, 2021, so the FDA had to make a final decision under priority review by January 16, 2022. However, Dr. Krause along with OVRR director Dr. Marion Gruber and CBER director Dr. Marks agreed that they could decide by mid-October 2021. Marks requested an even earlier decision date from OVRR, and Gruber and Krause concluded that they could possibly complete the review by September 15.

Marks then pushed for an even earlier decision deadline, resulting in Dr. Gruber highlighting all the required steps and issues for the FDA to address before granting approval based on the proper evaluations of effectiveness and safety. This timeline meant that even a September 15 deadline would prevent internal CBER vaccine testing that was "often performed at CBER before licensure of novel vaccines." The rapid approval would also prevent an FDA advisory committee meeting to discuss vaccine approval, which would have been feasible under the October deadline. In a July 15 email, Gruber told Marks, "it will not be possible to move the ADD [action due date] up further without cutting corners and lowering our review standards and that I would not be able to defend."[94] Dissatisfied with the message, Marks corresponded with acting FDA commissioner Woodcock to take over responsibility of the vaccine review from OVRR. They did so on July 19, removing Gruber and Krause. Krause testified that Woodcock and Marks expressed their desire to approve the Pfizer vaccine because states otherwise would not have been able to mandate vaccination. Krause explained that such a rationale was "completely outside of the purview of FDA" and strongly suggested political pressure from outside the agency "to complete the review more rapidly."[95]

In a September 2021 interview, Dr. Marks did not contradict Krause's testimony that quicker approval was meant to support faster policy action.[96] Marks insisted there was no external pressure driving the approval process; there was "an internal motivation here for those of us at the FDA to save lives," pointing to how COVID-19's deadliness drove his decision-making.

The day after approval of Pfizer-BioNTech's COVID-19 vaccine, the Department of Defense ordered the 2.3 million active and reserve members of the armed forces to get vaccinated, regardless of prior infection or risk level.[97] On September 9, 2021, President Biden similarly ordered vaccination for the 2.1 million civilian federal employees in the executive branch and millions of federal contractors.[98] The executive order stated that it was essential for employees to "take all available steps to protect themselves and avoid spreading COVID-19 to their co-workers and members of the public."

Through an Occupational Safety and Health Administration (OSHA) rule, Biden also required employers with at least one hundred employees to mandate workers get vaccinated or undergo weekly testing for COVID-19, affecting over 80 million workers.[99] Employers who did not comply would be subject to a $14,000 fine per violation. On November 4, CMS mandated vaccination for 17 million health care workers employed at hospitals and other institutions that got Medicare or Medicaid reimbursements.[100] *The New York Times* reported that Biden's mandates would cover two-thirds of the US workforce.[101] Announcing the moves on September 9, President Biden stated:

> This is not about freedom or personal choice. It's about protecting yourself and those around you—the people you work with, the people you care about, the people you love … We're going to protect vaccinated workers from unvaccinated co-workers.[102]

September 2021 was several months after the Provincetown breakthrough infection cases. Therefore, evidence showed that vaccinated individuals were still able to catch and transmit COVID-19. When infected, vaccination protected them against severe disease. This outcome matched previously recognized realities of vaccines for respiratory viruses with short incubation periods: they are meant to prevent severe disease, not mild illness and transmission. Vaccination would not eliminate COVID-19 circulation, meaning that most people would still get exposed to the virus.

By September 9, 2021, around 208 million Americans had received at least one COVID-19 vaccine dose, with over 177 million being fully vaccinated.[103] Most children had not yet been authorized to get a vaccine, while all adults were. Three-quarters (75.3 percent) of adults had at least one vaccine dose, while 64.5 percent completed their primary series—meaning one or two doses depending on the specific vaccine.

There had been around 40 million confirmed COVID-19 cases in the United States by September 9.[104] However, this is likely an underestimate as confirmed cases do not count people who got COVID-19 and were not hospitalized or did not otherwise report cases. Accounting for overlap between those who got vaccinated and those who got infected, many of the roughly 92 million eligible American adults who were not fully vaccinated and 64 million who were unvaccinated likely had infection-induced immunity.[105] Even though antibody/serology testing can detect people with previous infections, federal officials did not measure this phenomenon.[106]

While employers could allow unvaccinated individuals to get tested weekly, many states and private employers subsequently chose to impose their own mandates. By October 2021, over 1,900 Washington state workers quit or were fired due to vaccine mandates, and thousands of workers in New York City lost their jobs in 2021–22 due to the city's mandates for public and private employers.[107] Large companies like Citigroup, Google, United Airlines, and more announced they would fire unvaccinated employees.[108] Over 1,100 universities had some form of vaccine mandate for students and/or staff.[109] Many federal workers lost employment due to the mandate as well, including around 8,000 discharged military service members.[110]

The Supreme Court in *National Federation of Independent Business v. OSHA* (2022) ultimately struck down OSHA's rule requiring large employers to make their workers get vaccinated or test weekly under the rationale that the rule overstepped its legal authority.[111] Several lawsuits tied up the mandate for federal contractors nationwide until August 2022, and in various states thereafter due to court-issued injunctions.[112] Litigation similarly tied up the federal employee mandate from January 2022 through May 2023, but 93 percent of federal employees had already gotten at least one vaccine dose by January according to the Biden administration.[113] The vaccine mandates did go into effect for health care workers working at institutions that got Medicare/Medicaid reimbursements. The Biden administration later ended its remaining vaccine mandates in May 2023, citing significant declines in COVID-19 deaths and hospitalizations compared to 2021.[114]

In 2004, C-SPAN host Peter Slen asked NIAID director Dr. Anthony Fauci whether a woman who had the flu for fourteen days needed a flu vaccine, and he responded:

> Well no. If she got the flu for 14 days, she's as protected as anybody can be because the best vaccination is to get infected yourself … if she really has the flu, she

> definitely doesn't need a flu vaccine ... she doesn't need it ... the most potent vaccination is getting infected yourself.[115]

However, in an October 2021 CNN appearance, Dr. Fauci—who was then the chief medical advisor to President Biden—supported the vaccine mandate that made no exceptions for those with prior COVID-19 infection, including in low-risk populations.[116]

Federal policymakers' decision to mandate vaccination regardless of natural immunity was divorced from their chosen experts' advice and evidence on protection.[117] Dr. Offit was one of "a handful of immunologists, virologists, and vaccine experts" aiding CDC, NIH, and Biden administration officials to determine whether to count natural infection as a form of vaccination. He described the meeting as ending in a "split decision." People were split on letting natural immunity count, where he supported letting infection satisfy mandated vaccination. Three of the four experts supported counting natural immunity as at least one dose, but the administration overruled them.[118] Dr. Offit noted retrospectively, "it would have been reasonable not to mandate vaccination for people who had been previously infected, especially considering they might be barred from work for refusing vaccination. But hindsight is always 20/20."

The reasoning against counting natural infection included that thousands of Americans were dying from COVID-19 every week, vaccination could further boost natural immunity, people might fake a previous infection, and providing proof of immunity was an "administrative hurdle at a time when existing bureaucracy already overwhelmed many."[119] None of these reasons included evidence that people with infection-induced immunity required extra protection against COVID-19 or threatened others, and the tools existed to test for infection-induced protection. The meeting with outside experts took place after President Biden had issued his vaccine mandate. Thus, federal policy was made without supporting evidence regarding natural immunity nor deliberations with the expert advisors that considered the topic.

## Child Vaccination

While the FDA only authorized COVID-19 vaccination for those sixteen years old and above by the end of 2020, the agency issued an EUA permitting the Pfizer-BioNTech vaccine for children twelve to fifteen years old in May 2021.[120] On October 29, the FDA expanded this authorization to children five to eleven years old.[121] The CDC recommended that children aged twelve to fifteen and five to eleven years get vaccinated soon after each authorization.[122] Consequently, Louisiana, California and the District of Columbia (DC) announced plans to mandate vaccines for kids following full FDA approval.[123] However, none of them implemented their mandates, removing them in May 2022, February 2023, and November 2023, respectively.[124] Yet, smaller and more localized mandates did take place. For example, Hawaii required that high school athletes get vaccinated to participate in sports in August 2021.[125] Additionally, seventeen states successfully instituted bans on COVID-19 vaccine mandates for schools by November 2021, such as Texas, Florida, Michigan, Ohio, Arizona, and New Hampshire.[126]

The evidence underlying FDA emergency authorizations for children was weaker compared to the traditional approval process and the RCTs backing vaccine authorization for adults.[127] The clinical trial for five- to eleven-year-olds included 4,700 participants—a sample size too small to catch adverse events with risks of 1 in 5,000, which was the FDA's October 2021 calculated risk of vaccine-induced myocarditis (heart inflammation) for twelve- to fifteen-year-old boys.[128] The trial tested the impact of two doses of the Pfizer vaccine on antibody levels against COVID-19, and it tracked 4,600 participants for at least two months after their second dose. There were no cases of severe illness, hospitalization, or death.[129] Regarding such rare, severe outcomes, the FDA used its own assumption-based model to predict that the vaccine's benefits would outweigh its risks.[130] Yet, the model assumed myocarditis and pericarditis risk rates from a different age group (twelve- to fifteen-year-olds). Additionally, the clinical trial did not test for an impact on transmission, meaning it was not designed to test if vaccinating children would protect third parties.

The data backing the FDA's authorization for twelve- to fifteen-year-olds had smaller sample sizes. The agency determined effectiveness because the immune responses of 170 twelve- to fifteen-year-olds were at least as good as those of 190 sixteen- to twenty-five-year-olds following vaccination.[131] The FDA admitted, "data are not available to determine how long the vaccine will provide protection." The agency also examined randomized trial data in which zero out of roughly 1,100 vaccinated kids got COVID-19 compared to sixteen out of roughly 1,100 who got placebo. There were no reported cases of severe illness or death.[132] The FDA also admitted, "there are limited data to address whether the vaccine can prevent transmission of the virus from person to person." For safety, the agency reviewed several months of tracking data from the trial's 2,260 twelve- to fifteen-year-olds—a sample size too small to detect the age group's 1 in 5,000 risk of vaccine-induced myocarditis. Additionally, Pfizer allegedly hid a vaccine-caused severe adverse event for one twelve-year-old girl that left her wheelchair-bound and reliant on a feeding tube.[133]

Section 564 of the FD&C Act permits the FDA to issue an EUA for an unapproved product during a public health emergency given several conditions. The "totality of scientific evidence" must reasonably indicate that the product may be effective in treating a serious or life-threatening disease or condition and "there is no adequate, approved, and available alternative to the product for diagnosing, preventing, or treating such disease or condition."[134] Additionally, the product's "known and potential benefits" must "outweigh the known and potential risks."

Throughout the entirety of the pandemic, the monthly COVID-19 death rates for zero- to nine-year-olds and ten- to nineteen-year-olds have been less than 0.1 per 100,000 (cumulative rate of 0.3 per 100,000 from 2020 to mid-2024).[135] From May to October 2021, the monthly COVID-19 hospitalizations for zero- to nine-year-olds and ten- to nineteen-year-olds both ranged from one to seven per 100,000.[136] According to the CDC in March 2021, five- to seventeen-year-olds were half as likely to get COVID-19 as most older age groups, and significantly less likely to be hospitalized or die.[137] For example, 65- to 74-year-olds were 1,300 times more likely to die and 40 times more likely to be hospitalized than five- to seventeen-year-olds. A 2022 German analysis published in the *European Journal of Pediatrics* examined severe illness in children prior to vaccination from June 2020 through May 2021.[138] The researchers concluded that the severe disease and death burden of COVID-19 was low, and that this was "particularly the case for 5–11"-year-olds without comorbidities, and the risk of death for all children without comorbidities was 3 in 1,000,000.[139] While low, hospitalizations and deaths did occur among children—namely those with underlying conditions—leading figures like Dr. Offit to support widespread vaccination.[140] Yet, FDA and CDC actions did not specifically target the higher-risk groups more likely to benefit from vaccination.

Due to the extremely low risk of severe COVID-19 illness to children between the ages of five and fifteen, the EUA compared to traditional approval may not have been justified for the vast majority of children without serious underlying health conditions.[141] In September 2021, the UK's Joint Committee on Vaccination and Immunisation (JCVI) did not recommend healthy twelve- to fifteen-year-olds get the COVID-19 vaccine due to the relatively low benefits and the known risk of myocarditis.[142] The UK's chief medical officers (CMOs) overruled the JCVI, recommending that twelve- to fifteen-year-olds get a single dose of vaccine compared to the FDA's allowance of two doses.[143] The lead CMO Chris Whitty called the choice a "difficult decision" not to be seen as a "silver bullet" or quick solution. Making the shot available was based on the combination of reducing school disruption and a marginal health benefit. Whitty emphasized that the CMOs' decision was to extend an "offer" rather than a requirement. In February 2022, the JCVI advised "a non-urgent offer of two … doses" of the Pfizer-BioNTech vaccine for healthy five- to eleven-year-olds.[144] The "non-urgent" offer sharply contrasts with the FD&C Act's emergency requirements for an EUA along with the CDC's decision to recommend child vaccination regardless of differences in risk, such as whether a child was healthy or obese.

## There Is Never No Risk

While overall very effective, the COVID-19 vaccines—like nearly all treatments—were not without risk, and adverse events were especially prevalent in populations at low risk of severe illness from COVID-19. By February 2021, public reports had begun to document heart inflammation or myocarditis in young men that was induced by the mRNA vaccines and that required hospitalization.[145] By October 2021, Finland, Norway, and Sweden had suspended the use of the Moderna vaccine for males below the age of thirty.[146] According to June 2021 data available to the CDC's Advisory Committee on Immunization Practices (ACIP), the absolute risk of myocarditis following a second mRNA vaccine dose was one case for every 15,000–20,000 males aged twelve to twenty-four.[147]

Published in the *European Journal of Clinical Investigation* (*EJCI*), a 2022 systematic review of studies examined vaccine-induced myocarditis in young men. The authors concluded that the disease was "a rare but significant adverse event associated with COVID-19 vaccination, especially for men under 40."[148] While most studies note that the myocarditis risk from a COVID-19 infection is far greater than that from vaccination, this did not hold true when examining the second mRNA vaccine dose for young men specifically. The risk of myocarditis was rare but relatively high for men under the age of forty after receiving their second vaccine dose, especially from the Moderna product but also from Pfizer's shot.[149] One 2022 analysis in the American Heart Association's journal *Circulation* estimated that the myocarditis risk for men under forty years old after a second Moderna vaccine dose was six times greater than that from COVID-19 without vaccination.[150] Yet, this age group is broad, as the risk was highest for men aged twelve to twenty-four. The *EJCI* authors also reasoned that the risk of infection-induced myocarditis in studies "may be inflated and inaccurate" due to undercounting of COVID-19 cases.[151]

In April 2021, federal officials found the Johnson & Johnson vaccine to have a rare but serious side effect for women between the ages of eighteen and forty-eight: cerebral venous sinus thrombosis (CVST).[152] CVST is a type of blood clot that can cause seizures and death. This side effect also occurred in recipients of AstraZeneca's vaccine, although the shot was not authorized in the United States. Six reported cases of CVST included one death and another individual in critical condition. Consequently, the FDA and CDC briefly paused use of the J&J vaccine for a safety review, lifting it after ten days due to benefits outweighing risks.[153] The FDA also found the J&J vaccine to rarely cause a neurological disorder called Guillain-Barré syndrome (GBS) that can cause paralysis and permanent nerve damage.[154] Thus, the FDA attached a warning to the shot's fact sheet in July 2021 to account for both blood clots and GBS.[155] In December 2021, the CDC's ACIP recommended deprioritizing the J&J product compared to the mRNA vaccines.[156] In May 2022, the FDA restricted usage of the J&J vaccine to those eighteen and older who could not or would choose not to access other vaccines.[157] At that time, J&J had administered 18.7 million doses in the United States compared to over 550 million for Moderna and Pfizer.[158] J&J voluntarily withdrew its vaccine from the US market in May 2023 due in part to "no demand for new lots of the vaccine."[159]

In April 2024, *Vaccine* published the largest cohort study examining adverse events to date, including 99 million vaccinated individuals across eight countries.[160] Based on the individuals' electronic health records, they examined thirteen adverse events of special interest based on known safety signals—meaning observed adverse events suspected to be caused by the vaccines—from the Pfizer-BioNTech, Moderna, and AstraZeneca vaccines before and after vaccination. For the Pfizer and Moderna mRNA vaccines, the analysis found that they significantly increased the risk of the cardiovascular problems of myocarditis and pericarditis—inflammation of the sac surrounding the heart—after the first and second doses. Following the second dose of the Moderna shot, the risk of myocarditis was 6.1 times greater compared to baseline risks. These estimates likely undercount the risk of adverse cardiovascular events in young males given that the analysis did not stratify by age. The authors identified other statistically significant safety signals from the two mRNA vaccines, including but not limited to thrombocytopenia (low blood platelet levels), pulmonary embolism, splanchnic vein thrombosis (a form of blood clotting), and Bell's palsy. Overall and especially regarding the non-cardiovascular adverse events, the risks existed but were very rare.

As previously noted, natural/infection-induced immunity conferred significant protection against COVID-19, including severe illness, at a level potentially greater than vaccination. Additionally, data from a January 2022 *NEJM* analysis indicated that one dose of Pfizer or Moderna's mRNA vaccines could provide between roughly 85 percent and over 95 percent effectiveness against both hospitalization and death over the course of a month.[161] Thus, rare but known serious adverse events weighed more heavily for populations at low risk of serious COVID-19 complications—such as young people, healthy individuals, those previously infected, and/or people who received only a single mRNA vaccine dose.

While adverse events from the vaccines were rare, they could add to the risk from infection—rather than one substituting for the other—due to the inability of the vaccines to prevent infection and the absence of evidence of vaccination preventing transmission. For example, the American Heart Association in August 2022 wrote that the risk of vaccine-induced myocarditis was lower than infection-induced myocarditis but higher for men under forty receiving a second Moderna dose.[162] Yet, the risk from COVID-19 infection may add to the risk from vaccination for someone already at low risk and protected against severe illness (by vaccination or previous infection). For specifically a low-risk person with natural immunity, they may face the added risk of vaccine side effects. Nonetheless, federal officials did not recognize such nuance in their mandatory vaccination policy. Additionally, the FDA and CDC used data mining and statistics that potentially understated signals of rare vaccine risks, according to the inventor of such mining and statistical methods.[163]

Based on how the government funded the original trials and ultimately authorized and/or approved all products, federal policymakers had the power to require additional RCTs to gather evidence for the efficacy and safety of each vaccine dose for different demographic groups. The clinical trials that led to initial vaccine authorizations in the United States did not stratify by age, rather they examined all age groups except for most or all children. Considering that COVID-19 predominantly hospitalized and killed older Americans, the government could have required vaccine manufacturers to conduct additional trials for younger age groups with more participants and which lasted longer than a few months, as this group did not face the same severe danger as the elderly.

Protecting others was a major rationale underlying vaccine mandates; yet, the COVID-19 vaccine clinical trials tracked symptomatic infection but did not study transmission. According to epidemiologist and future CBER director Dr. Vinay Prasad, clinical trials could have studied transmission through examining the infection rates of people around participants.[164] Contrary to President Biden's claim about protecting the vaccinated from the unvaccinated, people who were vaccinated had robust protection from severe illness and death. Ultimately, federal policymakers chose not to use their authority to compel trials testing transmission, leaving the mandate impacting millions of Americans without a strong scientific foundation.

Given the public health emergency, millions of Americans benefited from the COVID-19 vaccines through preventing severe illness and death, especially among high-risk groups: the elderly, immunocompromised, overweight/obese, physically inactive, and others with underlying health conditions. Thus, the vaccines saved lives. However, one-size-fits-all federal vaccine policy did not follow the nuances of the evidence, and officials chose not to compel strong randomized trials for key areas of public health importance, such as vaccination of low-risk children and adults along with transmission.

## The Evidence-Notwithstanding Universal Booster Campaign

While the federal government did not strictly follow the evidence in the original vaccination campaign in 2021, its policies led to the fast creation of a vaccine that likely saved hundreds of thousands of American lives and millions globally.[165] However, the Biden administration pursued a universal booster campaign beginning in 2021 that increasingly relied on less evidence and caused net harm to low-risk subpopulations, such as young, healthy males. Federal leaders and public health officials also made unsubstantiated claims that industry could not legally make for medical products.

On August 18, five days before the FDA's August 23 approval of Pfizer-BioNTech's vaccine for those sixteen years and older, President Biden announced that the government would start offering COVID-19 booster shots (additional vaccine doses to "boost" immunity) by September 20 of that year for fully vaccinated adults.[166] Top public health officials backed this decision, such as acting FDA commissioner Janet Woodcock, CDC director Rochelle Walensky, NIH director Francis Collins, Biden's chief medical officer and NIAID director Anthony Fauci, and the chief science officer for the COVID-19 response and former FDA commissioner David Kessler.[167] Biden and these top officials made their decision prior to any FDA authorization or recommendations made by FDA or CDC advisory committees. According to former senior vaccine official Dr. Krause in his congressional testimony:

> While the announcements said that boosting would be subject to FDA and CDC review, setting a one-month deadline for an application that hasn't been received and for which data seemed very equivocal created the impression of pressure to achieve a certain outcome. Moreover, Dr. Woodcock was among those making the announcement, and she and Dr. Marks had already made it clear what would happen if anybody disagreed with her.[168]

In his remarks, Biden said: "You know, this shot will boost your immune response. It will increase your protection from COVID-19. And it's the best way to protect ourselves from new variants that could arise."[169] However, the original COVID-19 vaccines induced long-term protection against severe disease, and the risks of COVID-19 were especially low for younger and healthier Americans. Dr. Offit—who sat on the relevant FDA advisory committee—related that administration officials justified their decision by saying, "wait until you see the data coming out of Israel. Then you'll understand."[170]

The relevant Israeli study was observational, not an RCT or any other tightly controlled analysis.[171] The researchers examined Israelis aged sixty years and older and compared results of those who chose to get and not to get a third dose of the Pfizer-BioNTech vaccine after the Israeli government made them available. According to Dr. Offit, a central takeaway that the FDA advisory committee, VRBPAC, took from the study pertained to the 70- to 79-year-old group—representing three quarters of the study population. Around 7.5 percent of those who were unboosted and had a confirmed infection developed severe COVID-19 illness compared to 1.3 percent of those who got the booster.[172] However, the study defined severe illness as an elevated resting respiratory rate and low oxygen levels rather than hospitalization or death, differing from the United States' definition.[173]

While the difference was statistically significant, the analysis assumed that the population getting the booster was the same as the one that did not. Yet, this is not a scientifically valid assumption. As Dr. Offit explained, "it is likely that those who chose to be boosted were more attentive to their general health, more likely to wear masks and social distance, and less likely to engage in activities that put them at higher risk of Covid."[174] Confounding factors are why the FDA would not have authorized the original COVID-19 vaccines based on observational data rather than RCTs. Additionally, the study examined those aged sixty years and older, and the vast majority of the study population was at least seventy-five years old. Thus, the Israeli study did not back the Biden administration's decision to boost all adults.

Prior to the FDA advisory committee's vote, then-OVRR director Marion Gruber—a twenty-nine-year FDA veteran and director from 2011 to 2021—and then-deputy director Phil Krause resigned over White House political pressure for a near-universal booster policy.[175] In their September 2021 published article in *The Lancet*, Krause, Gruber, and their coauthors summarized the available studies they deemed relevant to boosting policy.[176] Like the Israeli study's weaknesses, they found that the observational studies backing boosting were "preliminary and difficult to interpret precisely due to potential confounding and selective reporting." They concluded that vaccinations continued to provide protection against severe disease, and "even if boosting were eventually shown to decrease the medium-term risk of serious disease, current vaccine supplies could save more lives if used in previously unvaccinated populations than if used as boosters in vaccinated populations."

While the White House campaigned for boosting all adults based on the Israeli data, the VRBPAC voted 16–2 against recommending authorization of a third dose of Pfizer vaccine for all Americans aged sixteen and older.[177] The committee unanimously voted to recommend authorization of boosters for Americans aged sixty-five and older and others at high risk for severe COVID-19. Without voting, the members also supported boosters for health care workers and others at high risk for exposure at their jobs. On September 22, the FDA provided an EUA for a third dose of the Pfizer-BioNTech vaccine in line with the advisory committee's official and unofficial recommendations for adults.[178]

Later in September 2021, the CDC's advisory committee, ACIP, unanimously voted to recommend Pfizer booster doses for those aged sixty-five and older along with adults residing in long-term care facilities and people aged fifty to sixty-four years with certain underlying medical conditions.[179] It deviated from the FDA's emergency authorization by not recommending people in high-risk jobs get a booster. However, CDC director Walensky overrode the advisory committee and backed booster shots for workers in jobs that the government deemed to be high risk for COVID-19 infection.[180] Walensky argued that her decision "best serve[d] the nation's public health needs" and was aligned with the FDA authorization.[181] Contrastingly, *The New York Times* reported that political pressures may have pushed Walensky to override the committee.[182] Dean of Brown University School of Public Health and future COVID-19 response coordinator Dr. Ashish Jha stated, "there's a complexity here, because Dr. Walensky was part of the White House announcement" that revealed Biden's plan to boost all adults.

In November 2021, the FDA de facto overrode its advisory committee's previous vote by expanding the authorization for booster doses from either Pfizer or Moderna to everyone eighteen years old and above.[183] The FDA did not consult their advisory committee and no RCTs backed this decision; rather, the evidence base consisted of the observational analyses previously described in *The Lancet* and antibody response data. In *The Washington Post*, Drs. Gruber, Krause, and Offit asserted, "the data simply does not show that every healthy adult should get a booster."[184] Adults, especially young adults, who received the first two doses were still strongly protected against severe disease and hospitalization. They wrote, "a healthy young person with two mRNA vaccine doses is extremely unlikely to be hospitalized with covid, so the case for risking any side effects—such as myocarditis—diminishes substantially." Rather than further vaccinating already-protected populations, they pushed federal officials to focus on increasing vaccine uptake among the unvaccinated.

The CDC followed the FDA on November 29, 2021, expanding its recommendations: "Everyone ages 18 and older should get a booster shot either when they are 6 months after their initial Pfizer or Moderna series or 2 months after their initial J&J vaccine."[185] In December 2021, the FDA further expanded the booster authorization to include sixteen- to seventeen-year-olds.[186] The agency again did not consult its advisory committee. In a subsequent response published in *The Washington Post*, Krause criticized the Biden administration for making "important decisions on vaccines without consulting independent panels of experts."[187] At the beginning of January 2022, the FDA authorized the Pfizer-BioNTech booster for all twelve- to fifteen-year-old children, including healthy kids. [188] By the end of the month, the FDA gave full approval for Moderna's vaccine for all adults.[189] On May 17, the agency further expanded emergency authorization for the Pfizer-BioNTech booster to all five- to eleven-year-olds.[190] Following each decision, the CDC recommended that all the authorized populations get a booster.[191]

The rapid expansion of booster authorizations and recommendations occurred as the Omicron variant of COVID-19 began to surge in the United States. Omicron was very contagious and evasive of any potential protection against mild illness from previous vaccinations. There were nearly 564,000 new weekly confirmed COVID-19 cases in the United States on December 1, 2021, spiking to almost 5.7 million weekly cases on January 17, 2022.[192] This is still the high point of weekly new COVID-19 cases since the pandemic began. More hospitalizations and deaths followed the cases. On December 1, 2021, there were nearly 46,700 new people in a hospital with COVID-19 every week; this number shot up to the pandemic peak of around 150,000 by mid-January.[193] Roughly 6,000 people died per week by December 1, 2021, increasing to around 15,000 by mid-January and over 19,000 by early-February.[194] This was the second deadliest point of the pandemic (the first was the previous winter). However, these spikes all fell by March–April and have never risen similarly since. By April 2022, weekly cases, new weekly hospitalizations, and weekly deaths plummeted to around 190,000, 11,000, and 4,600, respectively (See Figure 12).

The Omicron surge did not hurt the US population equally across demographic groups. Americans aged sixty-five and older dominated COVID-19 deaths during the Omicron wave.[195] In January 2022, 73.5 percent of the over 84,000 deaths involving COVID-19 were people aged sixty-five and older, 19.4 percent were fifty to sixty-four years old, 4.3 percent were forty to forty-nine years old, 1.8 percent were thirty to thirty-nine years old, 0.7 percent were eighteen to twenty-nine years old, and 0.2 percent were zero to seventeen years old.[196] These numbers do not differentiate whether individuals were obese/overweight, immunocompromised, inactive, or had any other underlying health condition. Unvaccinated people also disproportionately died. The death rates in January for boosted adults aged sixty-five and older and those vaccinated with no booster were 7 and 24 per 100,000, respectively, while the rate was 156 per 100,000 for the unvaccinated.[197]

For the vast majority of the population, vaccination without boosters, natural immunity, or some combination of the two still conferred significant protection against severe disease.[198] Also, while Omicron was very contagious, it was not as deadly as Delta.[199] As Dr. Offit explained, vaccination would not eliminate respiratory viruses with short incubation periods; rather, it would protect against severe illness and death.

Based on FDA authorizations and CDC recommendations, many universities required that all students be fully vaccinated—two mRNA doses or one dose of the J&J vaccine—and boosted.[200] Yet, in December 2021, the *NEJM* published Israeli data including almost 4.7 million people aged sixteen and above, finding ten cases of severe COVID-19 illness and no deaths among unboosted people aged sixteen to twenty-nine years with two vaccine shots.[201] Simultaneously, multiple analyses and foreign governments recognized an increased risk of heart inflammation for young adults, particularly men.[202]

A 2022 risk benefit analysis published in the BMJ's *Journal of Medical Ethics* found that COVID-19 booster mandates at universities "may result in a net harm to healthy young adults."[203] Examining young adults aged eighteen to twenty-nine, the authors estimated that for every hospitalization prevented, third-dose booster shots yielded 18.5 serious adverse events, 1.5–4.6 myopericarditis cases in males that usually require hospitalization, and 1,430–4,626 cases of reactogenicity at or below grade 3 that interfere with daily activities but do not usually require hospitalization.

Contrary to the argument that boosters were necessary to reduce transmission, the authors in the BMJ's *Journal of Medical Ethics* found that the third-dose booster, "at most," yielded only a transient and partial protection against infection that has limited secondary effects regarding transmission.[204] No RCTs had tested the boosters' effect on

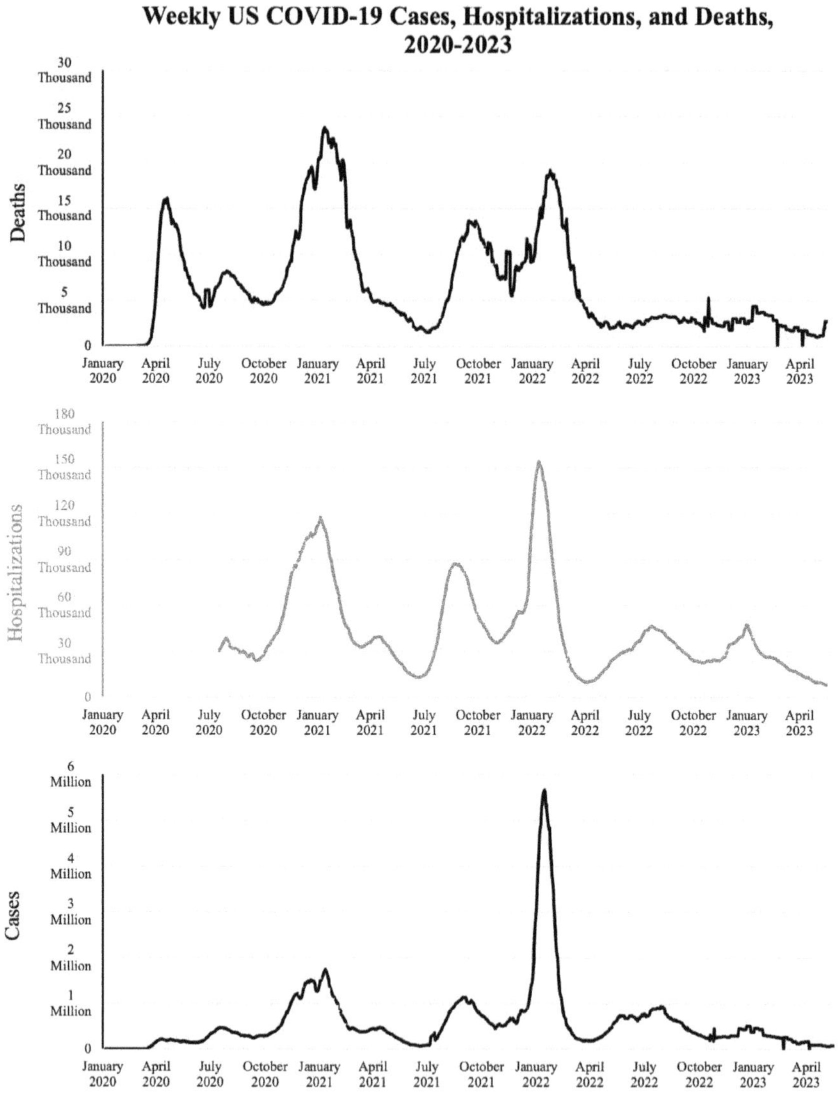


**Figure 12** Charts showing the changes in weekly confirmed COVID-19 cases, new hospital admissions, and confirmed deaths—including the spikes during the rise of the Omicron variant. Note that the hospitalization data begins in July 2020 due to a lack of earlier data. *Source*: Our World in Data, "COVID-19," Individual Datasets for Cases and Deaths & Hospitalizations, OWID's Technical Documentation, https://docs.owid.io/projects/etl/api/covid/.

transmission, and no analysis found significant, long-lasting reductions in infection. Thus, the authors noted that "repeated doses appear to provide diminishing benefits (in terms of reduced infection) per dose, especially among young adults."

On June 17, 2022, the FDA issued an EUA, allowing children as young as six months through four years to receive either the Pfizer-BioNTech or Moderna vaccines.[205] The agency also allowed all children above the age of six months to get the Moderna vaccine, as it had previously only been authorized for adults. Subsequently on June 18, the CDC agreed with its advisory committee and recommended that the nearly 20 million children between the ages of six months through five years get a COVID-19 vaccine.[206] The FDA determined efficacy of the Moderna vaccine for all age groups based on comparing antibody levels following vaccination of a few hundred young children to a similar number of young adults. Additionally, RCTs found that Moderna's shot had 50.6 percent and 36.8 percent relative efficacy against laboratory-confirmed infection for those aged six to twenty-three months and two to five years, respectively.[207] But, efficacy fell to 28.5 percent for two- to five-year-olds when including home testing. Relative efficacy was much higher for twelve- to thirteen-year-olds (93.3 percent), but this data was based on less-transmissible pre-Omicron strains. The Pfizer authorization was only based on antibody level comparisons between groups of a few hundred children and young adults, as the FDA deemed another COVID-19 case analysis "not to be reliable due to the low number of COVID-19 cases that occurred in study participants."[208] The same was true for Moderna's data for six- to eleven-year-olds. Safety analyses for both vaccines were based on populations of 3,000 or fewer participants.

An April 2022 CDC report based on national survey data found that by February 2022, around three quarters of all children had gotten COVID-19.[209] Yet, as epidemiologists Drs. Vinay Prasad and Alyson Haslam identified, the FDA relied upon studies that "included very few children" who previously had COVID-19.[210] Thus, the analyses did not factor in high levels of infection-induced immunity relevant when determining if emergency authorization rather than traditional approval was appropriate.

At the end of June 2022, Pfizer and Moderna presented evidence to the FDA's VRBPAC for new bivalent boosters designed to target not only the original COVID-19 strain but new variants.[211] VRBPAC member Dr. Offit explained that the data only showed increases in neutralizing antibodies that were "unlikely to be clinically significant." However, due to a sense of urgency around "immune-evasive strains" and the upcoming winter, the committee voted in favor of authorizing bivalent vaccines.[212]

When presenting evidence to the VRBPAC, Moderna and government scientists presented immunogenicity data (i.e., antibody levels) and intentionally omitted data that looked at actual infections.[213] While the actual data suffered from limitations (e.g., lack of blindness to treatment), it demonstrated that people who got the original booster had a lower COVID-19 infection rate than those who got the bivalent booster (1.9 percent to 3.2 percent). In January 2023, VRBPAC member Dr. Eric Rubin said that we're "not a group of children. We understand how to interpret these results." Fellow member Dr. Offit reacted, "you can't do this … It shook my faith in how these decisions were being made."

The FDA authorized both companies' bivalent boosters at the end of August 2022.[214] The agency authorized Pfizer's shot for those twelve years old and older and Moderna's shot for adults. Yet, neither company's data specifically for the new boosters came from humans; they were each based on immunogenicity data from eight to ten mice.[215] For human data, the FDA relied on studies of previous mRNA shots and investigational/unapproved BA.1-targeted vaccines (the bivalent boosters targeted the BA.4 and BA.5 lineages).

In advance of the agency's decision, FDA director Robert Califf tweeted: "Being vaccinated and boosted reduces your risk of dying or getting critically ill and going to the hospital. The updated booster also increases your chances of being in attendance at upcoming gatherings with family and friends."[216] However, he had no hard evidence to support his claims. In September 2022, the CDC agreed with its advisory committee, recommending that all Americans aged twelve and older get a bivalent booster shot (commonly the fourth recommended vaccine dose).[217] Following FDA authorizations, the agency extended this recommendation to everyone five years old and above the next month.[218] For children as young as six months, the FDA authorized and CDC recommended Moderna's and Pfizer's bivalent vaccines in December 2022, expanding the EUA to include booster doses for the age group in March and April 2023.[219]

In September 2022, Dr. Offit revealed that he would not get the new booster "until it is clear that people who have been primed, boosted, and naturally infected are nonetheless at high risk of serious illness when encountering the virus."[220] He also stated that the products were "grossly oversold" by advocates; such efforts to push the vaccine were led by government officials.[221]

The CDC and the White House misled the public and experts on the FDA's VRBPAC regarding the benefits of the bivalent booster. Making the public case for the shot, White House COVID-19 response coordinator Dr. Jha claimed that bivalent boosters "are substantial upgrades in our vaccines, in terms of their ability to prevent infection, prevent transmission and certainly to prevent serious illness."[222] Similarly, Pfzier claimed it provided better protection for both younger and older adults.[223] CDC director Walensky made similar claims about the bivalent boosters' improvements in September on MSNBC.[224] When prompted to respond to Dr. Offit's criticism that young, healthy people did not need a booster, CDC director Walensky stated, "we are simplifying our message ... you need to get your fall booster vaccine ... if you're over the age of 12 ... we've intentionally simplified the message so it's very very clear."

However, in October 2022, Dr. David Ho and several other researchers found no significant difference in the level of relevant antibodies generated by the bivalent booster compared to the monovalent booster (the previous vaccine).[225] These findings were supported by a similar study published the following day.[226] While claiming the superiority of the bivalent booster, the White House, FDA, CDC, and other public health officials did not have human data comparing the relative protective effects of the previous monovalent and new bivalent vaccines.[227] Additionally, the Omicron subvariants that the bivalent vaccine was meant to target represented under 25 percent of circulating strains by December 2022. Dr. Offit subsequently wrote: "I believe we should stop trying to prevent all symptomatic infections in healthy, young people by boosting them with vaccines containing mRNA from strains that might disappear a few months later."

By 2023, the federal government began officially pushing for an annual COVID-19 booster. In July 2023, new CDC director Mandy Cohen stated, "we anticipate that COVID will become similar to flu shots, where it is going to be you get your annual flu shot and you get your annual COVID shot."[228] On September 11—based on manufacturing and nonclinical immune response data—the FDA approved and authorized updated monovalent Pfizer and Moderna boosters, leading the CDC to recommend that everyone over the age of six months "get an updated COVID-19 vaccine to protect against the potentially serious outcomes of COVID-19 illness this fall and winter."[229] The shots were fully approved for everyone aged twelve and up, but only had emergency authorizations for those aged six months to eleven years old. The agency did not provide evidence that nearly all Americans required additional protection against severe disease.

Describing this "boostermania," Dr. Offit wrote that the government had shifted away "from the original goal of preventing severe disease in those at highest risk and drifted toward trying to prevent mild illness in everyone—which was, for all practical purposes, impossible."[230] Universal boosting policy stood at odds with other countries targeting severe illness and death. The WHO, UK, Germany, Finland, Norway, and Sweden all recommended boosting high-risk groups.[231] Yet, the FDA and CDC continued their universal boosting strategy in 2024 without randomized trials to support it, and the CDC recommended updated booster doses on June 27 prior to the eventual FDA approvals and authorizations on August 22.[232]

## Lack of Quality Evidence

The Biden administration did not compel RCTs to prove safety and efficacy for booster doses, instead relying on immunogenicity and limited observational data. In a June 8, 2020, opinion piece in *The New York Times* entitled "Could Trump Turn a Vaccine into a Campaign Stunt?," Drs. Ezekiel Emanuel and Paul Offit warned against President Trump's push for a quick vaccine due to the inability to meet robust standards of efficacy and safety.[233] They referenced how efficacy trials for the rotavirus and human papillomavirus vaccines took four and seven years, respectively. While the RCTs for the original COVID-19 vaccines eventually abated their concerns, they also warned against the "ominous" scenario that the COVID-19 vaccine could get EUA approval solely based on high levels of antibodies shown in immunogenicity data. They wrote:

> Even if a vaccine generates antibodies, it does not prove that the vaccine is effective at preventing infection; it only makes it more likely that the vaccine would be effective. Indeed, about half of the vaccines for other diseases that work and are on the market actually lack clear immunological correlates for protection, meaning they are effective but patients' antibodies, immune cells or other markers do not identify whether a patient is protected.[234]

Yet, the FDA relied upon such antibody data for approving and authorizing boosters including for low-risk groups like healthy young adults and children. Notably, Dr. Jha wrote on August 30, 2020, that issuing an EUA merely because the benefit of a vaccine is greater than the risk "is totally inappropriate," as vaccines are different from therapies in that they are given to healthy people and, thus, need to meet a higher bar.[235] Evidence in favor of boosters would also have the additional requirement of demonstrating that a particular population is in need of more protection than they already have from previous vaccination or infection.

Unlike randomized trials, observational studies test the existence of statistically significant correlations/associations rather than causal relationships.[236] They often suffer from serious limitations, such as confounding, multiplicity, and analytical variation. For example, a December 2021 Israeli study published in the *NEJM* examined two groups of adults aged fifty years and older that both received their first two doses, but only one received Pfizer's booster shot.[237] They found that the boosted group comparatively had an adjusted 90 percent relative reduction in mortality (unadjusted 94.6 percent reduction).

The study suffered from significant confounding bias. Examining the published study data, Drs. Tracy Høeg, Ram Duriseti, and Vinay Prasad published a correspondence in *NEJM*.[238] They calculated that the booster group had 94.8 percent lower mortality than the nonbooster group for deaths not related to COVID-19, which was practically the same as the unadjusted rate for deaths due to COVID. This demonstrated confounding from "healthy vaccine bias." People who received boosters were generally healthier than those who did not, as the vaccines would not dramatically reduce deaths from all causes. The authors of the Israeli study had access to this data but chose not to address it in their original publication, and they did not conduct any falsification test that would have exposed this confounding.

Another Israeli study published in April 2022 purported to show that adults aged sixty years and older who received a second Pfizer-BioNTech booster shot had lower hospitalization and mortality rates than those who only received one booster.[239] However, their data showed that differences in COVID-19 deaths began around eight to ten days after receiving the second booster. The RCT for the original Pfizer vaccine showed that the vaccine only lowered the occurrence of COVID-19 cases in comparison with a placebo group after around twelve days.[240] These results suggest confounding in the Israeli study. It is highly unlikely that a second booster would lower COVID-19 deaths among people with existing protection faster than it took the original vaccine to decrease infection itself among people without previous vaccinations.[241] Additionally, neither Israeli study examined data for the millions of Americans under the age of fifty whom the federal government recommended boosters for.

Moreover, observational studies are further limited due to the fact they often produce results that disagree with RCTs investigating the same questions. In a 2020 *JAMA* study, the authors identified 141 RCTs investigating clinical guidelines questions relating to different treatments in oncology.[242] They then created their own observational studies with data from the National Cancer Database (NCDB) that matched each RCT, and they investigated to what extent the RCT and observational results agreed. They found that the observational studies were not aligned with the RCTs 30.5 to 44.0 percent of the time depending on the type of analysis. While most observational data (52.8 to

56.9 percent) favored more aggressive treatment, the RCT results only agreed in four out of ten of these cases (40.0 to 41.2 percent).

The CDC recognized the weakness of the observational data backing boosters. During the ACIP meetings where the advisors voted whether and how to recommend boosters, agency employees graded the available evidence on vaccine effectiveness and safety. For example, in 2023 and 2024, the CDC graded the evidence type of observational studies as "low certainty."[243] Grades for all the presented evidence—including on hospitalization and death—were entirely "low" or "very low" certainty, with the latter especially applying to the evidence on boosting children. According to the agency, a low certainty grade meant the true effect of the vaccine "may be substantially different from the estimated effect," while a very low certainty grade meant "the true effect is likely to be substantially different."[244] Importantly, the evidence grades pertained to findings for (1) all adults and adolescents aged twelve and above and (2) infants and children aged six months to eleven years. There was not more specific grading of evidence for high- and low-risk groups by age and underlying health conditions.

The FDA could have required vaccine manufacturers to conduct RCTs for each booster as a prerequisite for authorization and approval. Alternatively, the agency could have authorized/approved boosters based on immunological and observational data for high-risk groups while requiring randomized trials for the rest of the population. The FDA also could have mandated trials designed to test the boosters' impact on transmission to identify any benefit to third parties, such as a low-risk individual benefitting a high-risk person by getting vaccinated. Agency leaders chose to not require any of these high-quality studies, opting to rely on low certainty data.

Agency decisions based on weak evidence followed the federal government purchasing booster doses in multiple billion-dollar deals with Moderna and Pfizer. The Biden administration purchased 200 million doses of the Moderna vaccine for $3.3 billion in June 2021 before FDA authorization of booster shots.[245] One month later in July, the government bought 200 million doses of the Pfizer-BioNTech vaccine for nearly $4.9 billion. Both of these purchases transferred billions of taxpayer funds to pharmaceutical companies in anticipation of boosters before public health officials had deemed such action necessary. These purchases were also meant to vaccinate children under the age of twelve. However, the FDA had also yet to authorize this action, and the purchases were far larger than what was required for just pediatric vaccination. Prior to authorization of the bivalent boosters in August 2022, the Biden administration purchased 105 million and 66 million doses of Pfizer's and Moderna's bivalent shots in June and July for $3.2 billion and over $1.7 billion, respectively.

## Distorted Public Messaging

Over the course of the booster campaign, federal and public health officials repeatedly spread misleading, false, and unsubstantiated claims. In February 2022, *The New York Times* reported how when the CDC published data to show booster effectiveness for adults younger than sixty-five, it left out data for those aged eighteen to forty-nine years (around two-thirds of the eighteen to sixty-four age range).[246] The limited comparison between 65-year-olds and 50- to 64-year-olds showed that the younger group benefited much less from booster shots and little overall.[247] Justifying the lack of transparency, CDC spokeswoman Kristen Nordlund said that the data is "not yet ready for prime time" and could be misinterpreted.[248] As a result, outside vaccine experts in the FDA and CDC advisory committees had to rely on Israeli data to give their recommendations, meaning that confounded observational data informed their advice relevant to universal boosting.

Following the FDA's approval and authorization of the 2023 booster, Dr. Jha went on mainstream television news shortly after leaving his post as White House COVID-19 response coordinator.[249] When a host asked him why healthy, young individuals who had received previous vaccinations and had COVID-19 three times should get the newest shot, Jha responded with three key arguments:

1. If you get vaccinated, COVID-19 infections will be much milder, and you'll be less likely to miss work.
2. The shot will make you less likely to spread it to others like your grandmother.
3. Getting the shot will reduce your chances of getting Long COVID.

However, Jha did not have strong evidence for these claims.[250] First, no randomized data demonstrated that vaccines would significantly reduce infection severity for already-protected low-risk groups, and the CDC graded the observational data as low certainty. Second, the FDA did not compel nor did Pfizer or Moderna voluntarily conduct any trials testing their boosters' impact on transmission. As vaccination did not prevent infection, unproven assurances may have provided vaccinated people a false sense of security—creating a substitution effect as with statins—incentivizing social behaviors that increased the risk of spreading the virus to high-risk groups.[251]

Third, there was no randomized trial data on boosters reducing the chance of getting Long COVID—a post-infection chronic condition that has not been strictly defined or well studied.[252] *JAMA* published a primary observational study that could support Jha's claim in 2022.[253] Long COVID prevalence among a cohort of 739 health care workers was 41.8 percent in the unvaccinated, 30.0 percent in those who had one vaccine dose, 17.4 percent in those who had two doses, and 16.0 percent in those who had three doses. The findings did not pertain to the 2023 booster, and the reduction in Long COVID became minimal by the third dose. But, the study had larger issues. For example, Long COVID was loosely defined as having at least one COVID-19 symptom (e.g., fatigue) persist for four weeks post infection, symptoms and duration were self-reported months or years after infection, most cases were pre-2022, there was no accounting for natural immunity, and the sample size was relatively small. Ultimately, a key figurehead of the public response to COVID-19 in the United States made statements about a medical intervention for which he lacked supporting data.

The argument in favor of universal boosting—as represented in the CDC's ACIP meetings that supported such recommendations—revealed dishonesty in the recommendation itself. During the September 2023 ACIP meeting where members voted to universally recommend the booster, proponents centrally argued that everyone wanting a vaccine should be able to get one regardless of the low certainty observational data.[254] Dr. Pablo Sanchez voted against the universal recommendation, bringing up the lack of evidence for children and the risk of side effects in young adults.[255] The counter viewpoint did not contest this, but claimed a universal recommendation would encourage the most people to get vaccinated.

The committee also highlighted that the majority of Americans have the risk factors of being overweight or obese. Yet, these people could have gotten vaccinated through a risk-based recommendation. Thus, the CDC recommendation instructed Americans above the age of six months to get boosted, yet the rationale behind the recommendation was not that robust evidence showed a need for low-risk groups.

Backing ACIP's rationale for universal boosting, Dr. Fauci stated in 2023, the "nuanced, totally correct way can also be the garbled-message way."[256] Fauci's statement mirrors then-CDC director Walensky's response to Dr. Offit about simplifying the message. Public health experts publicly and privately expressed this view: a nuanced, correct message may dissuade people with sufficiently high risk from getting the booster.[257] Therefore, federal policy universally recommended boosters for simplicity rather than accuracy, reflecting distrust that Americans would follow a risk-based recommendation. Yet, strategically employing dishonest messaging to the masses carries a high risk of fueling public distrust. Universal boosting failed to encourage widespread uptake, with only 21.6 percent and 23.0 percent of adults getting the 2023–24 and 2024–25 boosters, respectively, with lower rates for children (14.2 percent and 13.0 percent).[258]

Another key universal boosting campaign message was that an annual COVID-19 booster mirrored the annual flu shot. In September 2022, Dr. Fauci stated, "we likely are moving towards a path with a vaccination cadence similar to that of the annual influenza vaccine, with annual updated Covid-19 shots."[259] However, there are key differences between the viruses and vaccines. The FDA predicts specific influenza strains to target in the annual vaccine, and incorrectly predicting what strains will circulate has historically led to significant drop-off in protection against severe disease.[260] With COVID-19, millions of Americans with previous vaccinations and infections still enjoy protection against severe disease, especially in low-risk groups, due to T cells recognizing similar components of new strains. COVID-19 also has a larger age gradient than the flu, meaning that the risk of flu does not plummet for younger groups to the same extent as COVID-19.[261] Also, COVID-19 vaccines have been more reactogenic than flu shots and have known risks for low-risk groups, most prominently myocarditis in young men.[262]

Overall, as COVID-19 became less dangerous and Americans got protection via vaccination and/or infection, federal policy relied upon less and weaker evidence for vaccine authorizations, approvals, and recommendations. The agency utilized the EUA pathway rather than traditional approval to authorize vaccines with less evidence for low-risk populations, namely children.[263] While requiring RCTs to authorize the original vaccines, the FDA and CDC chose not to compel similar trials to authorize, approve, and recommend further doses for nearly all Americans, instead accepting immunogenicity and observational data.

Federal and public health officials promoted universal boosting with misleading, false, and unsubstantiated claims about benefits and risks. Thus, public officials acted as marketers of products for pharmaceutical companies without being subject to the same limitations. Federal law forbids companies from marketing their products based on unsubstantiated claims and for indications that they are not approved for.[264] There is no same restriction for public health officials. For example, neither Pfizer nor Moderna were legally permitted to say what Dr. Ashish Jha advertised: the vaccines "prevent transmission."[265] Nor could they repeat what CDC director Walensky told the US Senate in May 2021, "post vaccination ... you can't give it [COVID-19] to anyone else."[266]

From 2021 through 2023, Pfizer and Moderna—the providers of the vast majority of vaccine doses in the United States—made over $86 billion and nearly $39 billion in sales of their COVID-19 vaccines.[267] The US government's direct purchases of their vaccines accounted for nearly $25.3 billion (around 23 percent) of their 2021–22 global vaccine sales.[268]

The history of increasing industry influence over medical knowledge and government regulation over the last several decades shows government collaboration with industry and the adoption of industry interests as policy priorities. However, the COVID-19 pandemic represented a different phenomenon. The government not only vastly funded vaccine production and distribution in addition to guaranteeing patent monopolies, but federal officials acted as marketers on behalf of industry when robust evidence did not support their claims. The federal government carried the power of mandates and widespread influence that industry has never had on its own. This does not mean that federal policymakers made decisions out of explicit conflicts of interest with industry. Rather, their priorities aligned with vaccine manufacturers like Pfizer and Moderna regardless of their intentions.

A primary lesson from this COVID-19 case study is not *quid pro quo* industry corruption of government, but rather that the questions surrounding the reliability of medical knowledge do not just emerge from industry domination but also from government policy. Throughout most of this book, industry control of clinical research and its entanglements with key regulators in medical journals, clinical guidelines, and even the FDA have demonstrated significant flaws in the evidence base behind medical products in the United States. Government policy has played an instrumental role in allowing for this dynamic. Policymakers have actively weakened evidence standards and prioritized approval speed over guaranteeing safety and effectiveness prior to approval. They have chosen not to require clinical data transparency and high-quality trials.

The COVID-19 pandemic highlighted an additional wrinkle: the government has not just failed to stop industry from marketing medical products to the public with insufficient evidence, it has promoted unsubstantiated claims itself. The unreliability of medical knowledge is not solely a story of industry influence but also misuse of government power to further its own policy aims. The FDA actively chose not to use its power to make strong evidence-based decisions through compelling RCTs designed and powered to examine vaccine efficacy and safety for different demographic groups and indications like transmission. Increasing the trustworthiness of public health thus requires improving evidence standards for both industry and government.

The existence of a public health emergency especially empowered federal and public health officials, as the public entrusted them to lead the nation through a crisis by providing the most accurate, evidence-based, and honest information and recommendations. This dynamic is distinct from the pharmaceutical industry that is profit driven rather than a public servant, and the public is more inclined to distrust its messaging. Gallup polling shows that 60 percent of Americans viewed pharmaceutical companies negatively in September 2023, and a majority had held such negative views since 2016.[269] Consequently, public servants choosing not to prioritize honesty to the public helped decrease trust in the institutions meant to serve the public interest.

Loss of trust in public health has effects greater than just COVID-19. In 2019, a KFF survey found that 16 percent of American parents reported opposing public schools requiring children to receive measles, mumps, and rubella (MMR) vaccinations generally as a condition for attendance.[270] This number nearly doubled to 31 percent by 2023. Federal decision-making that fails to follow the science, Dr. Offit concludes, "only further erodes trust—not only from the public, but also from members of the scientific and medical community."[271]

11

# A Path Forward

*Health care has become yet another test of our democracy. Although success is in no way preordained, we, the citizens of that democracy, can rise to meet these immense challenges.*

—Dr. John Abramson[1]

Although there are severe issues with the medical knowledge that doctors and patients rely upon for the treatments they prescribe and use, these problems are the result of federal policy decisions. Thus, these issues are equally solvable through a new policymaking agenda. Public servants and elected representatives can guarantee the transparency of clinical trial data, the integrity of the evidence base, the reasonable safety and effectiveness of products, the independence of regulators, and the linkage of rewards for innovation with health outcomes rather than monopoly power. In light of the successes and failures from the COVID-19 vaccine rollout, legislators can push federal officials to remain honest and transparent with the American people to restore trust, so that society is collectively better prepared for future emergencies.

## The FDA Must Disclose the Metadata, CSRs, and De-identified Individual Participant Data for All Clinical Trials of Approved Medical Products

### Current Authority

Independent researchers, doctors, health care professionals, and the public do not have access to the most complete data from clinical trials. Rather, publicly available sources—namely registries and published articles in medical journals—contain limited summary data that does not allow for independent vetting of trial results presented by sponsors. However, the FDA has access to the protocols, CSRs, and IPD from clinical trial sponsors and investigators as part of the regulatory approval process. The agency maintains the largest collection of clinical trial data in the world.[2]

Under its existing statutory authority, the FDA can both prospectively release clinical trial data for medical products upon approval and retroactively release clinical trial data from previously approved products, including phase IV trials that further examine safety and efficacy.[3] This power stems from the Federal Housekeeping Statute or 5 US Code § 301:

> The head of an Executive department or military department may prescribe regulations for the government of his department, the conduct of its employees, the distribution and performance of its business, and the custody, use, and preservation of its records, papers, and property. This section does not authorize withholding information from the public or limiting the availability of records to the public.[4]

The law grants HHS, including the FDA, custody and use powers over all its "records, papers, and property." The Supreme Court upheld this reality in *Chrysler Corp. v. Brown* (1979) unless the disclosure violates substantive laws like the Trade Secrets Act (TSA) that explicitly bar specific disclosures.[5] The Court additionally made clear that federal agencies can disclose information both within and outside of FOIA exemptions, such as Exemption 4, as they are "an exception to the disclosure mandate of the FOIA and not a limitation on agency discretion."[6]

There are no laws, including the TSA, that explicitly prohibit the FDA from releasing the safety and efficacy information included in CSRs and de-identified IPD. The TSA prevents federal employees, officers, departments, and agencies from disclosing the following information when not authorized by law:

> Trade secrets, processes, operations, style of work, or apparatus, or to the identity, confidential statistical data, amount or source of any income, profits, losses, or expenditures of any person, firm, partnership, corporation, or association; or permits any income return or copy thereof or any book containing any abstract or particulars thereof to be seen or examined by any person except as provided by law.[7]

The FDA is authorized by law to disclose the safety and efficacy data it collects from clinical trials. Indeed, in the FDAAA, Congress gave HHS the mandate to "improve the transparency" of drug information and "allow patients and health care providers better access to [such] information" by creating a website that "improves communication of drug safety information to patients and providers."[8] For efficacy data, the law also allowed public disclosure of "other material determined appropriate by the [HHS] Secretary."[9] Therefore, the TSA's prohibitions would still not apply if such data were legally trade secrets.

However, the safety and efficacy data stored in CSRs and de-identified IPD also do not qualify as trade secrets. Under the Uniform Trade Secrets Act (UTSA), a trade secret is information that "derives independent economic value, actual or potential, from not being generally known [or ascertainable] to … other persons who can obtain economic value from its disclosure or use."[10] However, federal courts have repeatedly held that disclosure of the underlying safety and efficacy data from clinical trials would not cause meaningful competitive injury.[11] In *Public Citizen Health v. Dept. of Health* (1979), the US District Court for the District of Columbia reasoned that claims of data constituting trade secrets or confidential information are "frivolous" when the data does not regard "fees, payment schedules, or other commercial arrangements" along with "information about secret formulas or rare treatment methods."[12] As legal scholars Christopher Morten and Amy Kapczynski explain, "by its nature, safety and efficacy data has little or no direct value to brand-name competitors developing alternative compounds and thus will confer minimal or no competitive advantage."[13]

Ultimately, the FDA currently has the statutory authority to retroactively disclose clinical trial information already in its possession and prospectively disclose data for trials upon FDA approval. By disclosing the metadata, summary data, and de-identified IPD for FDA-approved medical products, the agency will allow independent researchers, health care professionals, and the public to know the true proven clinical value of the treatments that industry spends billions on marketing to them.

Such disclosure of clinical trial data would free up resources that the agency spends processing FOIA requests. From 2008 to 2017, the FDA spent $305 million dealing with FOIA requests, amounting to $2,653 per request.[14] Within a prospective disclosure system, the FDA can save money by requiring that manufacturers requesting approval submit de-identified data and proposed redactions.[15] The FDA would then only have to review the proposals. The EMA already implements this method.[16]

## Need for Congressional Action

While the FDA has the authority to disclose clinical trial data, it may choose not to do so. Along with how the FDA has not already instituted such regulations and the agency's historical deference to industry's objections to FOIA requests, the FDA has significant conflicts of interest with industry. Through the combination of factors like user fee funding and the revolving door, FDA senior officials have often shared priorities with industry. Moreover, the Supreme Court's *Loper* decision further highlights the likely need for congressional action, as FDA disclosure could cause lawsuits from companies seeking to prevent data transparency, disincentivizing agency action.[17]

Without an explicit congressional mandate, different iterations of the agency could also choose to institute different policies. The FDA under one presidential administration may choose to disclose the underlying clinical data for all FDA-approved medical products, and new agency leadership under another administration could suspend such a program. Different administrations may also vary in the level of transparency required, like how administrations have issued different executive orders regarding ethics requirements for appointed officials in executive agencies.

To ensure that the FDA discloses sufficient safety and efficacy data from clinical trials—namely CSRs and de-identified IPD—regardless of past policies, industry ties, and different administrations' priorities, Congress must pass legislation mandating such disclosure. Congressional action is not completely unprecedented, as Congress has mandated limited disclosure through both the 1997 FDAMA and 2007 FDAAA.

## Congress Must Create a National HTA Program

Without a national HTA program, clinical trial data transparency will not maximally lower costs and increase quality. Similarly to the UK, Canada, and Australia, Congress should legislate a national program appraising every FDA-approved medical product and intervention, products with new indications, and previously approved treatments with clinical significance. This federal body would buttress the FDA by showing not just that a medical product is safe and effective enough to be on the market, but whether it is better or worse in comparison to existing standards of care.

Unlike other nations, Congress should grant the body charged with conducting HTAs direct access to the underlying clinical trial data and the ability to conduct cost-effectiveness analyses. With this information, Congress can mandate that public insurers, such as Medicare and Medicaid, respect the recommendations from the HTAs. Thus, patients with public health insurance would have coverage of not just the highest quality treatments but also those that are the most cost-effective, saving costs for both patients and taxpayers.

Because most Americans (65.4 percent in 2023) have private health insurance rather than public insurance (36.3 percent), Congress can require private insurers to follow HTA recommendations, spreading the benefits to the most people.[18] However, even if such legislation is too unlikely to pass, private insurers could still benefit from accessing HTA reviews and recommendations. Like other wealthy nations, Congress should mandate that HTA assessments are made publicly available.

As Congress never repealed the authorization for the Office of Technology Assessment, Congress could simply appropriate funds to the OTA for a national HTA program.[19] Otherwise, the Congressional Research Service has noted that Congress could create a program within another legislative branch agency, such as the GAO or the CRS itself. Regardless of the new HTA program's location, Congress would need to properly fund it for effective appraisal of all new FDA-approved medical products. In 2024, the FDA approved fifty novel drugs along with thirty-three medical devices via premarket approval (not including the 510(k) pathway).[20]

## Congress Must Mandate Disclosure of Underlying Clinical Data to Medical Journals

Due to the medical profession's historic reliance on the published literature as the premier source of medical knowledge, improving the information in medical journals is the most effective way to provide doctors with the most accurate information. Such transparency is essential for the scientific community to effectively self-regulate. Thus, Congress must require that submitters of manuscripts for clinical trials provide peer reviewers and journal editors with access to the underlying data—including the complete trial protocol, full CSRs, and de-identified IPD. Disclosure must occur before article publication to ensure peer reviewers can use the data to vet submitted manuscripts.

While many published articles in medical journals follow regulatory approval, article publication also often precedes such approval.[21] Therefore, if Congress were to mandate that the FDA disclose safety and efficacy data upon approval, many published articles would not utilize the data. Even for articles following approval, there is no guarantee without legislation that peer reviewers and journal editors would always use FDA-disclosed data to vet manuscripts. Data disclosure is most impactful on medical knowledge prior to publication in peer-reviewed medical journals due to their gold-standard status among medical professionals. Therefore, legislative efforts to ensure effective clinical trial data transparency must address the journal publication and peer review process.

## Congress Must Revive and Revamp the National Guidelines Clearinghouse

Clinical guidelines critically direct clinicians' treatment decisions. However, COIs with industry, lack of access to clinical trial data, and insufficient evaluation of the available evidence have rendered many guidelines as poor sources of medical knowledge. Policymakers must use their authority to identify and promote quality guidelines to improve the standards of care that patients receive.

While most clinical guidelines are created by private organizations, the National Guidelines Clearinghouse allowed regulators to inform doctors of what guidelines met standards of quality. The Agency for Healthcare Research and Quality planned in 2017 for the NGC to assess to what extent guidelines met standards of trustworthiness.[22] Beforehand, the AHRQ had not made sure that the guidelines posted on the NGC website met the standards that the IOM had recommended in 2011.[23] Among randomly selected guidelines on the NGC in 2011, an estimated 35.1 percent of guidelines did not provide the evidence behind their recommendations.[24] Most guidelines (53.2 percent) did not disclose COIs; among those that did, 71.4 percent of chairs and 90.5 percent of cochairs had financial COIs. However, the 2017 policy shift never went into effect, as the NGC was shut down in 2018 due to a lack of funding.[25]

Congress must revive the NGC with adequate funding and mandate the clearinghouse to assess and identify which guidelines sufficiently meet quality standards, such as the IOM's 2011 recommendations. Thus, doctors, insurers, and other health care professionals could go to the NGC website and identify which guidelines are not written by authors with financial ties to industry. They could also see which guidelines both properly evaluate the evidence to make recommendations and make such evidence available to outside observers. For optimal impact, this reform must go alongside mandating disclosure and sharing of the underlying data behind clinical trials. Otherwise, guideline authors will not be able to truly vet the evidence, relying instead on limited summaries in published articles.

The NGC can also institute new, alternative metrics to assess the quality of CPGs. For example, rather than clinical guideline experts themselves only being subject experts in the relevant field, the NGC can incentivize guideline authors to include epidemiologists who are impartial specialists in evaluating evidence to find ways to address public health problems.[26] Thus, guideline authors would not only include individuals potentially tied to particular methods of care.

## Congress Must Create an Independent Healthy Study Review Board

While clinical trial data transparency produces many benefits—such as allowing peer reviewers and researchers to vet industry claims—it would not address industry sponsorship bias. Transparency shows the true results of a clinical trial after it has taken place, but it does not address issues with study design manipulation that make industry-sponsored research more likely to produce positive results. Therefore, Congress must create an independent health study review board (HSRB) to review and approve the study plans of clinical trials for all medical products prior to enrollment. HSRB approval must be a prerequisite for FDA approval.

While the FDA currently reviews the design of trials to ensure that they conform to federal law and meet good clinical practice (GCP) regulations—such as ensuring informed consent of participants—it does not ensure that trials are properly constructed to test the safety and efficacy of a product on target populations.[27] An independent board should consist of experts who examine key design components, such as having the trial's participant population reflect the target population. To ensure the integrity of board members, Congress must ban board members from working for industry for at least ten years prior to and following their employment on the board.

The HSRB should not approve phase III or IV clinical trials that use surrogate measures generally, and it should only allow surrogates in situations where (1) companies provide reasonable explanations that they cannot directly measure clinical outcomes and (2) the surrogate measures have been proven as validated correlates of important clinical outcomes. Many surrogate measures included on the FDA's Surrogate Endpoint Table lack evidence of strong correlations with relevant clinical outcomes, and this is especially true for cancer drugs.[28] Additionally, the rare allowances of validated surrogate endpoints should only pertain to products that treat life-threatening diseases and conditions for which there are no effective existing standards of care. Any clinical trials for products that are not treating life-threatening diseases and conditions, or where there are effective standards of care, must measure relevant clinical outcomes, as, for example, most surrogates do not prove that a cancer drug increases overall survival.[29]

Acceptable clinical trials must include other markers of high-quality testing, such as randomization, double-blinding, appropriate use of active and placebo comparators, and sufficient participant sizes. Nonrandomized trials are unreliable due to their inability to control for differences among treatment groups, and lack of double-blinding introduces bias among both participants and researchers alike. Active comparators should reflect best standards of care rather than products or doses that doctors do not currently use to treat their patients. Trials must have sufficiently large participant sizes; for example, the HSRB should not approve a trial design with a few hundred participants for a drug meant to treat millions of people. Such a trial would not be sufficiently powered to detect potential adverse events and safety signals. Additionally, trial participants must reflect the intended patient population. For example, a drug to treat Alzheimer's should not primarily include the youngest, healthiest possible participants, as this is not indicative of people with Alzheimer's.

In tandem with data transparency, this reform should greatly reduce industry-sponsorship bias. Board approval of study designs would reduce the ability for industry sponsors to use their leverage over CROs and their AMC competitors to control trial designs. While board approval would not stop selective publication of results in medical journals, data transparency for all FDA-approved products would allow researchers to access unpublished studies' data.

## Congress Must Strengthen the FDA's Evidence Requirements and Create a Separate Oversight Body

Over the last thirty years, the FDA has prioritized increasing the speed of medical product development, review, and approval over ensuring that such products are safe and effective. The agency has moved toward lifecycle regulation, where postmarketing studies replace sufficient proof of safety and efficacy before approval. The FDA must reshift its focus so that the vast majority of medical products are approved after proving safety and effectiveness. The agency should only accept lower standards of evidence for products that treat life-threatening diseases and conditions for which there are no effective existing standards of care.

Congress must reinstate the requirement that, at a minimum, products must have two clinical trials to receive FDA approval rather than one. Potential exceptions for one-trial-based approvals for life-threatening and serious conditions must have a timely second, high-quality postapproval trial. FDA regulators should not approve trials that deviate from HSRB-approved, high-quality designs so as not to compromise requirements like using clinical endpoints, randomization, double-blinding, and sufficiently large and representative participant populations. HSRB approval is only effective insofar as the FDA enforces adherence to the approved designs; thus, Congress must mandate that the FDA ensures compliance with stringent enforcement authorities.

FDA performance goals should not primarily be tied to the speed at which it reviews products and makes approval decisions. Rather, Congress should legislate annual performance reports pertaining to the agency's successes in ensuring safety and effectiveness of products first and foremost. Additionally, Congress should grant the FDA the mandate to hold duplicative products—those which are like existing treatments and for similar indications—to higher standards of evidence. The FDA should not approve products via traditional or accelerated approval where the evidence in favor is borderline or questionable and there is already an approved, similar product on the market.

Following the IOM's 2011 recommendations, Congress should eliminate the 510(k) pathway and replace it accordingly with a system that makes sure 99 percent of medical devices are not cleared without proving their safety and effectiveness.[30] Current standards of evidence for drugs are high compared to medical devices because substantial equivalence with a predicate device is not a test of safety and effectiveness, especially given that many predicate devices also utilize the 510(k) pathway. In the 2011 report, the IOM did not specify what the replacement system would exactly involve; however, it must include the ensuring of devices' "safety and effectiveness throughout their life cycle."[31] Thus, Congress must create an independent committee to expeditiously recommend specific alternatives to the 510(k) pathway that do not allow potentially harmful medical devices to be on the market without proving safety and effectiveness.

While the FDA must shift toward requiring proof of safety and effectiveness prior to approval, Congress must also enact changes that strengthen postmarketing surveillance. The HSRB must also approve the designs of postmarketing studies, and these trials cannot include signs of poor quality like lack of randomization and blinding, use of surrogate measures, and reliance on small, unrepresentative participant populations. Postmarketing trials are supposed to ensure that products should be on the market for their approved uses; therefore, regulators must require high-quality trials. Congress must command the FDA to pull a product off the market if they fail to prove their efficacy or safety or if they do not complete their trial within the initially required time frame unless the sponsor can prove that unexpected circumstances reasonably prevented them from doing so.

Congress must create a new department within the FDA to oversee postmarketing study requirements that is completely separate from the employees who approved the product. Regulators entrusted with monitoring whether marketed products are safe and effective should not have the potential for bias from having to admit they incorrectly granted an approval. Pointing out that the two FDA offices overseeing drug safety and working with industry to approve more drugs both exist within CDER, editor-in-chief of *The Lancet* Richard Horton wrote in 2004:

> Once a licensing approval has been made it is naturally in CDER's own interests to stand by its original decision. CDER's reputation would be damaged if its licensing judgments were constantly challenged by its own staff. This understandable but dangerous tendency to discourage dissent makes the Office of Drug Safety [now the Office of Surveillance and Epidemiology] … weak and ineffective. The inherent precedence that licensing of new drugs takes over safety evaluation is a serious flaw in FDA's complex regulatory structure.[32]

For pre- and post-marketing trials, the FDA must require that companies utilize independent investigators to conduct them and independent statisticians to analyze them. As Dr. Gøtzsche explains, "companies have every reason in the world to blindfold themselves by conducting poor studies, or fail to report them, or fail to even do them."[33]

## Congress Must Detach the FDA from Industry Capture

A regulatory agency charged with protecting the public interest should not be beholden to the very industries it regulates. Yet, the FDA relies on the companies it oversees for nearly half of its total funding, including 61.3 percent of its combined budgets for human drugs, biologics, and medical devices/radiological health in FY 2024.[34] Not only does industry provide the necessary funding for the FDA to operate, but it actively negotiates with the agency every five years on what legislative changes the FDA will ask Congress for within reauthorizations of user fee legislation. Since PDUFA I, industry funding of the FDA has exploded as the agency has adopted industry priorities of faster reviews and approvals, weakened standards of evidence, and greater collaboration between the agency and industry.

Congress must eliminate user fees so that the budget of the regulatory agency charged with ensuring the safety and effectiveness of medical products is not reliant on and negotiated with the companies it regulates. According to Dr. Drummond Rennie—who served as deputy editor at both *NEJM* and *JAMA*, "it is ludicrous to imagine that the FDA could truly work for the public if they continue to be paid not to."[35] In FY 2024, around $3.3 billion of the $6.9 billion FDA budget came from user fees.[36] Therefore, the government would have had to spend roughly 0.05 percent of total federal spending or 0.07 percent of revenue to replace industry funding.[37] This tiny amount relative to overall federal spending would allow for the FDA's financial independence from industry, and it would end the practice of the regulator negotiating with the regulated over its budget and priorities.

Furthermore, FDA employees, particularly senior officials, should not be allowed to seek future employment with the companies the public entrusts them with regulating. All FDA commissioners since the 1980s who have left government have gone on to make money from the pharmaceutical industry. Current federal regulations are extremely weak, imposing temporary bans on various lobbying activities, which do not include advising others on how to lobby. The only permanent ban, Section 207(a)(1), bars federal employees from communicating or appearing before the US government on government-related matters they were personally and substantially involved in.[38] This prohibition does not stop a former employee from working for a pharmaceutical company and using their experience to advise their lobbyists on how to secure better outcomes in the exact matters they worked on prior to leaving government service. These weak barriers also do nothing to address the financial incentives for government employees to not do anything in public service that may harm their chances of securing an industry job and earning large sums of money.

Thus, Congress must pass a lifetime ban on FDA commissioners and senior FDA employees from working for the industries they regulated. Working at the high levels of the FDA is a form of public service with immense consequences on the safety and effectiveness of products that Americans entrust the agency with protecting. General lifetime bans may not be feasible for the thousands of non-senior employees, because that may overly harm worker recruitment. So, Congress should pass lifetime restrictions solely regarding lobbying activities for such employees. These lobbying restrictions must include prohibitions on any aiding or advising of others' lobbying activities. While these restrictions may be hard to enforce, any effects of deterrence would benefit the public by stopping public servants from using their positions for personal profit and against the public interest. Additionally, many of these individuals (e.g., product reviewers) should face restrictions on working for industry generally, such as a ban of five to ten years.

Currently, Section 207 violations are felonies that can result in imprisonment up to five years, fines up to $50,000 per violation, or both.[39] Violations of these stricter regulations should also be felonies. However, imprisonment must be guaranteed to maximally deter misbehavior and prevent individuals from paying fines worth less than private salaries. Overall, these restrictions should sharply limit the revolving door, so that the same employees and same priorities are not shared by the regulators and the regulated.

Moreover, FDA advisory committee members should not have any financial COIs with industry that bias their voting behavior or weaken public trust. Current regulations provide the FDA with significant discretion over whether financial ties to industry constitute a COI and, if so, whether the government values the conflicted individuals' participation enough to waive any concerns. Additionally, FDA leadership successfully pushed for removal of the congressionally created caps on the number of COI waivers the agency could issue under the premise that it prevented them from recruiting qualified individuals.[40] Yet, this was not the case, as several analyses showed that significant minorities of medical experts had no ties to industry.[41] The FDA is fully capable of recruiting experts for its advisory committees that are independent of industry influence.

Thus, Congress must mandate that no voting members of advisory committees or any other influential individuals, such as speakers, who are not officially representing industry interests have any financial ties to industry. This restriction would include both general payments, like paid meals and consulting fees, along with research funding granted directly to a researcher or indirectly via their employer. Additionally, such restrictions would concern competing companies on top of the particular company whose product was under committee review. Such strict guidelines are necessary to ensure independent, unconflicted judgment from individuals with significant impact on FDA decision-making. COIs can produce dangerous approval recommendations, such as how conflicted FDA advisory committee members were essential in voting in favor of keeping Vioxx on the market after 30–60 thousand estimated American deaths and Merck itself pulled the drug from the market.[42]

## Congress Must Replace the Patent System

The aforementioned policy solutions are necessary to ensure the integrity of medical knowledge in the United States. Without transparency, product appraisals, reliable journals and guidelines, and an uncorrupted FDA with strong evidence standards,

Americans cannot fully know that the medical knowledge behind their health care is trustworthy. Just as Americans universally desire clean water, ensuring the reliability of medical products and treatments should be nonpartisan and uncontroversial.[43]

However, tackling the roots of the current system that incentivizes medical innovators to pursue profits detached from making Americans' healthier requires a much grander, more difficult solution. The patent system exacerbates the numerous problems with medical knowledge. Through rewarding innovation with monopoly pricing power, patents incentivize innovation to maintain market exclusivities over improving health outcomes. Companies can spend far less on slight modifications to existing products to extend patent protection compared to spending billions on identifying significant medical advancements. This government-protected monopoly power allows companies to charge exorbitantly high prices through denying market competition by generic manufacturers.

To profit, pharmaceutical and medical device companies must get doctors to prescribe and use their products even when the financial rewards from their patents are not tied to better health outcomes. This reality incentivizes them to bias the design, conduct, and focus of their trials to increase the chances of favorable outcomes. When trials do not yield results that help a company's bottom line, it can choose to not publish the results, biasing the pool of available evidence through selective publication. Companies also view their trials' data as marketing tools.[44] Thus, they maintain secrecy and keep control of trial data, suppressing the ability for other researchers to advance scientific knowledge. Peer reviewers of medical journals, clinical guideline writers, and independent experts cannot properly vet the results published in the existing literature.

Given these problems, Congress should replace the patent system with one that rewards improving health outcomes—not monopoly power—that prioritizes optimal study designs—not those that bias outcomes to enrich industry—that fosters sharing of knowledge—not secrecy—and that allows the most people to benefit from true innovation rather than only those with adequate health insurance coverage or who can afford monopoly prices. However, there is no perfect system in the real world. There are always benefits and flaws to each system, including the alternatives Chapter 9 discusses.

The contract-based system allows the public to directly finance research with the purpose of improving medical knowledge rather than maximizing profit. Public oversight would ensure that trial designs are high-quality, and regulations would mandate immediate sharing of research findings and clinical data as soon as possible. Government funding would eliminate the need for companies to recoup R&D losses through high prices, and contractors would immediately face competition. However, a primary limitation of this system is that it restricts innovation outside of the patent system to just the areas in which the government deems worthy of a contract. While public institutions' priorities may align better with public health than profit-seeking corporations in a patent model, this system is inherently restrictive. As such, one of the key proponents of a contract-based model, Dean Baker, envisions such a system living alongside and competing against the current patent system whereby it would win out over time by providing cheaper, effective treatments.[45] However, that would still leave the innovations of the patent system behind walls of biased trials, information secrecy, and high prices.

Contrastingly, the prize-based system directly ties financial rewards to improvements in health outcomes. Thus, industry efforts to bias trial designs would be counterproductive, as products not benefiting patients would earn less money. Unlike a contract-based system, prizes would replace patents, and the terms for eligibility to receive a prize could include the same restrictions that contracts can employ. The government can mandate that prize winners share and make publicly available all the clinical trial information upon approval, that study designs are approved by oversight bodies, and that products face competition immediately upon FDA approval. The government would not directly dictate in which areas R&D takes place, allowing for the more diverse array of private actors to compete and pursue ventures of interest. Yet, the prize system is limited by the power of a prize fund authority to determine when and to what degree a product benefits public health. Models like the Medical Innovation Prize Fund Act include both eligibility criteria and mandatory prize fund allocations to certain areas, like products that treat diseases with small patient populations. However, such models are inherently limited by human fallibility. The prize system can also disincentivize risky research, where companies are less likely to spend billions on R&D in areas where they deem success less likely even if success would greatly improve public health.

The publicly financed contract and prize systems need not be mutually exclusive. Together, they can eliminate some of each other's greatest flaws. A prize fund can serve as the central means to spur private innovation, as the government is not deciding who can conduct research. For specific areas of interest that require longer-term research, are risky, and/or are of substantial known public importance, the government can award competitive research contracts. Thus, the prize fund stops the government from monopolizing the decision-making on who conducts medical R&D, while contracts can guarantee that research that private actors fear will not yield prize rewards still takes place.

Furthermore, prize funds allow private actors to still compete with one another to produce the best discoveries that contracts would not, as the competition to get a contract takes place before any research is done. Competitive pressures would push researchers to develop products that best benefit public health, as health outcomes are the metric that decide prize amounts. However, as competition also breeds secrecy during the R&D process, contract-based research will better allow for the free sharing of information at all times of the research process rather than predominantly after FDA approval. Additionally, competition to win prizes may disincentivize research that takes many years to produce fruitful results; thus, public contracts can fill this void.

Both systems would allow regulators to incentivize and mandate high-quality, optimal designs for clinical research. For example, a prize system would not reward a company for discovering a new medication in which clinical trials only demonstrate significant benefit compared to placebo or anything that is not the current best standard of care in the respective field. They would only get substantial amounts of prize funds if the medication provides a substantial benefit over existing treatment. Additionally, the FDA or the aforementioned HSRB can oversee and approve study designs to ensure optimal construction. Likewise, publicly awarded contracts can involve requirements and regulations specific to the funded research, ensuring that only robustly designed trials get funding.

During the COVID-19 pandemic, the contract model would have led to open vaccine development with real-time information sharing for the pure purpose of quickly producing the most safe and effective product. Similarly, the prize fund system would have incentivized companies to compete strictly over quickly producing the most safe, effective vaccines possible, and clinical information would have become public following FDA approval. Without patent monopolies, these products could have immediately been accessible globally without requiring a TRIPS waiver. Additionally, direct contracts could have produced additional high-quality trials to assess vaccines' impacts across demographic groups and on viral transmission.

Prizes and contracts can also significantly increase the amount of mission-driven research conducted by nonprofits while still allowing for the for-profit motive to further spur innovation if policymakers deem it necessary. Eligibility for prize funds and public contracts can mandate that researchers belong to a nonprofit organization rather than a for-profit company. Therefore, the aim of researchers would legally be to provide the public service of furthering medical knowledge and improving public health rather than maximizing profit for owners and shareholders. Public funding would help ensure that these nonprofits have the resources they need to conduct their research. If public officials want to allow the for-profit model to exist to further incentivize research, both systems can allocate rewards and funding to for-profit companies while ensuring that a set percentage of funds goes toward nonprofits.

Along with better ensuring that medical research produces discoveries that improve public health, publicly funded prizes and contracts would significantly lower prices. Both systems get rid of patent monopolies; thus, inventions would immediately be subject to competition, driving the prices of lifesaving products dramatically lower than contemporary monopoly pricing. Currently, generics often can cost upward of 80–85 percent less than brand name products.[46] As of June 2025, it costs $22,712.73 for one hundred capsules ($227.13 per capsule) of Bausch Health's drug Syprine that patients use to treat Wilson's disease: a condition that causes dangerous levels of copper to build up in organs like the brain and liver.[47] Yet, the drug wholesaler Cost Plus Drugs sells the generic version (trientine HCl) at around $2.18 per capsule for ninety capsules, representing roughly 1.0 percent the cost of the Syprine.[48] The patent system is an exorbitant tax on Americans. Government gifting and enforcement of patent protections raised the cost of prescription drugs in 2022 alone by $430 billion if generics would have been 80 percent less expensive, which is the lower end of current general estimates.[49]

No system is perfect, and a prize-plus-contract system has limitations; however, they are significantly more manageable than the exorbitant costs of the current patent model. Naturally, public funding, regardless of the mechanism, means that government policymakers would make decisions about who gets taxpayer dollars for medical research. The prize system is relatively indirect, as the prize fund authority uses policymaker-crafted criteria to reward discoveries. Public contracts are much more direct, as officials choose who to fund before knowing the public health impacts of their research. Thus, skeptics may find concern in potential government abuse of power, ignorance, and/or inefficiency.

However, the patent system also involves decision-making by a concentrated group of individuals: predominantly corporate executives of large companies. Rather than serve the public interest, these corporate leaders make decisions to maximize profits through patent monopolies. For example, while the FDA approved Humira in December 2002, AbbVie spent its resources on filing 122 patents on the drug from 2014 onward as part of its strategy to prevent generic competition and maintain the power to charge monopoly prices.[50] In 2023, *The New York Times* reported that Humira generated over $208 billion in revenue since 2002; more than $114 billion (54.8 percent) came since 2016 after its patent exclusivity was originally set to expire.[51] Top corporate executives also prioritize enriching shareholders over investing in R&D, as the top 14 drug companies spent 105 percent of their net income on stock buybacks and dividends from 2013 to 2022—$72 billion more than R&D investment.[52]

Industry executives have knowingly harmed patients to generate profits. Merck executives knew that Vioxx caused severe cardiovascular events like heart attacks and strokes, yet they suppressed this information and pushed the product onto consumers, leading to estimated deaths of around 30–60 thousand Americans.[53] Four years before Merck pulled Vioxx from the market, on March 9, 2000, president of Merck Research Laboratories Edward Scolnick emailed the company's senior vice president of clinical sciences, Alan Nies, and others stating, "the CV [cardiovascular] events are clearly there … [i]t is a shame but it is a low incidence and it is mechanism based as we worried it was … [t]he class will do well and so will we."[54]

A 2020 *JAMA* article examined the twenty-six large pharmaceutical firms within the Global 500 or Fortune 1000 lists from 2003 to 2016, finding that twenty-two (84.6 percent) had paid penalties totaling more than $33 billion for illegal activities.[55] Some activities included failing to disclose negative information about a product, paying kickbacks to suppliers and customers, using deceptive marketing tactics, advertising products for unapproved uses, and defrauding government insurers.

While political corruption is a potential concern with public financing, this is true with any system relying on government actions, including the patent system. And, policymakers can create robust guardrails to maximally limit it. The patent system already incentivizes industry to spend billions on lobbying and campaign contributions to protect their monopoly pricing power. For example, PhRMA spent $72.6 million lobbying Congress in 2003 on efforts including blocking federal officials from negotiating drug prices for Medicare patients.[56] Such negotiations can halve drug costs, as the negotiating powers of the VA and DoD highlight.[57] PhRMA rewarded one of the leaders of the legislation, Rep. Billy Tauzin, with the role of PhRMA CEO and president, and he became the highest-paid health-law lobbyist in 2010.[58] To protect against similar levels of corruption among those awarding prize funds and granting public contracts, policymakers can legislate a lifetime or at least long-term (ten to fifteen years) ban on working for prize/contract recipients, in addition to prohibitions on holding financial COIs with recipients and industry more generally. Focusing funds on mission-driven nonprofits further reduces the risk of corruption due to limits on lobbying. But policymakers can also create an eligibility requirement that recipients of public funds cannot lobby outside of the necessary procedure of filing requests for contracts and prizes.

The principal argument in favor of the patent system is that monopoly pricing power is necessary to spur innovation, and any efforts to get rid of patents will hurt innovation.[59] However, as historian Jill Lepore wrote in *These Truths: A History of the United States*, "innovation might make the world a better place, or it might not; The point was, innovation was not concerned with goodness; It was concerned with novelty, speed, and profit."[60] To earn $208 billion, AbbVie prevented generic competition for Humira for twenty years following its approval in 2002 by filing and receiving 247 and 130 patents by 2021, respectively, along with engaging in a self-described "enhancement" strategy to modify aspects of the drug, like increasing its concentration, to "raise barriers to competitor ability to replicate."[61] From 2013 to 2022, AbbVie mirrored other large drug companies by investing $87 billion of its monopoly-derived revenue into stock buybacks and dividends, $25 billion more than in R&D and representing 137 percent of its net income.[62] The available evidence shows that innovation within the patent system is not concerned with improving public health as much as it is concerned with extending patent protections and maximizing profits.[63] New drugs often do not provide any significant added clinical benefit to existing standards of care. Manufacturers of most medical devices don't even prove the safety and effectiveness of their products to the FDA due to the 510(k) pathway.[64]

Furthermore, many innovations with immense public benefit have come from publicly funded research. The mRNA technology underlying both the Moderna and Pfizer vaccines came from decades of NIH-funded basic and applied research, allowing for the development of COVID-19 vaccines in under a year and likely saving hundreds of thousands of Americans and millions globally.[65] The development of the Moderna vaccine specifically was publicly funded as part of a public-private collaboration. A 2024 Policy Cures Research and Global Health Technologies Coalition report found that US government funding for global health research played a pivotal role in developing sixty-seven new technologies since 1999, such as twelve products to combat Ebola, twelve for tuberculosis, and eleven to fight malaria.[66]

While the government would have to spend billions more dollars to fully finance medical R&D, savings from lower prices would likely more than cover the cost. In 2020, the federal government would have had to spend roughly $183.6 billion more to cover the total cost of medical R&D.[67] In 2020, the US health care system spent $582 billion on prescription drugs, of which approximately $465.6 billion came from just branded drugs.[68] The FDA reports that generics typically cost 80–85 percent less than branded drugs; assuming an 80 percent cost decrease, Americans would have saved roughly $372.5 billion in 2020.[69] Thus, universal generic prices could have saved more than double the amount of money required to fund all medical R&D in 2020.

In 2022, 87 percent of prescription drug sales came from branded drugs even though 92 percent of drugs sold were generic.[70] Nearly $537 billion of $617 billion in drug costs were from just branded drugs. The United States would have saved roughly $430 billion assuming an 80 percent cost reduction via generics, far greater than the $251 billion the pharmaceutical industry spent—globally—on R&D in 2022.[71]

Critics of this proposal may question why in a current system debilitated by government failure, this reform may seemingly invoke more government as a solution. However, *the patent system is a failed government solution*. The nature of medical innovation and IP generally makes a true free market where innovators are sufficiently rewarded for their discoveries impossible. To address this market failure, the government can step in to guarantee that (1) innovators are incentivized to make discoveries, (2) such discoveries benefit the public health, and (3) the public has access to such beneficial innovations. The patent system—where the government uses the threat of the law to prevent any competition for two decades—only guarantees the first point. Drug and device manufacturers can use patents to not just recoup their losses, but earn substantial profits through monopoly power. However, these patented discoveries largely do not provide added clinical benefits to Americans. Government-enforced monopoly—the antithesis of a free market—makes these innovations, including those that provide added lifesaving benefits, inaccessible to many people due to high prices. Even when Americans can afford branded products, high prices place a strain on private and public insurers alike, raising the cost of premiums and the entire health care system.[72]

In contrast to government-enforced monopolies, a system of publicly funded prize funds and direct contracts would yield a more competitive and freer market while achieving all three goals. Thus, while this system would involve significantly more taxpayer funding upfront, it would not represent a government takeover of a currently free system. Rather—in an environment where a free market is not possible—this proposal would help put an end to a dangerous, expensive market failure that has produced crony capitalism at the expense of public health.

A key critique of adopting a new model is the idea that policymakers can simply reform the patent system. For example, various policy proposals would tighten requirements to receive patent protection and restrict the number of patents that a company can file for a particular product, limiting evergreening and shortening the time to generic competition.[73] Assuming these reforms are successful, they still fail to address the root issues of the patent system. Manufacturers still earn money based on achieving monopoly pricing power rather than improving health outcomes. Thus, the incentives still push them to distort medical knowledge, maintain secrecy, and spend billions marketing to doctors and patients even if their products are not better than existing treatments. While policymakers can improve the patent system, they cannot change its root incentive structure without switching to another model.

Ultimately, Congress must replace the patent system to make the purpose of medical research the advancement of scientific knowledge and public health rather than maximizing profits through monopolies that are the antithesis of a free market. Public funding through the combination of prize funds and contracts can strengthen the reliability of the knowledge behind the medical products that doctors and patients rely upon.

## Congress Must Increase Honesty and Transparency in Public Health and Mandate Trials

While the COVID-19 pandemic exemplified the current system's capacity to quickly produce effective vaccines that saved many lives, it also exposed the ability of government officials to make policy decisions without strong evidence and to dishonestly make unsubstantiated claims to the public. For example, CDC director Walensky implied that a young, healthy person who was previously vaccinated needed to get a booster shot to protect vaccinated third parties, like a family member, even though she lacked supporting trial evidence, and the vaccines were never approved for preventing transmission.[74]

The potential for this situation is likely unavoidable, as federal policymakers have wide latitude to make decisions producing great benefit or harm. Public officials are also largely freely able to make false statements. Along with public pressure, the remedy for misbehavior lies in the democratic process of directly electing politicians who also appoint, approve, and oversee executive branch officials. For example, the House Select Subcommittee on the Coronavirus Pandemic in 2024 investigated the behaviors of federal public health officials in relation to COVID-19, including Dr. Anthony Fauci.[75]

The executive branch's capacity to make beneficial or harmful decisions greatly increases during a public health emergency like the COVID-19 pandemic. Under Section 319 of the Public Health Service (PHS) Act, the HHS Secretary can declare a public emergency when (1) a disease or disorder represents such an emergency or (2) "a public health emergency, including significant outbreaks of infectious diseases or bioterrorist attacks, otherwise exists."[76] This declaration grants expanded powers to HHS, namely the ability to make grants, provide awards, enter into contracts, and conduct/support "investigations into the cause, treatment, or prevention of a disease or disorder."

Most relevant to the government's vaccination policies over the course of the COVID-19 pandemic, Section 564 of the FD&C Act allows the FDA to authorize an unapproved product during emergencies declared by HHS or other agencies like the Department of Homeland Security and DoD.[77] The government can make such emergency authorizations when the product may be effective in treating a serious or life-threatening disease or condition and "there is no adequate, approved, and available alternative to the product for diagnosing, preventing, or treating such disease or condition." The scope of the authorization should be based on "an assessment of the available scientific evidence." Such emergency powers are extremely important in emergencies, as fast-approaching dangers require fast-acting responses. With COVID-19 vaccines, the original EUAs for adults likely saved hundreds of thousands of American lives, especially among high risk groups like the elderly, unhealthy, and immunocompromised.[78]

Yet, federal policymakers did not target their emergency powers based on robust evidence to make COVID-19 vaccines available and recommended for high-risk individuals. Rather, they broadly mandated vaccinations and advocated universal boosting via one-size-fits-all policies. For example, mandated vaccination for federal workers and contractors and health care workers did not consider whether they had natural or infection-induced immunity that likely conferred greater protection than two-dose vaccinations.[79] There was also no high-quality evidence that the mandate would protect third parties. Rather than pursuing traditional approval, the FDA issued an emergency authorization for children, regardless of their risk, based on limited evidence and without demonstrating that COVID-19 constituted a significant danger to their health that met the statutory requirements for an EUA. And, the FDA authorized and CDC recommended repeated universal booster vaccinations based on no randomized clinical trials proving safety and efficacy at the same time as the danger of COVID-19 significantly decreased. Given increased mistrust in health institutions, officials must make honest, evidence-based decisions to earn and maintain the public's trust to reliably lead during crises.

Congress can pass measures to increase transparency, accountability, and honesty among federal employees. Such action will not eliminate all contributors to mistrust in public health institutions, but it will target key reasons for why such mistrust exists. First, statutory law currently does not explicitly mandate a consideration of how a public health emergency affects different groups with regards to the FDA's authority to issue an EUA. Thus, Congress must require that any EUA involve a detailed explanation for why the available evidence shows that (1) each group that the authorization allows to use the product is facing a serious or life-threatening condition or disease, (2) the product is safe and effective for each group, and (3) there is no adequate, approved, and available alternative regarding the relative risks and benefits for each group. While one may theoretically come up with an infinite number of different groups, the congressional mandate could specify major distinctions based on age, sex, and health status along with any other ones the FDA finds relevant to distinguish. Such transparency is additionally helpful, as medical researchers in a March 2024 report from the Georgetown University project PharmedOut noted that the contemporary standard for EUAs "is so vague that virtually any treatment can be approved under the political pressures of a pandemic or epidemic."[80]

Congress must similarly require that any CDC recommendations for authorized but not approved products have similar explanations. Thus, even if the FDA allows almost everyone to get an authorized product, the CDC would have to justify why it actively recommends usage among varying groups. This requirement would have forced the FDA and CDC to explain why the vaccine EUAs for the original and booster doses were necessary for old, young, unhealthy, and healthy people along with those who had previous vaccinations and/or natural immunity. While such a law would not have prevented the agencies from ultimately making the same decisions, it would have mandated an evidence-based explanation to the public for their unnuanced decision-making.

Furthermore, Congress can require that HHS more fully utilize its emergency powers for essential research. The NIH has significant resources—over $47 billion in 2024—and it uses most of this money to fund research.[81] The PHS Act grants HHS—which includes the NIH—expanded powers to conduct or support investigations into the treatment or prevention of diseases and disorders along with making grants, providing awards, and entering contracts.[82] Yet, during the COVID-19 pandemic, the FDA did not require that companies like Pfizer and Moderna conduct RCTs other than the original, short-term trials testing for safety and vaccine efficacy against symptomatic infection. No RCTs tested for the vaccines' effect on transmission or how they impacted different risk groups like younger adults versus the elderly or healthy adults compared to unhealthy adults. No RCTs were required for booster shots. The FDA had the power to require such trials for vaccine authorization and/or approval, and the NIH had the budget and emergency powers to finance these studies if policymakers wanted to guarantee they occurred rather than rely on industry. Consequently, Congress can mandate the FDA and NIH to use their emergency powers to require and finance randomized trials that cover all relevant indications whenever possible as a prerequisite for issuing EUAs.

In totality, it is likely impossible that, if all the reforms in this chapter became reality, the United States would suddenly have a perfect system of medical research and development. However, the current system does not reliably guarantee the safety and effectiveness of medical products. Industry dominates R&D and controls trial data, preventing independent vetting of the results yielded from its de facto self-examinations. Federal policymakers increasingly have weakened standards of evidence, while regulators have become entangled with the companies they are meant to oversee. Thus, these reforms would go a long way toward bettering public health and—as a direct consequence—deservedly improving public trust in American medical and public health institutions.

# Conclusion

The United States is an increasingly medicalized society. Health institutions and professionals treat increasing numbers of human conditions and behaviors as requiring treatment through various therapies, drugs, devices, and other medical products. An estimated 60–70 percent American adults in recent years have reported taking prescription drugs, or 158 to 184 million people in 2023.[1] This includes 55 percent of such adults who reported taking medication daily in 2021, and nearly half (48 percent) who disclosed taking more than one drug.[2] Additionally, the American Medical Association estimated in September 2021 that around 10 percent of all Americans will use an implanted medical device at some point in their lifetimes, equating to around 34.0 million Americans according to 2024 US Census Bureau estimates.[3] Simultaneously, the AMA posited that "fewer than 0.5% of these devices, however, are likely to have been tested in rigorous clinical trials" for safety and efficacy.[4]

In 2016, investigative reporters John Fauber and Kristina Fiore wrote a series of articles finding that expanded medical definitions for just eight relatively newly diagnosed conditions—prediabetes, low testosterone, intermittent explosive disorder, binge-eating disorder, female sexual arousal disorder, adult attention-deficit hyperactivity disorder (adult ADHD), overactive bladder disorder, and premenstrual dysphoric disorder—affected more than 77 percent of the US adult population.[5] All eight disorders were not part of mainstream medicine just twenty years prior, but with new definitions and lowered thresholds, millions of Americans suddenly had treatable conditions. Many of these changes came from mainstream medical institutions, such as clinical guidelines, which had significant ties to industry. For example, in 2013, the American Psychiatric Association revised the fourth edition of the *Diagnostic and Statistical Manual of Mental Disorders* (*DSM*), creating the new *DSM-5*. The new manual greatly expanded the number of Americans considered to have treatable conditions like adult ADHD, intermittent explosive disorder, and binge-eating disorder. Among the task force members who put together the *DSM-5*, 69 percent disclosed financial ties to the pharmaceutical industry.[6]

While Fauber and Fiore looked at relatively new medical conditions, millions more Americans have become treatment-eligible for other known conditions. As Chapter 4 discusses, changes in clinical treatment guidelines have recommended statins for millions of Americans for primary prevention. Roughly 20–30 million estimated Americans took statins for primary prevention in 2018–19 even though the treatment has not shown the ability to reduce the incidence of a single death, heart attack, or stroke for over 99 percent of these users if they took statins for 4.4 years.[7] Authors of key guidelines that have recommended greater statin usage for primary prevention for people at low-risk of heart disease, such as the 2013 American College of Cardiology and American Heart Association guidelines, also have had significant financial conflicts of interest with industry.[8]

Yet, while Americans get more medical treatments and the country spends more on health care than any other country, the United States achieves worse health outcomes, and Americans have a life expectancy that is over four years shorter than people in other wealthy nations.[9] Americans currently face health crises such as hundreds of thousands of annual cardiovascular disease deaths and a climbing obesity rate that is more than double that of comparable countries.[10] Additionally, prices for prescription drugs, medical devices, and other health interventions are far higher in the United States than in peer countries, where Americans often pay several times more for the same products.[11]

Given increasing medicalization and poor health outcomes, are the medical knowledge and institutions meant to promote effective and safe treatments reliable? Unfortunately, the available evidence resoundingly answers no. The research underlying medical products is predominantly funded, designed, and conducted by industry. Consequently, these trials churn out results significantly more favorable to industry than independently-run studies.[12] The very research agenda that such trials fulfill are whatever industry believes will reap maximum profits.

While the FDA approves products, the agency merely examines the results of industry self-examinations. Entrusting industry with such control over medical knowledge has not proven reliable. Roche's sponsorship of the clinical trials behind Tamiflu along with its control of the trial data misled the world into spending billions of dollars for a product with minimal benefit, especially in comparison to the company's more grand claims of Tamiflu's superiority.[13] Upon getting access to the clinical study reports of the Roche-sponsored trials, Tom Jefferson and the other Cochrane review authors found significant signs of bias.[14] These findings were not unique. In a 2008 Cochrane review examining the evidence behind using angiotensin-converting enzyme (ACE) inhibitors to treat primary hypertension, the authors concluded:

> Most of the trials in this review were funded by companies that make ACE inhibitors and serious adverse effects were not reported by the authors of many of these trials. This could mean that the drug companies are withholding unfavorable findings related to their drugs. Due to incomplete reporting of the number of participants who dropped out of the trials due to adverse drug reactions, as well as the short duration of these trials, this review could not provide a good estimate of the harms associated with this class of drugs. Prescribing the least expensive ACE inhibitor in lower doses will lead to substantial cost savings, and possibly a reduction in dose-related adverse events.[15]

While US lawmakers have technically increased clinical trial transparency, the advances have not made the underlying data from clinical trials accessible. The 1997 FDAMA and 2007 FDAAA made ClinicalTrials.gov the first national registry of clinical trials that allowed the public to access limited metadata and summary results in a searchable manner online. However, the available data on ClinicalTrials.gov are largely not more detailed than publicly available FDA review documents and do not include full CSRs and de-identified individual participant data.[16]

The only way to get the underlying clinical data from the FDA is retroactively through FOIA requests: a limited, lengthy, and costly avenue for researchers. The FDA has often sided with industry to deny and delay requests, as the agency attempted to delay access to clinical trial data behind Pfizer's COVID-19 vaccine by seventy-five years.[17] Even with the statutory authority to both prospectively and retroactively disclose clinical trial data, the FDA has imposed regulations onto itself, restricting its disclosure capacities and giving significant leeway to industry to block data releases.[18]

While the public entrusts the FDA with guaranteeing medical products' safety and effectiveness, doctors and medical professionals look to peer-reviewed medical journals as the key disseminators and gold standard of medical knowledge. Yet, these journals often serve as marketing arms of industry by publishing its trial results based on the limited summaries of data the companies choose to share with peer reviewers. Without access to the underlying data, journals cannot vet the information they publish. Thus, when industry largely funds, designs, and controls studies, medical journals serve as trusted stamps of approval for doctors who otherwise might be wary of industry-sponsored research.

Additionally, the authors of the published articles are frequently either employees of or have financial ties to industry. While journals largely require authors to disclose their financial interests—which does not stop COIs from occurring—they fail to do so for their editors even though investigations have found that at least around half of physician editors have received industry payments.[19] While payment amounts vary, the highest-paid editors have received millions of dollars in a single year from industry.

Many journals are not incentivized to reduce the level of industry control, as they can earn significant sums of money from article reprints, which sales representatives use to lobby physicians, along with advertising (to a lesser degree).[20] Journals are only as relevant as they publish relevant research, and industry has demonstrated a willingness to decrease the amount of manuscripts they submit to journals that impose restrictions. This was the case with *JAMA*'s 2005–13 policy of requiring industry-submitted research to include statistical analyses done by independent statisticians.[21]

Such weak peer review from medical journals provides industry with an undue influence over the dissemination of medical knowledge. Spending billions of dollars on direct-to-consumer advertising annually, manufacturers are able to push their products onto consumers who then ask for prescriptions from doctors.[22] Such advertising could be beneficial if the level of advertising dollars correlated with the added clinical benefit of a particular treatment; however, the opposite has been true.[23] Pharmaceutical companies spend more to advertise drugs with low-added clinical benefits compared to those with high-added benefits. Doctors are then not equipped to know the safety and effectiveness of drugs—especially in comparison to other methods of care—that are heavily advertised to their patients at the same time as drug representatives effectively lobby physicians' offices with reprints of medical journal articles.

As most doctors cannot realistically read thousands of medical journal articles, clinical practice guidelines synthesize and disseminate medical knowledge. However, they also suffer from lack of access to trial data and significant financial COIs. In 2011, the IOM concluded that guidelines generally suffer from poor quality, as they make recommendations from industry-sponsored studies with subpar designs, such as those using unrepresentative, small patient populations and poor comparators.[24] Aside from evidence limitations, many guideline recommendations lack significant substantiation. In 2001, the National Cholesterol Education Program recommended statin therapy for primary prevention in middle-aged women without actual clinical trial data pertaining to women.[25] The NCEP guidelines also nearly tripled the number of Americans recommended for statin therapy compared to the previous 1993 guidelines even though lifestyle modifications were significantly more powerful ways to reduce the risk of heart disease.[26]

Many organizations behind guidelines receive funding from companies that have an interest in their recommendations. For example, Eli Lilly provided more than 90 percent of the funding for the Surviving Sepsis Campaign that recommended usage of the company's drug Xigris, even though the evidence behind it was weak, and the company ultimately took it off the market in 2011.[27] There are also widespread COIs among guideline authors that often go unreported. Even though nearly three quarters of physician authors of major guidelines received payments from industry in 2020, only 37.4 percent reported their financial ties.[28]

Given industry control of research, lack of data transparency, and industry influence on medical journals and clinical guidelines, the FDA—with access to the underlying clinical trial data—is the central protector of the public by determining the safety and effectiveness of medical products. However, over the last forty years, the agency has shifted its priorities toward speedily reviewing medical products and away from ensuring that they are safe and effective. The FDA only requires a single clinical trial from industry to approve a product, and the agency has increasingly relied on unproven surrogate endpoints. Rather than focus on making sure drugs and devices are safe and effective before approval, the agency has embraced lifecycle regulation, where postmarketing studies are meant to provide such assurances after products are on the market. Yet, these trials often take years to occur if they happen at all, and they rely on the same poor-quality, industry-controlled designs like lack of randomization, blinding, and use of unproven surrogates. Over the last decade, the significant majority of novel drugs have used expedited pathways to FDA approval that involve shorter review times to critically appraise the evidence, greater FDA collaboration with industry, and more frequent use of surrogate endpoints that don't measure the clinical outcomes relevant to patients.[29]

However, the weakened evidence standards for pharmaceuticals are gold standard next to the lack of safety and effectiveness testing for most medical devices.

Ninety-nine percent of medical devices approved or cleared from 1976 to 2020 did not have to prove safety and effectiveness due to the 510(k) pathway that just requires new devices to prove that they are substantially equivalent to previous devices.[30] This has led to situations, such as with Penumbra's JET 7 catheter, where whole lines of products are continuously cleared based on one another without any single one proving they are safe and effective. or This has led to situations, such as with Penumbra's JET 7 catheter, where whole lines of products are continuously cleared based on one another without any single one proving they are safe and effective.[31] Additionally, medical devices recalled for causing serious injury and even death to patients are both often based on predicate devices that were similarly recalled and also used as the predicate for the FDA to clear future devices that end up being recalled.[32] For the small fraction of devices that need to get premarket approval from the FDA, device manufacturers—like drugmakers—sponsor and control the clinical trials along with owning the underlying data. The trials often suffer from lack of randomization, no blinding, surrogate endpoint usage, and small, unrepresentative sample sizes.

While most of the issues with weak standards of evidence for medical products come from congressionally passed legislation, the FDA has been a willing partner with industry due to regulatory capture. FDA employees regularly leave the agency to earn significant salaries working for pharmaceutical companies, and the federal laws restricting postemployment behavior are extremely weak. Every single FDA commissioner since the 1980s has gone on to make money from the pharmaceutical industry.[33] These former commissioners and other former FDA employees are free to use their experiences to help companies lobby the agency, and they can engage in direct lobbying themselves after waiting a few years. While FDA employees cannot accept gifts from companies during their tenure as public servants, the expert members of FDA advisory committees, who provide consequential recommendations to the FDA, often have significant COIs. In April 2024, the committee that recommended that the FDA approve the cardiac device TriClip had ten of its fourteen members receive payments directly or indirectly from the manufacturer.[34]

The 1992 PDUFA transformed the agency from a regulatory body funded by taxpayers to an agency that receives nearly half of its entire funding, including around 70 percent of its budget for human drugs, from the very companies it regulates.[35] Additionally, the FDA negotiates with industry on its recommendations to Congress regarding the new regulations and performance goals set with each five-year PDUFA reauthorization. The FDA files annual PDUFA performance reports demonstrating how well it meets industry priorities of faster product review times. Agency leaders have not derided such industry ties; rather, some have welcomed it. Former FDA commissioner Andrew von Eschenbach even indicated that barriers between industry and regulators are too strong.[36]

Given the numerous issues with medical knowledge, doctors stand as the last line of defense between patients and potentially ineffective, unsafe, or unnecessary treatments. Yet, they are often not trained to critically appraise the evidence. Rather, rigorous medical education focuses doctors' attention on absorbing large swaths of accepted medical knowledge and trusting sources of authority. Thus, physicians maintain high levels of trust in the institutions that have failed to uphold high standards of evidence: medical journals, clinical guidelines, and public health agencies.

At the same time, medical product companies—particularly the pharmaceutical industry—significantly influence doctors in every aspect of their education and careers, including premed, medical school, residency, fellowship, and continuing medical education. Influential physicians receive thousands of dollars from companies to promote their products to their colleagues. And, industry employs thousands of sales representatives to develop relationships with health care professionals, provide favors, present biased information, and ultimately increase industry sales. With all this industry influence, doctors must simultaneously attempt to provide the best care for their patients while working fifty hours per week on average, making it very difficult to conduct the additional job of scrutinizing the institutions and individuals that educate them.[37]

The patent model lies at the core of the entire system for medical products, rewarding innovators with government-enforced exclusivities and monopoly power for new discoveries. Patents do not tie financial rewards to health outcomes; rather, companies are rewarded for preventing competition for as long as possible and convincing the largest number of patients and doctors to use and prescribe their products. Thus, patents incentivize industry to conduct poorly designed, biased trials, hide the evidence from those trials, and dominate the sources that medical professionals rely upon most—medical journals and clinical guidelines—using their positive published pieces as proof to physicians of safety and effectiveness. Yet, most new drugs do not add any significant clinical benefit to existing therapies, most new devices do not even need to prove greater effectiveness, and companies spend more money marketing products that bring in the most sales but aren't the most beneficial relative to standard treatment.[38]

Incentives for industry to pursue obtaining and maintaining patents are strong to the extent that AbbVie has one of the best-selling drugs in the world, Humira, due to working to consistently expand its patent exclusivity length over the standard term of twenty years.[39] The vast majority of new patents have not been for novel treatments; they have been part of industry efforts to continuously extend patent protections for their products.[40] Along with not benefitting from a system that promotes the best medical discoveries for public health, patients face exorbitant costs due to manufacturer's ability to charge monopoly prices. The introduction of generics often reduces prices by 80 percent or more.[41]

Subservience to the patent model from federal government officials during the COVID-19 pandemic granted vaccine manufacturers immense profits and control over clinical trial data, which policymakers had the power to not allow. Taxpayers financed the underlying research behind the mRNA technology for both the Pfizer and Moderna vaccines.[42] Yet, Operation Warp Speed allowed both companies to earn billions of dollars not just from direct government purchases of the vaccines at well above cost, but from the ability to increase prices by as much as 4,000 percent once government stockpiles ran out.[43] Also, the government allowed private control over the clinical trial data when the vaccines were of immense public importance and millions of Americans would take them to prevent severe COVID-19 illness. Thus, Public Health and Medical Professionals for Transparency had to sue the FDA to get access to Pfizer's clinical trial data years after most Americans had already gotten vaccinated.[44]

Yet, a key lesson from the COVID-19 pandemic is that even though industry domination of medical research and development generally is a major issue, the use of government power to make policy based on weak evidence is both possible and dangerous. While the COVID-19 vaccine effectively protected millions of Americans from severe illness and death, particularly in high-risk groups, federal policymakers and public health officials chose to simplify their policies and messaging at the expense of truth and honesty.[45] Revealingly, when CDC director Walensky faced the criticism from Dr. Offit that young, healthy people did not need a vaccine booster, she did not substantively address the point. Rather, Walensky said, "we are simplifying our message ... you need to get your fall booster vaccine."[46]

Repeatedly throughout the pandemic, simplifying the message ignored scientific evidence where it existed and where it was lacking. When rolling out the vaccine mandate for federal employees, contractors, and health care workers, federal policymakers did not make any exceptions for people with infection-induced immunity even though such protection was stronger than that from the vaccine.[47] Based on small, limited studies, the FDA granted emergency use authorization for vaccines in children regardless of their health status even when children were at very low risk of severe COVID-19 illness. The FDA and CDC pushed universal booster shots regardless of age, health, and previously acquired immunity, even though most of the population was protected against severe illness and other countries were targeting booster vaccinations for high-risk groups. No randomized controlled trials testing relevant clinical outcomes for safety and efficacy backed universal boosting. The FDA even approved Pfizer-BioNTech's and Moderna's bivalent boosters, each based on antibody data from eight to ten mice and information about different vaccine products.[48]

Public health leaders, such as Dr. Ashish Jha, made public claims about the vaccines that were patently untrue and/or unsubstantiated, such as that someone getting a booster shot would protect their family by preventing transmission.[49] The FDA never compelled vaccine manufacturers to conduct any clinical trials proving that the vaccines prevent transmission. Virologists knew before the vaccine rollout that respiratory viruses such as COVID-19 had short incubation periods, and, thus, vaccines would serve to prevent severe disease rather than mild illness.[50] By summer 2021, breakthrough cases in Provincetown, Massachusetts proved that vaccinated individuals could get and spread the virus.[51] If pharmaceutical companies like Pfizer and Moderna marketed their products as government and public health officials like Dr. Fauci, CDC director Walensky, and Dr. Jha did, they could have been found liable for illegally marketing their products.

While the COVID-19 vaccines were safe for most Americans, they did present risks like any treatment, especially for specific groups. Young, healthy men—who were at extremely low risk of severe COVID-19 illness—faced vaccine mandates if they were in the federal workforce or went to many universities, even though they had a known risk of developing myocarditis. A *Journal of Medical Ethics* risk-benefit analysis found that university mandates—which followed CDC recommendations—presented a net harm to young men.[52] The vaccines cause other, rarer side effects for others within the general population. However rare, federal policymakers compelled people who were protected against severe illness to get unnecessary treatments that could cause harm. This decision was not made from an evaluation of the scientific evidence, rather, federal officials wanted to simplify their message.

As this book details, industry capture of the medical knowledge behind most drugs, devices, and other medical products has significantly harmed the reliability of US institutions. By choosing to adopt a one-size-fits-all approach and prioritize simplicity over an honest, transparent, and nuanced evaluation of the evidence, federal and public health officials only further reduced the reliability of institutions and, thus, the trust that many Americans have in the system. This legitimate mistrust can also fuel unreliable new sources of authority. For example, distrust in public health agencies increased public support for Dr. Robert Malone—who helped create the mRNA vaccine technology—and he made claims without robust evidence, like that COVID-19 vaccination caused one per 2,000–3,000 children to get hospitalized.[53] At the beginning of this book, I quoted Representative Dingell's concern that criticisms of public health officials would further undermine trust in public health institutions.[54] Perhaps, lack of faith in public health institutions, at least in part, is a result of their own actions.

Just as policy decisions can undermine trust, they can also rebuild it. Today, the reliability of the medical knowledge that all Americans rely upon for their health care is very weak. But, this current system and our entire situation is not preordained. It is the outcome of intentional policy decisions, and new policy decisions can redirect our course. Congress has the full authority to increase the transparency of medical knowledge, incentivize high-quality medical journals and guidelines, strengthen evidence standards, free the FDA from regulatory capture, and redirect the incentives of the entire medical research and development system to connect rewards for innovation directly with improvements in public health.

Perhaps these reforms can also help reverse the overmedicalization of American society. Industry has corrupted and dominated the research, regulatory processes, and education to promote their products to the most people to maximize profits over improving public health. While pharmaceuticals and medical devices save lives, several examples within this book, such as statin guidelines, highlight likely overmedicalization when other avenues to improve health, like lifestyle habits, are more potent but less profitable for industry. Indeed, nearly all medical and health services research focuses on new drugs and devices rather than the better delivery of health services.[55] Meanwhile, medical care only determines up to 20 percent of the social determinants of population health compared to 40 percent due to social and economic factors, 30 percent determined by health behaviors like diet and exercise, and 10 percent because of individuals' physical environments.[56]

In 2010, *JAMA Internal Medicine* introduced the "Less Is More" campaign. An April 2010 editorial opined:

> Our current health care system operates on the unspoken but widely prevalent belief that more care is always better than less and that new technology is always better than older methods. Yet, there are many cases in which these assumptions are wrong. Clearly, these erroneous assumptions negatively affect health by exposing patients to unnecessary harms of treatment and testing, with no expected benefit; they also increase the total cost of health care.[57]

In our current system, where innovation is only rewarded insofar as industry can make profits from patent monopolies regardless of public health benefit, medical research will be opposed to the concept of less is more. Less means less products sold and less profits made. But, in a world where medical knowledge is truly reliable and directed at areas best suited for the betterment of public health, perhaps Americans can trust that public health institutions, medical journals, clinical guidelines, and their doctors act in their best interest so that they can live healthy lives.

# Afterword: A New Regime

> *It's no secret that many of our institutions of democracy ... even of science and medicine are no longer transparent. As a consequence, they have become inefficient, dysfunctional, or corrupt. They've fallen captive to the profit-making industries, they have stagnated in bureaucratic secrecy, and, in siloing, they have lost touch with ordinary citizens.*
>
> —Robert F. Kennedy Junior[1]

A lifelong Democrat who ran both in the 2024 Democratic presidential primary and eventually in the general election as an independent, Robert F. Kennedy Jr. ultimately dropped out of the race in August 2024, endorsing and joining forces with Donald Trump.[2] Reflecting Trump's Make America Great Again (MAGA) slogan, Kennedy promised to Make America Healthy Again (MAHA).[3] After winning the 2024 presidential election, President-elect Trump announced his nomination of Kennedy to lead HHS, charging him with restoring "these Agencies to the traditions of Gold Standard Scientific Research, and beacons of Transparency, to end the Chronic Disease epidemic, and to Make America Great and Healthy Again!"[4]

Newly confirmed HHS Secretary Kennedy delivered his welcoming remarks to HHS staff on February 18, 2025.[5] Kennedy outlined severe issues with American public health institutions that have hurt public trust, promising to fix them. To address a growing chronic disease epidemic, Kennedy introduced three pillars of focus: undoing regulatory capture, radical transparency, and promoting gold-standard scientific research. To reclaim HHS from industry capture, Kennedy promised to remove conflicts of interest on advisory committees and shut the revolving door. To usher in radical transparency, the Secretary promised to make the "policy process so transparent that people won't even have to file a FOIA request." To promote high-quality science, Kennedy pushed commissioning research that would "satisfy all the stakeholders ... use protocols that we all agree on in advance and not alter the outcomes ... when ... they look inconvenient ... [and] depoliticize these issues and ... renew the search for existential truth."

I wrote most of this manuscript months prior to the 2024 election and much has changed in federal health care policy. Yet, the central issues this book identifies remain potent and dangerous. Kennedy's speech points to key issues this book raises, and the second Trump administration has ushered in significant changes to HHS. However, identifying issues and promising actions is one step; delivering solutions is another task entirely. Thus, this afterword will explore how the actions of the Trump administration and Kennedy-led HHS during their first six months relate to the major solutions and problems this book identifies.

## Staffing Reductions, Funding Cuts, and Consolidation

A major, official Trump administration initiative has been to reduce waste, fraud, and abuse throughout the federal government. The Department of Government Efficiency (DOGE)—an advisory entity rather than an official department—pushed extensive staffing and spending cuts across departments, including HHS. On February 11, President Trump signed an executive order to implement DOGE's "Workforce Optimization Initiative," including instructions for agency heads to "promptly undertake preparations to initiate large-scale reductions in force (RIFs)."[6]

The order also directed the Office of Management and Budget (OMB) to create a plan to reduce the federal workforce, including that "each agency hire no more than one employee for every four employees that depart." Consequently, the OMB directed federal agencies to "focus on the maximum elimination of functions that are not statutorily mandated" without harming the quality of "statutorily-required functions."[7] The OMB also told agencies to consolidate their structures, namely in duplicative, unnecessary, and noncritical areas.

Following the White House's and OMB's orders, HHS initially cut thousands of employees through initiatives like firing probationary employees, pushing early retirements, and offering $25,000 voluntary buyouts for federal workers.[8] On March 27, HHS announced another cut of 10,000 employees, claiming $1.8 billion in savings and downsizing the department from 82,000 to 62,000 employees.[9] The department also consolidated HHS's twenty-eight divisions into fifteen. Officially, these actions prioritized cutting unnecessary administrative roles and duplicative departments and agency functions.[10] The implementation of these changes depends on outcomes from various legal cases, with HHS finalizing some firings after a US Supreme Court decision, while Judge Melissa DuBose of the US District Court for the District of Rhode Island halted other terminations and the reorganization plan.[11]

President Trump's budget for FY 2026—a set of recommendations for Congress—would formalize HHS's restructuring, and it would cut the department's discretionary budget by $32.1 billion (25.2 percent).[12] While the proposal cuts only $272 million (3.9 percent) at the FDA, it slashes $19.1 billion (40.6 percent) at the NIH and $4.9 billion (53.3 percent) at the CDC. The NIH cuts would accompany reorganizing its twenty-seven institutes into eight. The administration justified halving the CDC budget by claiming it is returning the CDC to its core mission of addressing infectious diseases while other functions—like the National Institute for Occupational Safety and Health—move outside the agency as part of the consolidation.

While HHS has already taken significant action, the extent and effect of these cuts and consolidation actions will depend on the budget Congress passes. Additionally, Secretary Kennedy acknowledged HHS will have to correct mistakes.[13] In late February, Kennedy protected around 950 Indian Health Service workers after they had received layoff notices.[14] In June, *The Washington Post* reported that the Trump administration was scrambling to rehire laid-off employees and those who voluntarily resigned across the government, including HHS.[15] The CDC moved to reinstate over 450 employees that month.[16] Thus, the shroud of uncertainty makes detailing HHS's specific state after potential restructuring impossible.

Yet, the administration's general goal of HHS budget and staffing cuts will likely expand industry control of medical research. Industry currently dominates the medical research agenda in the United States, while the NIH has provided critical foundational research essential to private innovation. As Chapter 1 details, medical researchers and academics significantly shifted toward relying on industry in the 1980s, at least in part due to harder-to-get NIH research grants and federal funding constraints.[17] If the Trump administration successfully continues down this path—especially with a 40 percent cut to the NIH budget—this trend will likely continue. By April 2025, NIH cut around 1,200 employees, not counting incentivized retirements and resignations, which could further push researchers into industry's hands.[18] While Secretary Kennedy told Congress that he did not fire working scientists, the NIH did cut research contracts and the future is uncertain.[19]

With less money, the NIH would have less capacity to fund studies that industry would not. For example, Chapters 1 and 9 mention the 2002 Diabetes Prevention Program (DPP) study that tested the drug metformin against diet and exercise, finding that the latter was more effective in preventing the onset of type 2 diabetes.[20] In March 2025, NIH cut funding for the DPP, and the agency will have less resources to finance similar projects with less funding.[21]

Staffing and restructuring uncertainty also call into question Kennedy's call for radical transparency. While the administration has not proposed massive budget cuts to the FDA, it let go around 3,500 employees.[22] In April, HHS shut down entire FOIA offices, including at the FDA, for consolidation and fired many employees handling requests.[23] While HHS reinstated at least some of the staff, the disruption and reduced staff to handle FOIA requests will make it harder for researchers to get access to information like clinical trial data.[24] In an April 22 press conference, Secretary Kennedy promised to fully restore those FOIA offices and make it easier for people to get information, such as by posting releases from previous requests online for anyone to access.[25]

If true, Kennedy's FOIA plan would increase transparency; however, it does not approach having the FDA make underlying clinical trial data publicly available for FDA-approved products retroactively and prospectively. The data behind nearly all drug and device approvals would remain hidden from the public without a successful FOIA request. While promising to make FOIA requests easier, Kennedy has not addressed FDA deference to industry in blocking releases through a broad view of commercially confidential information. In his Senate Finance Committee confirmation hearing before becoming HHS secretary, Kennedy stated, "we should make sure that all the science is published with the raw data."[26] While he was specifically referring to NIH studies, he has the statutory authority to release data behind all FDA-approved products.

## Faster Approvals, AI, and COVID-19

The new FDA leadership has continued the general focus on faster approvals rather than stronger evidence standards, while simultaneously raising standards to approve COVID-19 vaccines. On June 10, 2025, FDA commissioner Marty Makary and CBER director Vinay Prasad published their "Priorities for a New FDA" in *JAMA* with the first listed priority to accelerate cures.[27] Pointing to expedited review processes during the COVID-19 pandemic, they "aim to pilot programs to deliver sponsors a decision in weeks" through allowing companies to submit more materials prior to trial completion, eliminating outdated regulatory processes, and then shortening the FDA review time after trial results are known.

Supporting the last point, on June, 17, the FDA announced the Commissioner's National Priority Voucher (CNPV) program, where the agency will review qualifying drugs in 1–2 months down from 10–12.[28] The Commissioner will give vouchers to companies for a company's specific investigational new drug or a drug at the company's discretion based on four criteria:

1. "Addressing a health crisis in the U.S."
2. "Delivering more innovative cures for the American people."
3. "Addressing unmet public health needs."
4. "Increasing domestic drug manufacturing as a national security issue."

Theoretically, enhanced communication between companies and the FDA along with submitting more application materials before filing the full application could account for much of the reduction in review times. However, the FDA will also convene a multidisciplinary review team for a single-day discussion to guide approval decisions. Additionally, the agency has not detailed guardrails to ensure drug companies receive a voucher based on merit rather than conflicts of interest. Neither has the FDA indicated how many vouchers it may provide.

Top HHS officials have also endorsed faster approvals and lower standards of evidence for cell and gene therapy, namely for rare and life-threatening diseases.[29] At a June 5 FDA roundtable, Commissioner Makary endorsed expedited approval programs, the Right to Try Act, and factoring postmarketing requirements in approval decisions. CBER director Vinay Prasad supported the use of both surrogate and clinical endpoints along with a variety of trial designs to go alongside randomized trials like real-world evidence. Secretary Kennedy referenced President Trump's executive order requiring the elimination of ten regulations for every one added and asked the panelists—industry and academic researchers—to suggest regulations to eliminate.

One major avenue that the new FDA will use to shorten review times is using artificial intelligence (AI). On May 8, 2025, Commissioner Makary announced a plan to have all FDA centers use AI by June 30:

> We need to value our scientists' time and reduce the amount of non-productive busywork that has historically consumed much of the review process. The agency-wide deployment of ... [AI] holds tremendous promise in accelerating the review time for new therapies.[30]

Among other uses, the FDA plans to use its AI program, "Elsa," to accelerate product reviews through summarizing "adverse events to support safety profile assessments."[31]

While AI usage does not lower evidence standards, it may hurt the validity of FDA reviews due to the technology's significant problems in producing accurate information. Ahead of schedule on June 2, the FDA launched Elsa to aid scientific reviewers. On June 3, NBC News reported that several FDA employees noted significant limitations to the tool.[32] One employee revealed that Elsa gave entirely or partially incorrect responses to questions about FDA-approved products and other public information. Providing false information matches the limitations of other AI models, otherwise known as "hallucinations."[33]

Other employees later told CNN that Elsa made up studies entirely, reflecting AI failures with the White House's release of The MAHA Report: a document outlining root causes of the childhood chronic disease epidemic.[34] The report authors used AI, leading to completely and partially inaccurate citations.[35] The report cited studies that did not exist, like a fake *JAMA Pediatrics* paper about changes in mental health and substance use during the COVID-19 pandemic among American adolescents.[36]

The FDA's focus on faster reviews and use of AI may present increasing danger when paired with lengthy product applications and fewer staff. Clinical study reports are thousands of pages, providing ample room for AI to make mistakes like it already has done. Even a minor data error could dramatically impact conclusions about safety and efficacy. Additionally, fewer staff increases reliance on AI. Therefore, if Elsa fails, there will likely be a weaker support structure to reasonably guarantee medical products' safety and effectiveness.

With immense processing power, AI could theoretically benefit the FDA, industry, and American people by speeding up regulatory and review processes without sacrificing evidence standards. Office of Drug Evaluation Sciences deputy director Jinzhong Liu claimed that Elsa allowed him to "perform scientific review tasks in minutes that used to take three days."[37] However, no publicly available testing results currently exist to prove AI's benefit to the FDA.

## COVID-19 Vaccines

In contrast to the FDA's primary focus on faster reviews, its leadership has prioritized enhanced evidence standards for COVID-19 vaccinations. On May 20, Commissioner Makary and Director Prasad published a new risk-based framework—comparable to peer nations—in *NEJM*.[38] Differing from the previous "one-size-fits-all regulatory framework," Makary and Prasad stated, "U.S. policy has sometimes been justified by arguing that the American people are not sophisticated enough to understand age- and risk-based recommendations. We reject this view." Opposing previous universal boosting, the FDA will approve COVID-19 vaccines based on immunogenicity data for people above the age of sixty-five and for all individuals aged six months and older if they have a CDC-defined high-risk condition for severe COVID-19 outcomes. This broad high-risk category could include 100–200 million Americans, as some of the CDC's conditions are diabetes, obesity, immunodeficiency, cancer, asthma, pregnancy, and certain mental health conditions like depression.

For all individuals aged between six months and sixty-four years without risk factors for severe COVID-19, the FDA will require "randomized, controlled trial data evaluating clinical outcomes" for approval. However, the FDA will only recommend the trials, so manufacturers would have to voluntarily conduct them. Given "global equipoise about yearly boosters for the 50–64-year-old" demographic, the agency especially recommends trials for this group. The FDA-preferred primary trial endpoint is symptomatic COVID-19 with secondary endpoints of severe COVID-19, hospitalization, and death. Participant follow-up should be at least six months.

Accordingly, the FDA approved Novavax's NUVAXOVID COVID-19 vaccine on May 19, 2025, and it approved Moderna's MNEXSPIKE shot on May, 30.[39] Both approvals pertain to individuals aged sixty-five and older, or those twelve to sixty-four years old with a high-risk condition for severe COVID-19. The twelve-year lower bound for age reflects the pediatric populations within completed studies. Additionally, Novavax and Moderna agreed to voluntary postmarketing commitments to complete randomized, placebo-controlled trials among adults aged fifty to sixty-four years without high-risk conditions for severe COVID-19 by July 31, 2026.

Given the new FDA framework, the CDC cannot recommend universal boosters for updated and new products. Additionally, on May 27, Secretary Kennedy alongside Commissioner Makary and NIH director Jay Bhattacharya announced that the CDC will no longer recommend that healthy children and healthy pregnant women get routine COVID-19 vaccinations.[40] Makary asserted, "there's no evidence healthy kids need it today and most countries have stopped recommending it for children." Indeed, peer countries like Australia and Finland do not recommend primary or booster doses for healthy children, instead targeting booster doses to elderly and high-risk groups.[41] The CDC now recommends that shared clinical decision-making decides whether kids get vaccinated, meaning conversations between doctors and parents.[42]

However, the decision did not include advice from the CDC's ACIP, and critics have pointed out that pregnancy is a listed risk factor for severe COVID-19.[43] In a CBS News interview, Makary defended not waiting for ACIP to meet:

> That panel has been a kangaroo court where they just rubber stamp every single vaccine put in front of them … [before the next meeting] we don't want an absolute recommendation for healthy kids … you look at the [meeting] minutes of the last couple years, they say we want a simple message for everybody … it was not a data-based conversation.[44]

Regarding healthy pregnant women, Makary pointed to a lack of RCTs and mixed observational study results. While the CDC lists pregnancy as a risk factor, he said official policy is for pregnant women to talk to their doctors. Reiterating Makary's ACIP criticism, Secretary Kennedy unilaterally fired all seventeen committee members on June 9.[45] Soon thereafter, Kennedy selected replacement members, including individuals with public opinions ranging from opposing universal boosting to believing the COVID-19 vaccines are ineffective and dangerous.[46]

Justifying the significantly different evidence standards for cell and gene therapy compared to COVID-19 vaccination, CBER director Prasad explained how the former concerns severe cases often with small sample sizes where randomized trials are less practical, while the latter involves low-risk, healthier populations with millions of people.[47] However, the agency has not addressed the general degradation of evidence standards for most drugs and the nearly universal lack of safety and efficacy testing for devices while it prioritizes faster approvals. The FDA has also not demonstrated a new approach to ensure trial integrity and timely completion of postmarketing studies.

## Combatting Regulatory Capture

While also embracing further collaboration with industry, HHS has taken limited action to address the regulatory capture of the FDA. Describing their priorities for the FDA, Makary and Prasad argued for developing a "close relationship" with industry. To provide guidance and predictability, they argue the FDA "must become a user-friendly FDA that partners with industry rather than takes a receive-only posture … [but] guard against a cozy relationship that has characterized the agency in the past and led to allegations of industry capture."[48]

Regarding the former, the FDA has not only prioritized faster reviews and enhanced communications with industry, but the FDA announced a national listening tour from at least June to September with closed-door meetings "directly with pharmaceutical and biotech CEOs."[49] According to the agency itself, the meetings are meant to directly get "input from biotechnology and pharmaceutical leaders on how the FDA can modernize its regulatory framework to better support innovation and patient access to safe and effective therapies." The June 17 national voucher program announcement followed several of these meetings.

With the latter, on April 17, Commissioner Makary announced a ban on employees of regulated companies from serving on FDA advisory committees as nonvoting members, aiming to "restore impeccable integrity to the process and avoid potential conflicts of interest."[50] Industry employees can only attend meetings like the public. Makary said that such industry involvement "represents a cozy relationship … [and] the FDA has a history of being influenced unduly by corporate interests." The rule had an immediate impact, as the FDA previously recognized, "almost without exception, FDA's Advisory Committees have industry representatives who act on behalf of regulated industry at committee meetings."[51]

Yet, no current policy tackles the significant financial COIs between voting committee members and industry, along with the agency's power to infinitely provide waivers allowing conflicted individuals to serve on advisory committees.[52] However, the agency did not waive disclosed conflicts for VRBPAC members meeting to recommend a viral strain for 2025–26 COVID-19 vaccines to target.[53] Additionally, Makary and Prasad assert the agency "will take conflict of interest seriously" and stress they will "never forget one of the worst self-inflicted wounds of US health care—the FDA's illegal approval of oxycontin … the immediate hiring of the former FDA regulator by Purdue Pharma, and a subsequent epidemic that killed approximately 1 million people in the US.[54] Yet, no official policy from the current administration would have stopped the ten directly conflicted members on the joint FDA advisory committee in 2005 from keeping Vioxx on the market after it killed an estimated 30,000–60,000 Americans and Merck had pulled it from the market.[55]

Secretary Kennedy has yet to fulfill his promise to shut the revolving door, and it is unknown how he could accomplish this goal without Congress. Title 18 Section 207 of the US code still provides very limited regulation of lobbying activities for former government employees that does not impact indirect, lobbying-support roles.[56] Congress would need to legislate stricter limits. While the president can issue executive orders demanding ethics pledges from executive branch officials, President Trump both rescinded President Biden's order and has yet to issue his own.[57]

While it remains to be seen if top FDA officials will work for industry in the future, several have past ties. FDA commissioner Makary served on the board of pharmaceutical company Harrow Health and as the chief medical officer for Sesame, a telehealth company that offers GLP-1 weight-loss medications.[58] Deputy commissioner for Human Foods Kyle Diamantas worked as a corporate lawyer defending FDA-regulated companies; for example, he unsuccessfully defended Abbott Laboratories from claims that its baby formula caused severe health issues, including death.[59] Deputy general counsel and chief counsel for Food, Research, and Drugs Robert Foster worked for biopharmaceutical companies MiNK Therapeutics and SaponiQx as director of Legal and Business Affairs and "Senior Counsel and Corporate Strategy," respectively.[60] He also served on the board of biotechnology company Autonomous Therapeutics.

Furthermore, HHS has not expressly targeted user fees; rather, the White House wants to increase them, and staffing cuts may increase industry leverage. In a September 2024 *Wall Street Journal* piece, Kennedy advocated for reforming PDUFA, deriding FDA reliance on user fees as putting "bureaucrats' purse strings in the hands of the pharmaceutical industry."[61] As HHS secretary, he has taken no formal action on this issue, but the firing of 3,500 FDA employees included those in charge of negotiating with industry for a 2027 PDUFA reauthorization.[62] Lack of experienced negotiators may give greater leverage to industry to reap policy favors in exchange for more funding. However, previous negotiations have benefitted industry, so new negotiators could also have the opposite effect. Additionally, while President Trump's budget proposal decreases overall FDA funding, it increases user fee funding to $3.6 billion—up from $3.3 billion (47.8 percent) in FY 2024—meaning industry payments would finance 52.9 percent of the agency's budget.[63]

## Issues Not Addressed

Neither the administration nor Congress has seriously addressed key issues of this book on top of the aforementioned lack of tackling industry domination of medical research, promoting clinical trial transparency, fixing poor evidence standards for drugs and devices, and ending regulatory capture at the FDA. For example, the administration has put forth no reforms to address the lack of transparency and effective peer review with the medical journals and clinical guidelines that health care professionals rely upon. Regarding industry influence, on a May 27, 2025, podcast episode, Secretary Kennedy suggested he would create in-house agency journals for NIH scientists and potentially NIH-funded researchers to publish in, barring them from publishing with journals like *NEJM*, *The Lancet*, and *JAMA* "because they're all corrupt."[64] Kennedy explained:

> If you want to publish in a journal, you have to pay $10,000 to get the study published. So, the pharmaceutical company concocts a study that shows the outcome that they want that statins work or that SSRIs work … and then … they pay to get that published and they order reprints from the journal … and then they give them to the pharmaceutical reps.[65]

Yet, HHS has not suggested plans to improve the quality of journals or guidelines for privately funded research that directs doctors' decision-making regarding industry's medical products, such as revitalizing the National Guideline Clearinghouse. HHS has the power to publicly grade journals and guidelines on standards of trust, like those the IOM suggested in 2011.[66] Such reform is essential given how the scientific community privately regulates itself, and industry has corrupted this system.

Unsurprisingly, the government has taken no action to deal with the underlying patent system for medical innovation that focuses on producing treatments to secure and maintain monopoly pricing power rather than better health outcomes. As Chapter 11 discusses, smaller congressional and regulatory actions can increase transparency, evidence standards, and the overall integrity of medical knowledge. However, only changing the patent system will tackle the root causes incentivizing industry to bias studies, keep knowledge secret, push products with limited to no added benefits to existing treatments, and charge exorbitantly high prices.

## The Situation

Over the first half-year of the Trump administration and Kennedy-led HHS, the most significant changes have been cutting agency staff and budgets along with consolidation. These initiatives will likely bolster industry domination of medical research and—without further action—hurt transparency for the medical knowledge behind products. While the FDA has raised standards for COVID-19 vaccine approvals, its priorities at large continue the decades-long prioritization of faster approvals with a unique focus on AI, whose effect remains to be seen. Even though Secretary Kennedy has promised to end the regulatory capture of the FDA, action has been very limited thus far, with no official policy tackling financial COIs among advisory committee voting members, the revolving door, and user fees. Ultimately, the administration has another few years to address the major issues this book highlights.

Regardless of its policies, the current government has identified true, systemic issues in the current system of medical knowledge. In its May 2025 report, the MAHA Commission derided the "Corporate Capture and the Revolving Door" of the federal regulatory agencies, along with the industry domination of scientific research that has a "deep and widespread influence."[67] It points specifically to industry sponsorship bias, corruption of the academic literature, lobbying expenditures, funding of medical providers, financing of medical education, and support for patient advocacy groups. It recommends NIH funding for studies testing the health impacts of lifestyle modifications along with greater FDA surveillance of drugs' safety and effectiveness.[68]

Yet, much of the public debate surrounding the administration's actions revolves around either (1) recognizing these massive issues and endorsing the government's vision of change or (2) criticizing government policies while defending the current institutions.[69] As I detail, there are significant limitations to how the administration has addressed these issues. Additionally, I do not cover many of the Trump administration's health care policies at the focus of intense partisan debate—such as cuts to Medicaid and other health programs—which do not tie to this book.[70] Yet, regardless of one's views on these various policies, there are significant issues with the system of medical knowledge in the United States. There are not only two options: fully endorsing the administration and recognizing the problems or completely opposing the government and denying the issues.

The current system of medical knowledge is not reliable. Industry has captured and dominated medical research, and federal policymakers and regulators have adopted corporate priorities. Accordingly, the United States is an increasingly medicalized society while suffering worse health outcomes and far higher prices than other nations. Partisan affiliation does not negate these realities. Yet, this situation is neither final nor preordained. Americans can fix this broken system of knowledge underlying the health care we all rely upon. The first step is recognizing that the issues exist.

# Notes

## Introduction

1 House Select Subcommittee on the Coronavirus Pandemic, "Investigating the Origins of COVID-19," 2023, https://www.youtube.com/watch?v=g4rF91BeSJU.
2 Ibid, 1:29:30–1:30:41.
3 WHO, "WHO COVID-19 Dashboard: Number of COVID-19 Deaths Reported to WHO (Cumulative Total)," World Health Organization Data, May 18, 2025, https://data.who.int/dashboards/covid19/deaths?n=o; CDC, "United States COVID-19 Hospitalizations, Deaths, Emergency Department (ED) Visits, and Test Positivity by Geographic Area," Covid Data Tracker, May 24, 2025, https://covid.cdc.gov/covid-data-tracker.
4 Alec Tyson and Brian Kennedy, "Public Trust in Scientists and Views on Their Role in Policymaking: Appendix: Detailed Charts and Tables," Pew Research Center, November 14, 2024, https://www.pewresearch.org/science/2024/11/14/public-trust-in-scientists-and-views-on-their-role-in-policymaking/.
5 Ashley Kirzinger et al., "KFF COVID-19 Vaccine Monitor September 2023: Partisanship Remains Key Predictor of Views of COVID-19, Including Plans to Get Latest COVID-19 Vaccine," KFF, September 27, 2023, https://www.kff.org/health-misinformation-and-trust/poll-finding/kff-covid-19-vaccine-monitor-september-2023/.
6 Audrey Kearney et al., "KFF Tracking Poll on Health Information and Trust: January 2025," KFF, January 28, 2025, https://www.kff.org/health-information-trust/poll-finding/kff-tracking-poll-on-health-information-and-trust-january-2025/.
7 Ibid., 10.
8 Ibid., 47.
9 Kearney et al., "KFF Tracking Poll on Health Information and Trust."
10 "State of Texas v. Pfizer, Inc.: Plaintiff's Original Petition," Ken Paxton: Attorney General Of Texas, November 30, 2023, https://www.texasattorneygeneral.gov/sites/default/files/images/press/Pfizer%20Vaccine%20Petition%20Filed.pdf.
11 "Assessing America's Vaccine Safety System's Part I," 2024, 4, https://www.congress.gov/118/chrg/CHRG-118hhrg54866/CHRG-118hhrg54866.pdf.
12 CDC, "Understanding the Opioid Overdose Epidemic," CDC: Overdose Prevention, June 9, 2025, https://www.cdc.gov/overdose-prevention/about/understanding-the-opioid-overdose-epidemic.html.
13 NIH, "Drug Overdose Deaths: Facts and Figures," National Institute on Drug Abuse, August 2024, https://nida.nih.gov/research-topics/trends-statistics/overdose-death-rates#Fig3.
14 Duff et al., "The Opioid Crisis in the United States: A Brief History," Congressional Research Service, November 30, 2022, https://crsreports.congress.gov/product/pdf/IF/IF12260.

15 Bertha Madras et al., "President's Commission on Combating Drug Addiction and the Opioid Crisis," November 1, 2017, https://trumpwhitehouse.archives.gov/sites/whitehouse.gov/files/images/Final_Report_Draft_11-15-2017.pdf; Amy Howe, "Justices Put Purdue Pharma Bankruptcy Plan on Hold," SCOTUSblog, August 10, 2023, https://www.scotusblog.com/2023/08/justices-put-purdue-pharma-bankruptcy-plan-on-hold/.
16 Anne Estrup Olesen et al., "Different Effects of Morphine and Oxycodone in Experimentally Evoked Hyperalgesia: A Human Translational Study," *British Journal of Clinical Pharmacology* 70, no. 2 (2010): 189–200, https://doi.org/10.1111/j.1365-2125.2010.03700.x; John Abramson, *Sickening: How Big Pharma Broke American Health Care and How We Can Repair It* (Boston, MA: Mariner Books, 2022), 156.
17 Government Accountability Office, "Prescription Drugs: OxyContin Abuse and Diversion and Efforts to Address the Problem," December 2003: 17, https://www.gao.gov/assets/gao-04-110.pdf.
18 Barry Meier, "In Guilty Plea, OxyContin Maker to Pay $600 Million," *The New York Times*, May 10, 2007, sec. Business, https://www.nytimes.com/2007/05/10/business/11drug-web.html; David Armstrong and Jeff Ernsthausen, "Data Touted by OxyContin Maker to Fight Lawsuits Doesn't Tell the Whole Story," ProPublica, September 9, 2019, https://www.propublica.org/article/data-touted-by-oxycontin-maker-to-fight-lawsuits-doesnt-tell-the-whole-story.
19 "Purdue Settles OxyContin Charge for $600M," CNN Money, May 10, 2007, https://money.cnn.com/2007/05/10/news/companies/oxycontin/index.htm.
20 Meier, "In Guilty Plea, OxyContin Maker to Pay $600 Million."
21 Armstrong and Ernsthausen, "Data Touted by OxyContin Maker to Fight Lawsuits Doesn't Tell the Whole Story"; Jeremy Hill et al., "Sacklers to Exit from Complex Purdue Bankruptcy with Billions," Bloomberg, September 1, 2021, https://www.bloomberg.com/news/features/2021-09-01/sackler-family-exits-bankruptcy-trial-over-purdue-pharma-s-oxycontin.
22 CBS News, "Purdue Pharma Continued Deceptive Sales Practices for OxyContin after 2007, Whistleblower Says," CBS Mornings, June 20, 2018, https://www.cbsnews.com/news/oxycontin-purdue-whistleblower-says-drug-maker-continued-deceptive-sales-practices/.
23 US Department of Justice, "Press Release: Opioid Manufacturer Purdue Pharma Pleads Guilty to Fraud and Kickback Conspiracies," Office of Public Affairs, November 24, 2020, https://www.justice.gov/opa/pr/opioid-manufacturer-purdue-pharma-pleads-guilty-fraud-and-kickback-conspiracies; US Department of Justice, "Press Release: Justice Department Announces Global Resolution of Criminal and Civil Investigations with Opioid Manufacturer Purdue Pharma and Civil Settlement with Members of the Sackler Family," Office of Public Affairs, October 21, 2020, https://www.justice.gov/opa/pr/justice-department-announces-global-resolution-criminal-and-civil-investigations-opioid.
24 Brian Mann and Martha Bebinger, "Purdue Pharma, Sacklers Reach $6 Billion Deal with State Attorneys General," NPR, March 3, 2022, https://www.npr.org/2022/03/03/1084163626/purdue-sacklers-oxycontin-settlement.
25 Harrington, United States Trustee, Region 2 v. Purdue Pharma L. P. et al., 603 U.S. (US Supreme Court 2024).
26 Office of the Attorney General, "Attorney General Bonta Helps Secure $7.4 Billion from Purdue Pharma and the Sackler Family for Fueling the Opioid Crisis," State of

California Department of Justice, January 23, 2025, https://oag.ca.gov/news/press-releases/attorney-general-bonta-helps-secure-74-billion-purdue-pharma-and-sackler-family; Meredith Deliso, "States Agree to $7.4 Billion Settlement with Purdue Pharma in Opioid Litigation," ABC News, June 16, 2025, https://abcnews.go.com/US/states-agree-74-billion-settlement-purdue-pharma-opioid/story?id=122892221.

27 Abramson, *Sickening*, 155.

28 Government Accountability Office, "Prescription Drugs: OxyContin Abuse and Diversion and Efforts to Address the Problem."

29 Madras et al., "President's Commission on Combating Drug Addiction and the Opioid Crisis," 21.

30 Chris McGreal, "Big Pharma's Response to the Opioid Epidemic: Pay But Deny," *The New York Review*, November 11, 2019, https://www.nybooks.com/online/2019/11/11/big-pharmas-response-to-the-opioid-epidemic-pay-but-deny/.

31 Sarah Zhang, "The One-Paragraph Letter from 1980 That Fueled the Opioid Crisis," *The Atlantic* (blog), June 2, 2017, https://www.theatlantic.com/health/archive/2017/06/nejm-letter-opioids/528840/.

32 Jane Porter and Jick Hershel, "Addiction Rare in Patients Treated with Narcotics," *New England Journal of Medicine* 302, no. 2 (January 10, 1980): 123, https://doi.org/10.1056/NEJM198001103020221.

33 Zhang, "The One-Paragraph Letter from 1980 That Fueled the Opioid Crisis"; Madras et al., "President's Commission on Combating Drug Addiction and the Opioid Crisis."

34 Abigail Zuger, "A Doctor's Guide to What to Read on the Opioid Crisis," *The New York Times*, December 17, 2018, sec. Books, https://www.nytimes.com/2018/12/17/books/review/opioid-abuse-drug-dealer-anna-lembke.html.

35 Madras et al., "President's Commission on Combating Drug Addiction and the Opioid Crisis," 19.

36 Jane C. Ballantyne and Jianren Mao, "Opioid Therapy for Chronic Pain," *New England Journal of Medicine* 349, no. 20 (November 13, 2003): 1943–53, https://doi.org/10.1056/NEJMra025411.

37 Peter Whoriskey, "Rising Painkiller Addiction Shows Damage from Drugmakers' Role in Shaping Medical Opinion," *The Washington Post*, December 30, 2012, https://www.washingtonpost.com/business/economy/2012/12/30/014205a6-4bc3-11e2-b709-667035ff9029_story.html.

38 Sanford H. Roth et al., "Around-the-Clock, Controlled-Release Oxycodone Therapy for Osteoarthritis-Related Pain: Placebo-Controlled Trial and Long-Term Evaluation," *Archives of Internal Medicine* 160, no. 6 (March 27, 2000): 853–60, https://doi.org/10.1001/archinte.160.6.853.

39 Whoriskey, "Rising Painkiller Addiction Shows Damage from Drugmakers' Role in Shaping Medical Opinion."

40 Jerry Mitchell, "How the FDA Helped Pave the Way for an Opioid Epidemic," *The Clarion-Ledger*, January 26, 2018, https://www.clarionledger.com/story/news/2018/01/26/opioid-epidemic-how-fda-helped-pave-way/950561001/.

41 Caitlin Esch, "How One Sentence Helped Set Off the Opioid Crisis," Marketplace, December 13, 2017, https://www.marketplace.org/2017/12/13/opioid/; Andrew Kolodny, "How FDA Failures Contributed to the Opioid Crisis," *AMA Journal of Ethics* 22, no. 8 (August 2020): E743–50, https://doi.org/10.1001/amajethics.2020.743.

42 Kolodny, "How FDA Failures Contributed to the Opioid Crisis," 745.

43 Ibid; Curtis Wright, "Exhibit 4: Medical Officer Review, Integrated Summary of Efficacy, Oxycodone Controlled Release, NDA 20553, Curtis Wright, M.D. and Medical Officer Review, OxyContin Study 0402B-Cancer Pain, Curtis Wright, M.D.," Regulations.gov, June 9, 2015.
44 Madras et al., "President's Commission on Combating Drug Addiction and the Opioid Crisis."
45 Whoriskey, "Rising Painkiller Addiction Shows Damage from Drugmakers' Role in Shaping Medical Opinion."
46 Daniel C. Beachler et al., "An Evaluation of the Effect of the OxyContin Reformulation on Unintentional Fatal and Nonfatal Overdose," *The Clinical Journal of Pain* 38, no. 6 (June 2022): 396–404, https://doi.org/10.1097/AJP.0000000000001034; NIH, "Drug Overdose Deaths: Facts and Figures."
47 Jason Lazarou, Bruce H. Pomeranz, and Paul N. Corey, "Incidence of Adverse Drug Reactions in Hospitalized Patients: A Meta-Analysis of Prospective Studies," *JAMA* 279, no. 15 (April 15, 1998): 1200–5, https://doi.org/10.1001/jama.279.15.1200.
48 Denise Grady, "Study Says Thousands Die From Reaction to Medicine," *The New York Times*, April 15, 1998, https://www.nytimes.com/1998/04/15/us/study-says-thousands-die-from-reaction-to-medicine.html.
49 FDA, "Preventable Adverse Drug Reactions: A Focus on Drug Interactions," US Food & Drug Administration, March 6, 2018, https://www.fda.gov/drugs/drug-interactions-labeling/preventable-adverse-drug-reactions-focus-drug-interactions.
50 Linda T. Kohn et al., *To Err Is Human: Building a Safer Health System* (Washington, DC: National Academies Press, 2000), https://doi.org/10.17226/9728.
51 Office of Inspector General, "Adverse Events in Hospitals: National Incidence Among Medicare Beneficiaries," US Department of Health and Human Services, November 2010, https://oig.hhs.gov/oei/reports/oei-06-09-00090.pdf.
52 John T. James, "A New, Evidence-Based Estimate of Patient Harms Associated with Hospital Care," *Journal of Patient Safety* 9, no. 3 (2013): 122–8, https://doi.org/10.1097/PTS.0b013e3182948a69.
53 Martin A. Makary and Michael Daniel, "Medical Error—the Third Leading Cause of Death in the US," *BMJ* 353, no. 8056 (May 3, 2016): i2139, https://doi.org/10.1136/bmj.i2139.
54 Office of Science & Data Policy, "Trends in Prescription Drug Spending, 2016–2021," ASPE, September 2022, https://aspe.hhs.gov/sites/default/files/documents/88c547c976e915fc31fe2c6903ac0bc9/sdp-trends-prescription-drug-spending.pdf.
55 NIH, "Drug Overdose Deaths: Facts and Figures."
56 Wise Diagnostic Content Team, "Overmedication of America: Prescription Drug Use on the Rise," Wise Diagnostic Systems, September 6, 2022, https://blog.wisedx.com/blog/overmedication-of-america-prescription-drug-use-on-the-rise; Matej Mikulic, "Total Number of Medical Prescriptions Dispensed in the U.S. from 2009 to 2022," Statista, May 22, 2024, https://www.statista.com/statistics/238702/ us-total-medical-prescriptions-issued/; IQVIA, "The Use of Medicines in the U.S. 2023: Usage and Spending Trends and Outlook to 2027," IQVIA Institute, May 2, 2023, https://www.iqvia.com/insights/the-iqvia-institute/reports-and-publications/reports/the-use-of-medicines-in-the-us-2023.

57 "Richest Countries in the World: How They Stack Up in GDP in 2024?," Global Citizen Solutions, June 6, 2024, https://www.globalcitizensolutions.com/richest-countries-in-the-world/.
58 Shameek Rakshit and Matthew McGough, "How Does U.S. Life Expectancy Compare to Other Countries?," Peterson-KFF Health System Tracker, January 31, 2025, https://www.healthsystemtracker.org/chart-collection/u-s-life-expectancy-compare-countries/.
59 Jacob Bor et al., "Excess US Deaths before, during, and after the COVID-19 Pandemic," *JAMA Health Forum* 6, no. 5 (May 23, 2025): e251118, https://doi.org/10.1001/jamahealthforum.2025.1118.
60 Christopher B. Forrest et al., "Trends in US Children's Mortality, Chronic Conditions, Obesity, Functional Status, and Symptoms," *JAMA*, July 7, 2025, https://doi.org/10.1001/jama.2025.9855.
61 Munzira Z. Gunja, Evan D. Gumas, and Reginald D. Williams II, "U.S. Health Care from a Global Perspective, 2022: Accelerating Spending, Worsening Outcomes," The Commonwealth Fund, January 31, 2023, https://doi.org/10.26099/8ejy-yc74; Roosa Tikkanen and Melinda K. Abrams, "U.S. Health Care from a Global Perspective, 2019: Higher Spending, Worse Outcomes?," The Commonwealth Fund, January 30, 2020, https://doi.org/10.26099/7avy-fc29.
62 Ashley Kirzinger et al., "Public Opinion on Prescription Drugs and Their Prices," KFF, August 21, 2023, https://www.kff.org/health-costs/poll-finding/public-opinion-on-prescription-drugs-and-their-prices/.
63 Rakshit and McGough, "How Does U.S. Life Expectancy Compare to Other Countries?"
64 Andrew W. Mulcahy, Daniel Schwam, and Susan L. Lovejoy, "International Prescription Drug Price Comparisons: Estimates Using 2022 Data," RAND *Corporation*, February 1, 2024, https://doi.org/10.7249/RRA788-3.
65 ASPE, "Comparing U.S. and International Market Size and Average Pricing for Prescription Drugs, 2017–2022," Issue Brief, Assistant Secretary of Planning and Evaluation, December 2024, https://aspe.hhs.gov/sites/default/files/documents/4326cc7fe43bc11770598cf2a13f478c/international-market-size-prices.pdf.
66 Dana Goldman and Darius Lakdawalla, "The Global Burden of Medical Innovation," USC-Brookings Schaeffer Initiative for Health Policy, January 30, 2018, https://www.brookings.edu/articles/the-global-burden-of-medical-innovation/.
67 Dana O. Sarnak et al., "Paying for Prescription Drugs around the World: Why Is the U.S. an Outlier?," Commonwealth Fund, October 5, 2017, https://www.commonwealthfund.org/sites/default/files/documents/___media_files_publications_issue_brief_2017_oct_sarnak_paying_for_rx_ib_v2.pdf.
68 Martin Wenzl and Elias Mossialos, "Prices for Cardiac Implant Devices May Be up to Six Times Higher in the US than in Some European Countries," *Health Affairs* 37, no. 10 (2018): 1570–7, https://doi.org/10.1377/hlthaff.2017.1367.
69 Junxiu Liu et al., "Trends in Food Sources and Diet Quality among US Children and Adults, 2003–2018," *JAMA Network Open* 4, no. 4 (April 12, 2021): e215262, https://doi.org/10.1001/jamanetworkopen.2021.5262; Steven H. Woolf et al., "How Are Income and Wealth Linked to Health and Longevity," Urban Institute, April 2015, https://www.urban.org/sites/default/files/publication/49116/2000178-How-are-Income-and-Wealth-Linked-to-Health-and-Longevity.pdf; Neil J. MacKinnon et al., "Mapping Health Disparities in 11 High-Income Nations," *JAMA Network Open* 6, no. 7 (July 7, 2023): e2322310, https://doi.org/10.1001/jamanetworkopen.2023.22310.

## 1 Industry Control

1 Lisa Bero, "Industry Influence on Research: A Cycle of Bias," in *The Commercial Determinants of Health* (New York, NY: Oxford University Press, 2023): 188.
2 Hamilton Moses et al., "The Anatomy of Medical Research: US and International Comparisons," *JAMA* 313, no. 2 (January 13, 2015): 174–89, https://doi.org/10.1001/jama.2014.15939.
3 Stephan Ehrhardt, Lawrence J. Appel, and Curtis L. Meinert, "Trends in National Institutes of Health Funding for Clinical Trials Registered in ClinicalTrials.Gov," *JAMA* 314, no. 23 (December 15, 2015): 2566–7, https://doi.org/10.1001/jama.2015.12206.
4 Leonardo M. Siena et al., "Industry Involvement and Transparency in the Most Cited Clinical Trials, 2019–2022," *JAMA Network Open* 6, no. 11 (November 14, 2023): e2343425, https://doi.org/10.1001/jamanetworkopen.2023.43425.
5 "U.S. Investments in Medical and Health Research and Development: 2016–2020," Research!America, January 2022, https://www.researchamerica.org/wp-content/uploads/2022/09/ResearchAmerica-Investment-Report.Final_.January-2022-1.pdf.
6 NIH, "Basic Research—Digital Media Kit," National Institutes of Health, June 2, 2022, https://stagetestdomain3.nih.gov/news-events/basic-research-digital-media-kit; Francisco Moris and Christopher Pece, "Definitions of Research and Development: An Annotated Compilation of Official Sources," US National Science Foundation, May 19, 2022, https://ncses.nsf.gov/pubs/ncses22209.
7 Hussain S. Lalani, Jerry Avorn, and Aaron S. Kesselheim, "US Taxpayers Heavily Funded the Discovery of COVID-19 Vaccines," *Clinical Pharmacology & Therapeutics* 111, no. 3 (July 9, 2021): 542–4, https://doi.org/10.1002/cpt.2344; Mrinalika Roy, "Moderna Receives $483 Million BARDA Award for COVID-19 Vaccine Development," *Reuters*, April 16, 2020, https://www.reuters.com/article/idUSKBN21Y3DZ/.
8 Edward W. Zhou, Matthew J. Jackson, and Fred D. Ledley, "Spending on Phased Clinical Development of Approved Drugs by the US National Institutes of Health Compared with Industry," *JAMA Health Forum* 4, no. 7 (July 14, 2023): e231921, https://doi.org/10.1001/jamahealthforum.2023.1921.
9 Ekaterina Galkina Cleary et al., "Comparison of Research Spending on New Drug Approvals by the National Institutes of Health vs the Pharmaceutical Industry, 2010–2019," *JAMA Health Forum* 4, no. 4 (April 28, 2023): e230511, https://doi.org/10.1001/jamahealthforum.2023.0511.
10 FDA, "Development & Approval Process | Drugs," US Food & Drug Administration, August 8, 2022, https://www.fda.gov/drugs/development-approval-process-drugs.
11 Thomas Bodenheimer, "Uneasy Alliance—Clinical Investigators and the Pharmaceutical Industry," *New England Journal of Medicine* 342, no. 20 (May 18, 2000): 1539–44, https://doi.org/10.1056/NEJM200005183422024; Robert Steinbrook, "Gag Clauses in Clinical-Trial Agreements," *New England Journal of Medicine* 352, no. 21 (May 26, 2005): 2160–2, https://doi.org/10.1056/NEJMp048353.
12 Abramson, *Sickening*, 111; Jill A. Fisher and Corey A. Kalbaugh, "United States Private-Sector Physicians and Pharmaceutical Contract Research: A Qualitative Study," ed. Joseph S. Ross, *PLoS Med* 9, no. 7 (July 24, 2012): e1001271, https://doi.org/10.1371/journal.pmed.1001271; X. Mona Guo and Emma L. Barber, "The Invisible Hand of Industry," *Clinical Obstetrics & Gynecology* 65, no. 2 (June 2022): 260–7, https://doi.org/10.1097/GRF.0000000000000697.

13 Bodenheimer, "Uneasy Alliance—Clinical Investigators and the Pharmaceutical Industry"; Peter C. Gøtzsche, *Deadly Medicines and Organised Crime: How Big Pharma Has Corrupted Healthcare*, Kindle Edition (London, UK: Radcliffe Publishing, 2013), 57.
14 Frank Davidoff et al., "Sponsorship, Authorship, and Accountability," *New England Journal of Medicine* 345, no. 11 (September 13, 2001): 825–7, https://doi.org/10.1056/NEJMed010093.
15 Barbara J. Culliton, "The Academic-Industrial Complex: A Host of New Agreements for Industrial Sponsorship of Academic Research Are the Focus of a Growing Debate," Science 216, no. 4549 (May 28, 1982): 960, https://doi.org/10.1126/science.11643748; Institute of Medicine, *Funding Health Sciences Research: A Strategy to Restore Balance* (The National Academies Press, 1990), https://doi.org/10.17226/1625; Abramson, Sickening, 109–13.
16 Culliton, "The Academic-Industrial Complex."
17 Gøtzsche, *Deadly Medicines and Organised Crime*, 57.
18 Gemma Mitchell, Matthew Lesch, and Jim McCambridge, "Alcohol Industry Involvement in the Moderate Alcohol and Cardiovascular Health Trial," *American Journal of Public Health* 110, no. 4 (April 2020): 485–8, https://doi.org/10.2105/AJPH.2019.305508.
19 NIH Advisory Committee to the Director (ACD), "ACD Working Group for Review of the Moderate Alcohol and Cardiovascular Health Trial," National Institutes of Health, June 2018: 3, https://acd.od.nih.gov/documents/presentations/06152018Tabak-B.pdf.
20 Mitchell, Lesch, and McCambridge, "Alcohol Industry Involvement in the Moderate Alcohol and Cardiovascular Health Trial."
21 Justin E. Bekelman, Yan Li, and Cary P. Gross, "Scope and Impact of Financial Conflicts of Interest in Biomedical Research: A Systematic Review," *JAMA* 289, no. 4 (January 22, 2003): 454–65, https://doi.org/10.1001/jama.289.4.454.
22 Andreas Lundh et al., "Industry Sponsorship and Research Outcome," ed. Cochrane Methodology Review Group, *Cochrane Database of Systematic Reviews 2017*, no. 2 (February 16, 2017): Article MR000033, https://doi.org/10.1002/14651858.MR000033.pub3.
23 Siena et al., "Industry Involvement and Transparency in the Most Cited Clinical Trials, 2019–2022."
24 Moses et al., "The Anatomy of Medical Research."
25 "U.S. Investments in Medical and Health Research and Development: 2016–2020."
26 Sanne Magnan, "Social Determinants of Health 101 for Health Care: Five Plus Five," National Academy of Medicine, October 9, 2017, https://nam.edu/social-determinants-of-health-101-for-health-care-five-plus-five/#:~:text=Medical%20care%20is%20estimated%20to,socioeconomic%20factors%2C%20and%20environmental%20factors.
27 Alice Fabbri et al., "The Influence of Industry Sponsorship on the Research Agenda: A Scoping Review," *American Journal of Public Health* 108, no. 11 (November 1, 2018): e9–16, https://doi.org/10.2105/AJPH.2018.304677.
28 Bero, "Industry Influence on Research: A Cycle of Bias," 189.
29 Diabetes Prevention Program Research Group, "Reduction in the Incidence of Type 2 Diabetes with Lifestyle Intervention or Metformin," *New England Journal of Medicine* 346, no. 6 (February 7, 2002): 393–403, https://doi.org/10.1056/NEJMoa012512.

30 D. N. Lathyris et al., "Industry Sponsorship and Selection of Comparators in Randomized Clinical Trials," *European Journal of Clinical Investigation* 40, no. 2 (January 13, 2010): 172–82, https://doi.org/10.1111/j.1365-2362.2009.02240.x.
31 Audrey D. Zhang et al., "Assessment of Clinical Trials Supporting US Food and Drug Administration Approval of Novel Therapeutic Agents, 1995–2017," *JAMA Network Open* 3, no. 4 (April 21, 2020): e203284, https://doi.org/10.1001/jamanetworkopen.2020.3284.
32 Jeffrey M. Rothenstein et al., "Company Stock Prices before and after Public Announcements Related to Oncology Drugs," *JNCI: Journal of the National Cancer Institute* 103, no. 20 (September 26, 2011): 1507–12, https://doi.org/10.1093/jnci/djr338.
33 Higgins et al., "Chapter 7: Considering Bias and Conflicts of Interest among the Included Studies," *Cochrane Handbook for Systematic Reviews of Interventions* (Cochrane Collaboration, 2023), https://training.cochrane.org/handbook/current/chapter-07.
34 Candice Estellat, "Lack of Head-to-Head Trials and Fair Control Arms: Randomized Controlled Trials of Biologic Treatment for Rheumatoid Arthritis," *Archives of Internal Medicine* 172, no. 3 (February 13, 2012): 237–44, https://doi.org/10.1001/archinternmed.2011.1209.
35 Ibid.
36 "Chapter 7: Considering Bias."
37 David J. Graham et al., "Risk of Acute Myocardial Infarction and Sudden Cardiac Death in Patients Treated with Cyclo-Oxygenase 2 Selective and Non-selective Non-steroidal Anti-inflammatory Drugs: Nested Case-Control Study," *The Lancet* 365, no. 9458 (February 5, 2005): 475–81, https://doi.org/10.1016/S0140-6736(05)17864-7; David Graham, "Testimony of David J. Graham, MD, MPH," U.S. Senate Committee on Finance, November 18, 2004, https://www.finance.senate.gov/imo/media/doc/111804dgtest.pdf.
38 Harlan M Krumholz et al., "What Have We Learnt from Vioxx?," *BMJ* 334, no. 7585 (January 18, 2007): 120–3, https://doi.org/10.1136/bmj.39024.487720.68.
39 Abramson, *Sickening*, 113–14.
40 Donald Light, ed., *The Risks of Prescription Drugs* (New York City: Columbia University Press, 2010): 15–16.
41 Ibid., 15.
42 Ibid.; Abramson, *Sickening*, chap. 6.
43 Fred E. Silverstein et al., "Gastrointestinal Toxicity with Celecoxib vs Nonsteroidal Anti-inflammatory Drugs for Osteoarthritis and Rheumatoid Arthritis: The CLASS Study: A Randomized Controlled Trial," *JAMA* 284, no. 10 (September 13, 2000): 1247–55, https://doi.org/10.1001/jama.284.10.1247.
44 Peter Lurie and Allison Zieve, "Sometimes the Silence Can Be like the Thunder: Access to Pharmaceutical Data at the FDA," *Law and Contemporary Problems* 69, no. 3 (Summer 2006): 85–97, https://www.jstor.org/stable/27592139.
45 Light, *The Risks of Prescription Drugs*, 82.
46 Ibid.; Abramson, *Sickening*, 31–3, 114.
47 Light, *The Risks of Prescription Drugs*, 82.
48 A. Hrobjartsson et al., "Observer Bias in Randomised Clinical Trials with Binary Outcomes: Systematic Review of Trials with Both Blinded and Non-blinded Outcome Assessors," *BMJ* 344, no. 7848 (February 27, 2012): e1119, https://doi.org/10.1136/

bmj.e1119; Asbjørn Hróbjartsson et al., "Observer Bias in Randomized Clinical Trials with Measurement Scale Outcomes: A Systematic Review of Trials with Both Blinded and Nonblinded Assessors," *Canadian Medical Association Journal* 185, no. 4 (March 5, 2013): E201–11, https://doi.org/10.1503/cmaj.120744.

49 Gøtzsche, *Deadly Medicines and Organised Crime*, 45.

50 Rotem Botvinik-Nezer et al., "Variability in the Analysis of a Single Neuroimaging Dataset by Many Teams," *Nature* 582, no. 7810 (May 20, 2020): 84–8, https://doi.org/10.1038/s41586-020-2314-9.

51 Gøtzsche, *Deadly Medicines and Organised Crime*, 45.

52 Ibid., 46.

53 Mayookha Mitra-Majumdar and Aaron S. Kesselheim, "Reporting Bias in Clinical Trials: Progress toward Transparency and Next Steps," *PLoS Med* 19, no. 1 (January 19, 2022): e1003894, https://doi.org/10.1371/journal.pmed.1003894.

54 Erick H. Turner et al., "Selective Publication of Antidepressant Trials and Its Influence on Apparent Efficacy," *New England Journal of Medicine* 358, no. 3 (January 17, 2008): 252–60, https://doi.org/10.1056/NEJMsa065779.

55 William J. Canestaro et al., "Favorable and Publicly Funded Studies Are More Likely to Be Published: A Systematic Review and Meta-Analysis," *Journal of Clinical Epidemiology* 92 (August 22, 2017): 58–68, https://doi.org/10.1016/j.jclinepi.2017.08.004.

56 Glen I. Spielmans and Peter I. Parry, "From Evidence-Based Medicine to Marketing-Based Medicine: Evidence from Internal Industry Documents," *Journal of Bioethical Inquiry* 7 (January 21, 2010): 13–29, https://doi.org/10.1007/s11673-010-9208-8.

57 Jeremy Olson, "U Doctor Scrutinized over Drug Research," Twin Cities, March 18, 2009, https://www.twincities.com/2009/03/18/u-doctor-scrutinized-over-drug-research/.

58 John Tumas, "FW: Meta Analyses," March 23, 2000, https://www.industrydocuments.ucsf.edu/drug/docs/#id=spkw0221.

59 Olson, "U Doctor Scrutinized over Drug Research."

60 Spielmans and Parry, "From Evidence-Based Medicine to Marketing-Based Medicine."

61 Steve Litherland, "RE: 2 EPS Abstracts for APA," December 6, 1999, https://www.industrydocuments.ucsf.edu/drug/docs/#id=yhlw0221.

62 John Tumas, "RE: 2 EPS Abstracts for APA," December 6, 1999, https://www.industrydocuments.ucsf.edu/drug/docs/#id=yhlw0221.

63 Dawn I. Velligan et al., "Does Cognitive Function Improve with Quetiapine in Comparison to Haloperidol?," *Schizophrenia Research* 53, no. 3 (January 15, 2002): 239–48, https://doi.org/10.1016/S0920-9964(01)00268-7.

64 Tumas, "RE: 2 EPS Abstracts for APA," December 6, 1999.

65 Gøtzsche, *Deadly Medicines and Organised Crime*, 75; Christopher J. Derry, Sheena Derry, and R. Andrew Moore, "Sumatriptan (Oral Route of Administration) for Acute Migraine Attacks in Adults," *Cochrane Database of Systematic Reviews* 2012, no. 2 (February 15, 2012): Article CD008615, https://doi.org/10.1002/14651858.CD008615.pub2.

66 Peer Carsten Tfelt-Hansen, "Unpublished Clinical Trials with Sumatriptan," *The Lancet* 374, no. 9700 (October 31, 2009): 1501–2, https://doi.org/10.1016/S0140-6736(09)61906-1.

67 "Ownership of Data—Federal Policies," The Office of Research Integrity, accessed June 21, 2025, https://ori.hhs.gov/education/products/rcradmin/topics/data/tutoria

l_2.shtml; "Data Ownership," The Office of Research Integrity, accessed June 21, 2025, https://ori.hhs.gov/content/Chapter-6-Data-Management-Practices-Data-ownership; NIH, "Clinical Trial Requirements for Grants and Contracts," Grants & Funding, July 26, 2017, https://grants.nih.gov/policy/clinical-trials.htm; National Institutes of Health, "NIH Policy on the Dissemination of NIH-Funded Clinical Trial Information," Federal Register, September 21, 2016, https://www.federalregister.gov/documents/2016/09/21/2016-22379/nih-policy-on-the-dissemination-of-nih-funded-clinical-trial-information.

68 "Patent and Trademark Law Amendments Act of 2007," Pub. L. No. 96–517, US Code (1980), https://www.govinfo.gov/content/pkg/USCODE-2011-title35/html/USCODE-2011-title35-partII-chap18.htm; Gregory A. Petsko, "Who Owns the Data?," *Genome Biology* 6, no. 4 (March 31, 2005): Article 107, https://doi.org/10.1186/gb-2005-6-4-107.

69 National Research Council, *Access to Research Data in the 21st Century: An Ongoing Dialogue among Interested Parties: Report of a Workshop* (Washington, DC: National Academies Press, 2002): 1–4, https://doi.org/10.17226/10302.

70 Spielmans and Parry, "From Evidence-Based Medicine to Marketing-Based Medicine," 14.

71 Michelle M. Mello, Brian R. Clarridge, and David M. Studdert, "Academic Medical Centers' Standards for Clinical-Trial Agreements with Industry," *New England Journal of Medicine* 352, no. 21 (May 26, 2005): 2202–10, https://doi.org/10.1056/NEJMsa044115.

72 PhRMA, "Principles on Conduct of Clinical Trials of Clinical Trial Results," Pharmaceutical Research and Manufacturers of America, October 14, 2020: 17, https://cdn.aglty.io/phrma/global/resources/import/pdfs/PhRMAPrinciples%20of%20Clinical%20Trials%20FINAL.pdf.

73 Ibid., 19–20.

74 Peter Doshi et al., "Rapid Response: Open Letter to the CEOs of Pfizer and Moderna," Comment on "Covid-19: Researchers Face Wait for Patient Level Data from Pfizer and Moderna Vaccine Trials," August 31, 2022, https://www.bmj.com/lookup/doi/10.1136/bmj.o1731.

75 Food and Drug Administration, "21 CFR 20.61—Trade Secrets and Commercial or Financial Information Which Is Privileged or Confidential," Code of Federal Regulations, April 16, 2024, https://www.ecfr.gov/current/title-21/chapter-I/subchapter-A/part-20/subpart-D/section-20.61.

76 Institute of Medicine, *Sharing Clinical Trial Data*.

77 Amsterdam University of Applied Sciences, "(Statistical) Analysis Plan," June 12, 2023, https://www.amsterdamuas.com/uv-openscience/toolkit/planning/sap/sap.html.

78 Suzie Cro et al., "Evidence of Unexplained Discrepancies between Planned and Conducted Statistical Analyses: A Review of Randomised Trials," *BMC Medicine* 18 (May 29, 2020): Article 137, https://doi.org/10.1186/s12916-020-01590-1.

79 Institute of Medicine, *Sharing Clinical Trial Data*.

80 US Department of Health and Human Services et al., "Guidance for Industry: Providing Clinical Evidence of Effectiveness for Human Drug and Biological Products," FDA, May 1998, https://www.fda.gov/media/71655/download.

81 Institute of Medicine, *Sharing Clinical Trial Data*.

82 Center for Drug Evaluation and Research, "Guideline for Industry: Structure and Content of Clinical Study Reports," FDA, July 1996: 1, https://www.fda.gov/regulatory-information/search-fda-guidance-documents/e3-structure-and-content-clinical-study-reports.
83 "Food and Drug Administration Amendments Act of 2007," Pub. L. No. 110–85 (2007), https://www.congress.gov/bill/110th-congress/house-bill/3580?q=%7B%22search%22%3A%5B%22cite%3APL110-85%22%5D%7D&s=5&r=1.
84 US National Library of Medicine, "How to Submit Your Results," ClinicalTrials.gov, June 2023, https://classic.clinicaltrials.gov/ct2/manage-recs/how-report.
85 Amy Kapczynski and Christopher J. Morten, "The Big Data Regulator, Rebooted: Why and How the FDA Can and Should Disclose Confidential Data on Prescription Drugs and Vaccines," *California Law Review* 109, no. 2 (2021): 493–558, https://doi.org/10.15779/Z380K26C1T.
86 Emily Huddle, "FDA's New Integrated Review Template and Implications for Regulatory Intelligence," Regulatory Focus, March 22, 2021, https://www.raps.org/News-and-Articles/News-Articles/2021/3/FDAs-new-integrated-review-template-and-implicatio.
87 Janet Woodcock, Peter Stein, and Kevin Bugin, "Integrated Drug Reviews at the US Food and Drug Administration," *JAMA Internal Medicine* 180, no. 9 (July 27, 2020): 1248–50, https://doi.org/10.1001/jamainternmed.2020.1981.
88 Matthew Herder, Christopher J. Morten, and Peter Doshi, "Integrated Drug Reviews at the US Food and Drug Administration—Legal Concerns and Knowledge Lost," *JAMA Internal Medicine* 180, no. 5 (March 2, 2020): 629–30, https://doi.org/10.1001/jamainternmed.2020.0074; Kapczynski and Morten, "The Big Data Regulator, Rebooted," 513–14.
89 FDA, "FDA's Labeling Resources for Human Prescription Drugs," US Food & Drug Administration, April 4, 2024, https://www.fda.gov/drugs/laws-acts-and-rules/fdas-labeling-resources-human-prescription-drugs.
90 FDA, "Frequently Asked Questions about Labeling for Prescription Medicines," US Food & Drug Administration, April 1, 2024, https://www.fda.gov/drugs/fdas-labeling-resources-human-prescription-drugs/frequently-asked-questions-about-labeling-prescription-medicines.
91 Ashley M. Hopkins, Andrew Rowland, and Michael J. Sorich, "Data Sharing from Pharmaceutical Industry Sponsored Clinical Studies: Audit of Data Availability," *BMC Medicine* 16 (September 28, 2018): Article 165, https://doi.org/10.1186/s12916-018-1154-z.
92 Institute of Medicine, *Sharing Clinical Trial Data: Maximizing Benefits, Minimizing Risk* (Washington, DC: National Academies Press, 2015), 91, https://doi.org/10.17226/18998.
93 "Clinical Trials Phases Defined," University of Cincinnati College of Medicine, accessed June 21, 2025, https://med.uc.edu/depart/psychiatry/research/clinical-research/crm/trial-phases-1-2-3-defined; NIH, "NIH Clinical Research Trials and You: The Basics," National Institutes of Health, October 3, 2022, https://www.nih.gov/health-information/nih-clinical-research-trials-you/basics.
94 Peter C. Gøtzsche, "Why We Need Easy Access to All Data from All Clinical Trials and How to Accomplish It," *Trials* 12, no. 1 (November 23, 2011): Article 249, https://doi.org/10.1186/1745-6215-12-249.

95 Liebson Philip R., "Muraglitazar and the FDA: What Constitutes Drug Safety?," *Preventive Cardiology* 9, no. 2 (January 29, 2007): 110–14, https://doi.org/10.1111/j.1520-037X.2000.5474.x.
96 Steven E. Nissen, "Effect of Muraglitazar on Death and Major Adverse Cardiovascular Events in Patients with Type 2 Diabetes Mellitus," *JAMA* 294, no. 20 (November 23, 2005): 2581–6, https://doi.org/10.1001/jama.294.20.joc50147.
97 Nicholas S. Downing et al., "Postmarket Safety Events among Novel Therapeutics Approved by the US Food and Drug Administration between 2001 and 2010," *JAMA* 317, no. 18 (May 9, 2017): 1854–63, https://doi.org/10.1001/jama.2017.5150.
98 Gøtzsche, "Why We Need Easy Access to All Data from All Clinical Trials and How to Accomplish It."
99 "Federal Food, Drug, and Cosmetic Act," 21 U.S.C. § 331—Prohibited acts (2022), https://www.law.cornell.edu/uscode/text/21/331; Gail A. Van Norman, "Off-Label Use vs Off-Label Marketing of Drugs," *JACC: Basic to Translational Science* 8, no. 2 (2023): 224–33, https://doi.org/10.1016/j.jacbts.2022.12.011.
100 Van Norman, "Off-Label Use vs Off-Label Marketing of Drugs," 225.
101 Lawrence Hurley, "US High Court Leaves Intact $142 Million Verdict against Pfizer," *Reuters*, December 9, 2013, sec. Healthcare & Pharmaceuticals, https://www.reuters.com/article/business/healthcare-pharmaceuticals/us-high-court-leaves-intact-142-million-verdict-against-pfizer-idUSBRE9B80K1/.
102 John Abramson, "Expert Report of John Abramson, MD.," August 11, 2008, 35, https://www.industrydocuments.ucsf.edu/drug/docs/#id=kyhw0217.
103 Ibid, 4.
104 K. C. Gorson et al., "Gabapentin in the Treatment of Painful Diabetic Neuropathy: A Placebo Controlled, Double Blind, Crossover Trial," *Journal of Neurology, Neurosurgery & Psychiatry* 66, no. 2 (February 1, 1999): 251–2, https://doi.org/10.1136/jnnp.66.2.251; Abramson, *Sickening*, 28.
105 Miroslav Backonja et al., "Gabapentin for the Symptomatic Treatment of Painful Neuropathy in Patients with Diabetes Mellitus: A Randomized Controlled Trial," *JAMA* 280, no. 21 (December 2, 1998): 1831–6, https://doi.org/10.1001/jama.280.21.1831.
106 Abramson, *Sickening*, 33.
107 Abramson, "Expert Report of John Abramson, MD," 67.
108 Jeffrey S. Barkin, "Report on the Use of Neurontin for Bipolar and Other Mood Disorders," July 25, 2008, 2, https://www.industrydocuments.ucsf.edu/drug/docs/#id=gxjm0223.
109 Yogendra Kumar Gupta, Meenakshi Meenu, and Prafull Mohan, "The Tamiflu Fiasco and Lessons Learnt," *Indian Journal of Pharmacology* 47, no. 1 (February 2015): 11–16, https://doi.org/10.4103/0253-7613.150308.
110 Laurent Kaiser et al., "Impact of Oseltamivir Treatment on Influenza-Related Lower Respiratory Tract Complications and Hospitalizations," *Archives of Internal Medicine* 163, no. 14 (July 28, 2003): 1667–72, https://doi.org/10.1001/archinte.163.14.1667.
111 Vinayak K. Prasad and Adam S. Cifu, *Ending Medical Reversal: Improving Outcomes, Saving Lives* (Baltimore: Johns Hopkins University Press, 2015): 136–7.
112 Peter Doshi, Tom Jefferson, and Chris Del Mar, "The Imperative to Share Clinical Study Reports: Recommendations from the Tamiflu Experience," *PLoS Med* 9, no. 4 (April 10, 2012): e1001201, https://doi.org/10.1371/journal.pmed.1001201; "Drug

Label: Tamiflu (Oseltamivir Phosphate) Capsules and Oral Suspension," US Food & Drug Administration, March 2011, https://www.accessdata.fda.gov/drugsatfda_docs/label/2011/021087s056_021246s039lbl.pdf; Ele Ibarra-Pratt to Joanna McNamara, "NDA 21-087 TAMIFLU (Oseltamivir Phosphate) MACMIS ID#8675," April 14, 2000, https://web.archive.org/web/20090710121114/https://www.fda.gov/downloads/Drugs/GuidanceComplianceRegulatoryInformation/EnforcementActivitiesbyFDA/WarningLettersandNoticeofViolationLetterstoPharmaceuticalCompanies/UCM166329.pdf.

113 "About Us," *Cochrane*, 2024, https://www.cochrane.org/about-us.

114 Tom Jefferson et al., "Neuraminidase Inhibitors for Preventing and Treating Influenza in Healthy Adults," ed. The Cochrane Collaboration, *Cochrane Database of Systematic Reviews* 2005, no. 2 (April 20, 2005): Article CD001265, https://doi.org/10.1002/14651858.CD001265.

115 Doshi, Jefferson, and Del Mar, "The Imperative to Share Clinical Study Reports."

116 Associated Press, "Drug Manufacturer Says U.S. Wants to Increase Tamiflu Stockpile," Fox News, January 31, 2006, https://www.foxnews.com/story/drug-manufacturer-says-u-s-wants-to-increase-tamiflu-stockpile.

117 Richard Van Noorden, "Report Disputes Benefit of Stockpiling Tamiflu," *Nature*, April 10, 2014, https://doi.org/10.1038/nature.2014.15022.

118 Andrew Jack, "Tamiflu: 'A Nice Little Earner,'" *BMJ* 348, no. 7953 (April 9, 2014): g2524, https://doi.org/10.1136/bmj.g2524.

119 "WHO Model List of Essential Medicines," World Health Organization, August 2017, https://www.who.int/publications/i/item/eml-20.

120 P. Doshi, "Neuraminidase Inhibitors—the Story behind the Cochrane Review," *BMJ* 339, no. 7734 (December 8, 2009): b5164, https://doi.org/10.1136/bmj.b5164.

121 Doshi, Jefferson, and Del Mar, "The Imperative to Share Clinical Study Reports."

122 Abramson, *Sickening*, 128.

123 Tom Jefferson et al., "Neuraminidase Inhibitors for Preventing and Treating Influenza in Adults and Children," *Cochrane Database of Systematic Reviews* 2018, no. 1 (April 10, 2014): Article CD008965, https://doi.org/10.1002/14651858.CD008965.pub4.

124 Abramson, *Sickening*, 128; "WHO Model List of Essential Medicines."

## 2 Less Opaque Is Still Opaque

1 Trudo Lemmens and Candice Telfer, "Access to Information and the Right to Health: The Human Rights Case for Clinical Trials Transparency," *American Journal of Law & Medicine* 38, no. 1 (2012): 63–112, https://papers.ssrn.com/sol3/papers.cfm?abstract_id=1932436.

2 Kay Dickersin and Drummond Rennie, "Registering Clinical Trials," *JAMA* 290, no. 4 (July 23, 2003): 516–23, https://doi.org/10.1001/jama.290.4.516.

3 R. J. Simes, "Publication Bias: The Case for an International Registry of Clinical Trials," *Journal of Clinical Oncology* 4, no. 10 (October 1, 1986): 1529–41, https://doi.org/10.1200/JCO.1986.4.10.1529.

4 Daniel L. Shaw and Joseph S. Ross, "US Federal Government Efforts to Improve Clinical Trial Transparency with Expanded Trial Registries and Open Data Sharing,"

*American Medical Association Journal of Ethics* 17, no. 12 (December 2015): 1152–9, https://journalofethics.ama-assn.org/sites/joedb/files/2018-05/pfor1-1512.pdf.

5 US Department of Health & Human Services, "A Timeline of HIV and AIDS," HIV.gov, accessed April 17, 2024, https://www.hiv.gov/hiv-basics/overview/history/hiv-and-aids-timeline.

6 Deborah G. Katz et al., "The AIDS Clinical Trials Information Service (ACTIS): A Decade of Providing Clinical Trials Information," *Public Health Reports* 117, no. 2 (2002): 123–30, https://doi.org/10.1016/S0033-3549(04)50118-8.

7 Lemmens and Telfer, "Access to Information and the Right to Health."

8 "Health Omnibus Extension of 1988," Pub. L. No. 100–607, U.S. Code (1988), https://www.congress.gov/bill/100th-congress/senate-bill/2889/text.

9 Katz et al., "The AIDS Clinical Trials Information Service (ACTIS)."

10 Julian Ring, "30 Years Ago, One Decision Altered the Course of Our Connected World," *NPR*, April 30, 2023, sec. National Security, https://www.npr.org/2023/04/30/1172276538/world-wide-web-internet-anniversary.

11 CDC, "Notices to Readers AIDS Clinical Trials Information Service," MMWR, September 13, 1991, https://www.cdc.gov/mmwr/preview/mmwrhtml/00015127.htm.

12 Katz et al., "The AIDS Clinical Trials Information Service (ACTIS)."

13 Lemmens and Telfer, "Access to Information and the Right to Health"; Shaw and Ross, "US Federal Government Efforts to Improve Clinical Trial Transparency with Expanded Trial Registries and Open Data Sharing."

14 "Food and Drug Administration Modernization Act of 1997," Pub. L. No. 105–15 (1997), https://www.congress.gov/bill/105th-congress/senate-bill/830/text?q=%7B%22search%22%3A%5B%22cite%3APL105-115%22%5D%7D&r=1&s=2.

15 "Investigational Drugs and Biologics," UVA: Office of the Vice President for Research, accessed June 21, 2025, https://med.virginia.edu/clinicalresearch/protocol-manager/set-up-study/compliance/investigational-new-drug-ind/.

16 Institute of Medicine, *Developing a National Registry of Pharmacologic and Biologic Clinical Trials: Workshop Report* (Washington, DC: National Academies Press, 2006): 63–80, https://doi.org/10.17226/11561.

17 Ibid.

18 "Press Release: National Institutes of Health Launches 'ClinicalTrials.Gov,'" NIH, April 29, 2004, https://www.nlm.nih.gov/archive/20040831/news/press_releases/clntrlpr00.html.

19 Robert Steinbrook, "Registration of Clinical Trials—Voluntary or Mandatory?," *New England Journal of Medicine* 351, no. 18 (October 28, 2004): 1820–2, https://doi.org/10.1056/NEJMp048264.

20 Food and Drug Administration Amendments Act of 2007.

21 Ibid., 904.

22 US National Library of Medicine, "How to Submit Your Results."

23 Deborah A. Zarin et al., "Trial Reporting in ClinicalTrials.Gov—The Final Rule," *New England Journal of Medicine* 375, no. 20 (November 17, 2016): 1998–2004, https://doi.org/10.1056/NEJMsr1611785.

24 Food and Drug Administration Amendments Act of 2007: 911.

25 "FDAAA 801 and the Final Rule," ClinicalTrials.gov, January 9, 2024, https://clinicaltrials.gov/policy/fdaaa-801-final-rule#submit-results-info.

26 Tony Tse, Rebecca J. Williams, and Deborah A. Zarin, "Reporting 'Basic Results' in ClinicalTrials.Gov," *Chest* 136, no. 1 (2009): 295–303, https://doi.org/10.1378/chest.08-3022; Food and Drug Administration Amendments Act of 2007: 914.
27 Tony Tse and Rebecca J. Williams, "ClinicalTrials.Gov to Include Basic Results Data," *NLM Technical Bulletin*, no. 364 (October 21, 2008): e15, https://www.nlm.nih.gov/pubs/techbull/so08/so08_clinicaltrials.html.
28 "Clinical Trials Registration and Results Information Submission," Health and Human Services Department, September 21, 2016, https://www.federalregister.gov/documents/2016/09/21/2016-22129/clinical-trials-registration-and-results-information-submission.
29 For a fuller list of changes, check here: https://prsinfo.clinicaltrials.gov/FinalRuleChanges-12Dec2016.pdf.
30 Zarin et al., "Trial Reporting in ClinicalTrials.Gov—The Final Rule."
31 National Institutes of Health, "NIH Policy on the Dissemination of NIH-Funded Clinical Trial Information."
32 Naomi Reice Buchwald, "Seife v. U.S. Department of Health & Human Services, No. 1:18-Cv-11462-NRB: Document 65," United States District Court for the Southern District of New York, February 24, 2020, https://law.yale.edu/sites/default/files/area/center/isp/65._order_on_sj_copy.pdf.
33 Deborah A. Zarin et al., "Update on Trial Registration 11 Years after the ICMJE Policy Was Established," *New England Journal of Medicine* 376, no. 4 (January 26, 2017): 383–91, https://doi.org/10.1056/NEJMsr1601330.
34 Hiroki Saito and Christopher J. Gill, "How Frequently Do the Results from Completed US Clinical Trials Enter the Public Domain?—A Statistical Analysis of the ClinicalTrials.Gov Database," ed. Vasee Moorthy, *PLoS ONE* 9, no. 7 (July 15, 2014): e101826, https://doi.org/10.1371/journal.pone.0101826.
35 Andrew P. Prayle, Matthew N. Hurley, and Alan R. Smyth, "Compliance with Mandatory Reporting of Clinical Trial Results on ClinicalTrials.Gov: Cross Sectional Study," *BMJ* 344, no. 7838 (January 3, 2012): d7373, https://doi.org/10.1136/bmj.d7373.
36 Nicholas J. DeVito, Seb Bacon, and Ben Goldacre, "Compliance with Legal Requirement to Report Clinical Trial Results on ClinicalTrials.Gov: A Cohort Study," *The Lancet* 395, no. 10221 (February 1, 2020): 361–9, https://doi.org/10.1016/S0140-6736(19)33220-9.
37 Charles Piller, "FDA and NIH Let Clinical Trial Sponsors Keep Results Secret and Break the Law," Science, January 13, 2020, https://www.science.org/content/article/fda-and-nih-let-clinical-trial-sponsors-keep-results-secret-and-break-law.
38 Charles Piller, "Clinical Scofflaws?," Science, January 13, 2020, https://www.sciencemag.org/news/2020/01/clinical-scofflaws?.
39 Deborah A. Zarin et al., "10-Year Update on Study Results Submitted to ClinicalTrials.Gov," *New England Journal of Medicine* 381, no. 20 (November 13, 2019): 1966–74, https://doi.org/10.1056/NEJMsr1907644; University of Oxford, "Who's Sharing Their Clinical Trial Results?," FDAAA Trials Tracker, accessed July 14, 2025, https://fdaaa.trialstracker.net/.
40 Zarin et al., "10-Year Update on Study Results Submitted to ClinicalTrials.Gov."
41 Piller, "FDA and NIH Let Clinical Trial Sponsors Keep Results Secret and Break the Law."

42 Jacqueline R. Berman, "Fourteen Years Later, FDA Flexes Its Clinicaltrials.Gov Enforcement Authority," *Morgan Lewis* (blog), May 3, 2021, https://www.morganlewis.com/blogs/asprescribed/2021/05/fourteen-years-later-fda-flexes-its-clinicaltrials-gov-enforcement-authority.
43 FDA, "ClinicalTrials.Gov—Notices of Noncompliance and Civil Money Penalty Actions," US Food & Drug Administration, April 11, 2025, https://www.fda.gov/science-research/fdas-role-clinicaltrialsgov-information/clinicaltrialsgov-notices-noncompliance-and-civil-money-penalty-actions.
44 University of Oxford, "Who's Sharing Their Clinical Trial Results?"
45 Abramson, *Sickening*, 213.
46 Lisa M. Schwartz et al., "ClinicalTrials.Gov and Drugs@FDA: A Comparison of Results Reporting for New Drug Approval Trials," *Annals of Internal Medicine* 165, no. 6 (June 14, 2016): 421–30, https://doi.org/10.7326/M15-2658.
47 "Proceedings and Debates of the 112th Congress, Second Session," *Congressional Record* 158, no. 71 (May 17, 2012), https://www.congress.gov/112/crec/2012/05/17/CREC-2012-05-17.pdf.
48 James Love, "BIO Memo Opposing Transparency of Drug Development Costs, Sales, Prices, and Clinical Trial Outcomes," *Knowledge Ecology International* (blog), May 21, 2012, https://www.keionline.org/21844.
49 Kapczynski and Morten, "The Big Data Regulator, Rebooted."
50 Department of Health and Human Services (HHS), "34 CFR § 5.20—Requirements for Making FOIA Requests," Code of Federal Regulations, April 16, 2024, https://www.ecfr.gov/current/title-45/subtitle-A/subchapter-A/part-5.
51 Office of Information Policy (OIP), "Frequently Asked Questions," FOIA.gov, accessed June 21, 2025, https://www.foia.gov/faq.html#:~:text=Exemption%201%3A%20Information%20that%20is,disclosure%20by%20another%20federal%20law.
52 Office of Information Policy, "Department of Justice Guide to the Freedom of Information Act—Exemption 4," US Department of Justice, December 16, 2021: 263, https://www.justice.gov/archive/oip/foia_guide09/exemption4.pdf.
53 Alexander C. Egilman et al., "Systematic Overview of Freedom of Information Act Requests to the Department of Health and Human Services from 2008 to 2017," *Research Integrity and Peer Review* 4 (December 9, 2019): Article 26, https://doi.org/10.1186/s41073-019-0086-2.
54 Chrysler Corp. v. Brown, 441 U.S. 281 (US Supreme Court 1979).
55 Ibid., 282.
56 Food and Drug Administration, "21 CFR 20.61—Trade Secrets and Commercial or Financial Information Which Is Privileged or Confidential," Code of Federal Regulations, April 16, 2024, https://www.ecfr.gov/current/title-21/chapter-I/subchapter-A/part-20/subpart-D/section-20.61.
57 Ibid.
58 Ibid.
59 "Executive Order 12600—Predisclosure Notification Procedures for Confidential Commercial Information," Office of the Federal Register, June 23, 1987, https://www.archives.gov/federal-register/codification/executive-order/12600.html.
60 Food and Drug Administration, "21 CFR 20.61—Trade Secrets and Commercial or Financial Information Which Is Privileged or Confidential."
61 Kapczynski and Morten, "The Big Data Regulator, Rebooted," 523.

62 Jesse M. Furman, "Seife v. Food & Drug Administration," United States District Court for the Southern District of New York, No. 1:2017cv03960: Document 129, March 27, 2019, https://law.justia.com/cases/federal/district-courts/new-york/nysdce/1:2017cv03960/474913/129/.
63 Lurie and Zieve, "Sometimes the Silence Can Be like the Thunder."
64 Food Marketing Institute v. Argus Leader Media, 588 U.S. (US Supreme Court 2019).
65 US Department of Justice, "Exemption 4 after the Supreme Court's Ruling in Food Marketing Institute v. Argus Leader Media," Office of Information Policy, October 4, 2019, https://www.justice.gov/oip/exemption-4-after-supreme-courts-ruling-food-marketing-institute-v-argus-leader-media.
66 Food Marketing Institute v. Argus Leader Media, 588 US, 2.
67 Stephen Breyer, Food Marketing Institute v. Argus Leader Media, 588 U.S. (US Supreme Court 2019): 4.
68 "HHS Fiscal Year Freedom of Information Annual Report" (US Department of Health & Human Services, 2020–2025), each report available at: 2024: https://www.hhs.gov/foia/reports/annual-reports/2024/index.html; 2023: https://www.hhs.gov/foia/reports/annual-reports/2023/index.html; 2022: https://www.hhs.gov/foia/reports/annual-reports/2022/index.html; 2021: https://www.hhs.gov/foia/reports/annual-reports/2021/index.html; 2020: https://www.hhs.gov/foia/reports/annual-reports/2020/index.html; 2019: https://www.hhs.gov/foia/reports/annual-reports/2019/index.html.
69 Egilman et al., "Systematic Overview of Freedom of Information Act Requests to the Department of Health and Human Services from 2008 to 2017."
70 Kapczynski and Morten, "The Big Data Regulator, Rebooted," 521.
71 Jenna Greene, "'Paramount Importance': Judge Orders FDA to Hasten Release of Pfizer Vaccine Docs," *Reuters*, January 7, 2022, https://www.reuters.com/legal/government/paramount-importance-judge-orders-fda-hasten-release-pfizer-vaccine-docs-2022-01-07/.
72 Mark Pittman, "Public Health and Medical Professionals for Transparency v. Food and Drug Administration, No. 4:21-Cv-1058-P: Document 35," United States District Court for the Northern District of Texas Fort Worth Division, January 6, 2022, https://web.archive.org/web/20240923095918/https://www.fdanews.com/ext/resources/files/2022/01-07-22-PittmanFOIAOrder.pdf?1641590012.
73 Kapczynski and Morten, "The Big Data Regulator, Rebooted," 521–2.
74 FDA, "FOIA Fees," US Food & Drug Administration, June 10, 2023, https://www.fda.gov/regulatory-information/freedom-information/foia-fees.
75 Food and Drug Administration, "21 CFR Part 314—Applications for FDA Approval to Market a New Drug," Code of Federal Regulations, April 16, 2024), https://www.ecfr.gov/current/title-21/chapter-I/subchapter-D/part-314; Food and Drug Administration, "21 CFR 601.51—Confidentiality of Data and Information in Applications for Biologics Licenses," Code of Federal Regulations, April 16, 2024, https://www.ecfr.gov/current/title-21/chapter-I/subchapter-F/part-601/subpart-F/section-601.51.
76 Margaret Kwoka, "FOIA, Inc.," *Duke Law Journal* 65, no. 7 (2016): 1361–437, https://scholarship.law.duke.edu/dlj/vol65/iss7/2.
77 "News Update," EU Clinical Trials Register, accessed June 21, 2025, https://www.clinicaltrialsregister.eu/.
78 "Instructions for Clinical Trial Registration and Reporting," Karolinska Institutet, accessed June 21, 2025, https://staff.ki.se/media/110085/download.

79 EMA, "European Medicines Agency Policy on Access to Documents: POLICY/0043," European Medicines Agency, October 4, 2018, https://www.ema.europa.eu/en/documents/other/policy-43-european-medicines-agency-policy-access-documents_en.pdf.
80 Jean-Marc Ferran and Sarah J. Nevitt, "European Medicines Agency Policy 0070: An Exploratory Review of Data Utility in Clinical Study Reports for Academic Research," *BMC Medical Research Methodology* 19 (November 5, 2019): Article 204, https://doi.org/10.1186/s12874-019-0836-3.
81 EMA, "External Guidance on the Implementation of the European Medicines Agency Policy on the Publication of Clinical Data for Medicinal Products for Human Use," European Medicines Agency, October 15, 2018, https://www.ema.europa.eu/en/documents/regulatory-procedural-guideline/external-guidance-implementation-european-medicines-agency-policy-publication-clinical-data-medicinal-products-human-use-version-14_en.pdf.
82 Ibid.
83 David F. López, "Clinical Data Publication Procedural Timelines," EMA Webinar, May 16, 2023, https://www.ema.europa.eu/en/documents/presentation/presentation-cdp-procedural-timelines_en.pdf.
84 EMA, "External Guidance on the Implementation of the European Medicines Agency Policy on the Publication of Clinical Data for Medicinal Products for Human Use"; Institute of Medicine, *Sharing Clinical Trial Data*, 70.
85 Anaya Rehman and Evan Richardson, "Streamline Clinical Data Publication under EMA Policy 0070," Certara, February 14, 2025, https://www.certara.com/blog/streamline-clinical-data-publication-under-ema-policy-0070/.
86 Lincoln Tsang and Hannah Kerr-Peterson, "Relaunch of the EMA's Policy on the Proactive Publication of Clinical Data," Ropes & Gray, May 25, 2023, https://www.ropesgray.com/en/insights/alerts/2023/05/relaunch-of-the-emas-policy-on-the-proactive-publication-of-clinical-data.
87 López, "Clinical Data Publication Procedural Timelines."
88 European Medicines Agency, "Clinical Data Publication (Policy 0070) Webinar—Step 2," YouTube, November 22, 2024, at 04:36 and 16:28, https://www.youtube.com/watch?v=WUps1nBuFFo&t=374s.
89 Kapczynski and Morten, "The Big Data Regulator, Rebooted," 519.
90 Barbara M. Undark, "Canada Makes Clinical Trial Data Available to Public," *The Transmitter*, October 16, 2019, https://www.spectrumnews.org/news/canada-makes-clinical-trial-data-available-to-public/.
91 Alexander C. Egilman et al., "Transparency of Regulatory Data across the European Medicines Agency, Health Canada, and US Food and Drug Administration," *Journal of Law, Medicine & Ethics* 49, no. 3 (2021): 456–85, https://doi.org/10.1017/jme.2021.67.
92 Ibid.
93 Scott Gottlieb, "FDA News Release: FDA Commissioner Scott Gottlieb, M.D., on New Steps FDA Is Taking to Enhance Transparency of Clinical Trial Information to Support Innovation and Scientific Inquiry Related to New Drugs," FDA, January 16, 2018, https://web.archive.org/web/20240306125943/https://www.fda.gov/news-events/press-announcements/fda-commissioner-scott-gottlieb-md-new-steps-fda-taking-enhance-transparency-clinical-trial.

94 "FDA Statement: FDA Continues to Support Transparency and Collaboration in Drug Approval Process as the Clinical Data Summary Pilot Concludes," FDA, March 26, 2020, https://web.archive.org/web/20250202093251/https://www.fda.gov/news-events/press-announcements/fda-continues-support-transparency-and-collaboration-drug-approval-process-clinical-data-summary; "FDA Concludes the Clinical Data Summary Pilot Program," CenterWatch, March 29, 2020, https://www.centerwatch.com/articles/24610-fda-concludes-the-clinical-data-summary-pilot-program.

95 "FDA Statement: FDA Continues to Support Transparency and Collaboration in Drug Approval Process as the Clinical Data Summary Pilot Concludes."

96 "Health Technology Assessment Body," European Medicines Agency, accessed June 21, 2025, https://www.ema.europa.eu/en/glossary/health-technology-assessment-body#:~:text=A%20public%20organisation%20that%20provides,medicines%20that%20have%20been%20authorised.

97 USC Schaeffer & Aspen Institute Advisory Panel, "Health Technology Assessment for the U.S. Healthcare System Background Paper," USC Schaeffer, 2019, https://schaeffer.usc.edu/wp-content/uploads/2024/10/Health-Technology-Assessment-for-the-U.S.-Healthcare-System_Background-Paper.pdf.

98 National Institute of Health and Care Excellence, "NICE Health Technology Evaluation Topic Selection: The Manual | 1 Summary of the Topic Selection Process," NICE, January 31, 2022, https://www.nice.org.uk/process/pmg37/chapter/summary-of-the-topic-selection-process.

99 National Institute of Health and Care Excellence, "NICE Health Technology Evaluation Topic Selection: The Manual | 2 Identifying Priorities for the Health and Care System," NICE, January 31, 2022, https://www.nice.org.uk/process/pmg37/chapter/identifying-priorities-for-the-health-and-care-system.

100 Amyas Morse, "Access to Clinical Trial Information and the Stockpiling of Tamiflu," National Audit Office, May 21, 2013: 17–20, https://www.nao.org.uk/wp-content/uploads/2013/05/10155-001_Access-to-clinical-trial-info-and-the-stockpiling-ofTamiflu_21-May.pdf.

101 USC Schaeffer & Aspen Institute Advisory Panel, "Health Technology Assessment for the U.S. Healthcare System Background Paper."

102 Ibid.

103 "National Committee for the Evaluation of Medical Devices and Health Technologies (CNEDiMTS*)," Haute Autorité de Santé, March 6, 2024, https://www.has-sante.fr/jcms/c_2036238/en/national-committee-for-the-evaluation-of-medical-devices-and-health-technologies-cnedimts.

104 USC Schaeffer & Aspen Institute Advisory Panel, "Health Technology Assessment for the U.S. Healthcare System Background Paper."

105 Kapczynski and Morten, "The Big Data Regulator, Rebooted," 517, 519; FDA, "Driving Biomedical Innovation: Initiatives to Improve Products for Patients," Food and Drug Administration, October 2011, https://www.celebrationofscience.org/assets/Uploads/DrivingBiomedicalInnovation-ImprovingProductsforPatients.pdf.

106 John F. Sargent Jr., "The Office of Technology Assessment: History, Authorities, Issues, and Options," Congressional Research Service, April 29, 2020, https://sgp.fas.org/crs/misc/R46327.pdf.

107 "Office of Technology Assessment Act," Pub. L. No. 92–484, U.S. Code (1972), https://www.govinfo.gov/content/pkg/STATUTE-86/pdf/STATUTE-86-Pg797.pdf.

108 USC Schaeffer & Aspen Institute Advisory Panel, "Health Technology Assessment for the U.S. Healthcare System Background Paper."
109 Sargent Jr., "The Office of Technology Assessment: History, Authorities, Issues, and Options"; Gregory C. Kunkle, "New Challenge or the Past Revisited?," Princeton University, 1995, https://www.princeton.edu/~ota/ns20/nchal_f.html.
110 Jennifer Wong, "The History of Technology Assessment and Comparative Effectiveness Research for Drugs and Medical Devices and the Role of the Federal Government," *Biotechnology Law Report* 33, no. 6 (December 22, 2014): 221–48, https://doi.org/10.1089/blr.2014.9967; Office of Technology Assessment, *Health Care Technology and Its Assessment in Eight Countries* (United States Congress, 1995): 1291–300, https://www.princeton.edu/~ota/disk1/1995/9562/956211.PDF.
111 USC Schaeffer & Aspen Institute Advisory Panel, "Health Technology Assessment for the U.S. Healthcare System Background Paper"; AHRQ, "Technology Assessment Program," Agency for Healthcare Research and Quality, January 2013, https://www.ahrq.gov/research/findings/ta/index.html.
112 Amanda K. Sarata, "Funding for ACA-Established Patient-Centered Outcomes Research Trust Fund (PCORTF) Extended through FY2029," Congressional Research Service, February 6, 2020, https://crsreports.congress.gov/product/pdf/IN/IN11010.
113 Ethan M. Balk et al., "Long-Term Health Outcomes in Obstructive Sleep Apnea: A Systematic Review of Comparative Studies Evaluating Positive Airway Pressure and the Validity of Breathing Measures as Surrogate Outcomes," Agency for Healthcare Research and Quality, December 1, 2022, https://www.ahrq.gov/sites/default/files/wysiwyg/research/findings/ta/sleep-apnea/sleep-apnea-report.pdf.
114 USC Schaeffer & Aspen Institute Advisory Panel, "Health Technology Assessment for the U.S. Healthcare System Background Paper"; ICER, "Guide to Understanding Health Technology Assessment (HTA)," Institute for Clinical and Economic Review, August 2018, https://icer.org/wp-content/uploads/2020/10/ICER-Guide-to-Understanding-Health-Technology-Assessment-6.19.18.pdf.
115 Praveen Thokala, Josh J. Carlson, and Mike Drummond, "HTA'd in the USA: A Comparison of ICER in the United States with NICE in England and Wales," *Journal of Managed Care & Specialty Pharmacy* 26, no. 9 (August 28, 2020): 1162–70, https://doi.org/10.18553/jmcp.2020.26.9.1162.

## 3 False Prophets and the Role of Medical Journals

1 Monica Mihaela Marta, "A Brief History of the Evolution of the Medical Research Article," *Medicine and Pharmacy Reports* 88, no. 4 (September 28, 2015): 567–70, https://doi.org/10.15386/cjmed-560.
2 Saeed Safari, Alireza Baratloo, and Mahmoud Yousefifard, "Medical Journalism and Emergency Medicine," *Emergency* (Tehran, Iran) 3, no. 3 (July 5, 2015): 83–6, https://www.ncbi.nlm.nih.gov/pmc/articles/PMC4608339/; Andreas Gipper, "Latin Translations of Scientific Journals in the Seventeenth Century," in *In die falsche Richtung?*, vol. 10, ed. Julia Heideklang, Jan Shavrin, and Anja Wolkenhauer (Berlin, Heidelberg: J.B. Metzler, 2025), 109–24, https://doi.org/10.1007/978-3-662-71231-3_5.
3 Marta, "A Brief History of the Evolution of the Medical Research Article."

4 Safari, Baratloo, and Yousefifard, "Medical Journalism and Emergency Medicine."
5 Scott H. Podolsky, Jeremy A. Greene, and David S. Jones, "The Evolving Roles of the Medical Journal," *New England Journal of Medicine* 366, no. 16 (April 19, 2012): 1457–61, https://doi.org/10.1056/NEJMp1113567.
6 Ibid.
7 JAMA, "A Conversation with Dr Kirsten Bibbins-Domingo, JAMA's New Editor in Chief," AMA Ed Hub, July 5, 2022, https://edhub.ama-assn.org/jn-learning/video-player/18707306.
8 J. H. Salisbury, "The Subordination of Medical Journals to Proprietary Interests," *Journal of the American Medical Association* XLVI, no. 18 (May 5, 1906): 1337–8, https://doi.org/10.1001/jama.1906.62510450011001d.
9 JAMA, "A Conversation with Dr Kirsten Bibbins-Domingo, JAMA's New Editor in Chief."
10 D. L Sackett et al., "Evidence Based Medicine: What It Is and What It Isn't," *BMJ* 312, no. 7023 (January 13, 1996): 71–2, https://doi.org/10.1136/bmj.312.7023.71; Iqbal Ratnani et al., "Evidence-Based Medicine: History, Review, Criticisms, and Pitfalls," *Cureus* 15, no. 2 (February 21, 2023): e35266, https://doi.org/10.7759/cureus.35266.
11 Ibid.; Achilleas Thoma and Felmont F. Eaves, "A Brief History of Evidence-Based Medicine (EBM) and the Contributions of Dr David Sackett," *Aesthetic Surgery Journal* 35, no. 8 (July 10, 2015): NP261–3, https://doi.org/10.1093/asj/sjv130.
12 Gordon Guyatt et al., "Evidence-Based Medicine: A New Approach to Teaching the Practice of Medicine," *JAMA* 268, no. 17 (November 4, 1992): 2420–5, https://doi.org/10.1001/jama.1992.03490170092032.
13 Benjamin Djulbegovic and Gordon H. Guyatt, "Progress in Evidence-Based Medicine: A Quarter Century On," *The Lancet* 390, no. 10092 (July 22, 2017): 415–23, https://doi.org/10.1016/S0140-6736(16)31592-6.
14 Ibid.
15 Committee on Standards for Developing Trustworthy Clinical Practice Guidelines, Board on Health Care Services, and Institute of Medicine, *Clinical Practice Guidelines We Can Trust*, ed. Robin Graham et al. (Washington, DC: National Academies Press, 2011), https://doi.org/10.17226/13058.
16 Michael LeFevre, "From Authority- to Evidence-Based Medicine: Are Clinical Practice Guidelines Moving Us Forward or Backward?," *The Annals of Family Medicine* 15, no. 5 (September 2017): 410–12, https://doi.org/10.1370/afm.2141.
17 Bernard Lo et al., *Conflict of Interest in Medical Research, Education, and Practice* (Washington, DC: National Academies Press, 2009): 2 https://doi.org/10.17226/12598.
18 Kristine Rasmussen et al., "Collaboration between Academics and Industry in Clinical Trials: Cross Sectional Study of Publications and Survey of Lead Academic Authors," *BMJ* 363, no. 8170 (October 3, 2018): k3654, https://doi.org/10.1136/bmj.k3654.
19 Siena et al., "Industry Involvement and Transparency in the Most Cited Clinical Trials, 2019–2022."
20 "Disclosure of Financial and Non-Financial Relationships and Activities, and Conflicts of Interest," ICMJE, accessed June 13, 2024, https://www.icmje.org/recommendations/browse/roles-and-responsibilities/author-responsibilities--conflicts-of-interest.html.

21 Rafael Dal-Ré, Arthur L. Caplan, and Ana Marusic, "Editors' and Authors' Individual Conflicts of Interest Disclosure and Journal Transparency. A Cross-Sectional Study of High-Impact Medical Specialty Journals," *BMJ Open* 9, no. 7 (July 23, 2019): e029796, https://doi.org/10.1136/bmjopen-2019-029796.
22 Rafael Dal-Ré and Ana Marušić, "Are Journals Following the ICMJE Recommendations Complying with Conflicts of Interest Disclosure Policies," *European Journal of Internal Medicine* 57 (August 1, 2018): e17–19, https://doi.org/10.1016/j.ejim.2018.07.025.
23 Jessica J. Liu et al., "Payments by US Pharmaceutical and Medical Device Manufacturers to US Medical Journal Editors: Retrospective Observational Study," *BMJ* 359, no. 8127 (October 26, 2017): j4619, https://doi.org/10.1136/bmj.j4619.
24 Waqas Haque et al., "Conflicts of Interest of Editors of Medical Journals," ed. Neil R. Smalheiser, *PLoS ONE* 13, no. 5 (May 18, 2018): e0197141, https://doi.org/10.1371/journal.pone.0197141.
25 National Institutes of Health, "Financial Conflicts of Interest Tutorial," https://grants.nih.gov/grants/policy/coi/tutorial2018/FINANCIAL-CONFLICT-OF-INTEREST.pdf.
26 Haque et al., "Conflicts of Interest of Editors of Medical Journals."
27 Victoria S. S. Wong, Lauro Nathaniel Avalos, and Michael L. Callaham, "Industry Payments to Physician Journal Editors," ed. Barbara Mintzes, *PLoS ONE* 14, no. 2 (February 7, 2019): e0211495, https://doi.org/10.1371/journal.pone.0211495.
28 Dal-Ré, Caplan, and Marusic, "Editors' and Authors' Individual Conflicts of Interest Disclosure and Journal Transparency. A Cross-Sectional Study of High-Impact Medical Specialty Journals."
29 "Instructions for Authors," JAMA Network Open, accessed April 22, 2024, https://jamanetwork.com/journals/jamanetworkopen/pages/instructions-for-authors.
30 Richard Horton, "Offline: What Is Medicine's 5 Sigma?," *The Lancet* 385, no. 9976 (April 11, 2015): 1380, https://doi.org/10.1016/S0140-6736(15)60696-1.
31 Emma Parish, Theodora Bloom, and Fiona Godlee, "Statins for People at Low Risk," *BMJ* 351, no. 8018 (July 21, 2015): h3908, https://doi.org/10.1136/bmj.h3908.
32 "Journals Stating That They Follow the ICMJE Recommendations," ICMJE, accessed April 21, 2025, https://web.archive.org/web/20250421163702/https://www.icmje.org/journals-following-the-icmje-recommendations/.
33 "About ICMJE," ICMJE, accessed April 22, 2024, https://www.icmje.org/about-icmje/#:~:text=The%20current%20members%20of%20the,Korean%20Medical%20Science%2C%20%D8%A7%D9%84%D9%85%D8%AC%D9%84%D8%A9%20%D8%A7%D9%84%D8%B7%D8%A8%D9%8A%D8%A9.
34 Catherine De Angelis et al., "Clinical Trial Registration: A Statement from the International Committee of Medical Journal Editors," *New England Journal of Medicine* 351, no. 12 (September 16, 2004): 1250–1, https://doi.org/10.1056/NEJMe048225.
35 Ibid.
36 Christine Laine et al., "Update on Trials Registration: Clinical Trial Registration: Looking Back and Moving Ahead," ICMJE, June 2007, https://www.icmje.org/news-and-editorials/clincial_trial_reg_jun2007.html.
37 Darren B. Taichman et al., "Data Sharing Statements for Clinical Trials: A Requirement of the International Committee of Medical Journal Editors," *Annals of Internal Medicine* 167, no. 1 (June 6, 2017): 63–5, https://doi.org/10.7326/M17-1028.

38 "Clinical Trials," ICMJE, accessed April 22, 2024, https://www.icmje.org/recommendations/browse/publishing-and-editorial-issues/clinical-trial-registration.html#:~:text=Data%20sharing%20statements%20must%20indicate,(e.g.%2C%20study%20protocol%2C%20statistical.
39 Darren B. Taichman et al., "Sharing Clinical Trial Data: A Proposal From the International Committee of Medical Journal Editors," *Annals of Internal Medicine* 164, no. 7 (January 26, 2016): 505–6, https://doi.org/10.7326/M15-2928.
40 Taichman et al., "Data Sharing Statements for Clinical Trials."
41 Dan L. Longo and Jeffrey M. Drazen, "Data Sharing," *New England Journal of Medicine* 374, no. 3 (January 21, 2016): 276–7, https://doi.org/10.1056/NEJMe1516564.
42 Hopkins, Rowland, and Sorich, "Data Sharing from Pharmaceutical Industry Sponsored Clinical Studies."
43 Jennifer Miller et al., "Sharing of Clinical Trial Data and Results Reporting Practices among Large Pharmaceutical Companies: Cross Sectional Descriptive Study and Pilot of a Tool to Improve Company Practices," *BMJ* 366, no. 8208 (July 10, 2019): l4217, https://doi.org/10.1136/bmj.l4217.
44 Natansh D. Modi et al., "Audit of Data Sharing by Pharmaceutical Companies for Anticancer Medicines Approved by the US Food and Drug Administration," *JAMA Oncology* 8, no. 9 (July 28, 2022): 1310–16, https://doi.org/10.1001/jamaoncol.2022.2867.
45 FDA, "Frequently Asked Questions about Labeling for Prescription Medicines," US Food & Drug Administration, April 1, 2024, https://www.fda.gov/drugs/fdas-labeling-resources-human-prescription-drugs/frequently-asked-questions-about-labeling-prescription-medicines.
46 Karthik Murugiah et al., "Availability of Clinical Trial Data From Industry-Sponsored Cardiovascular Trials," *Journal of the American Heart Association* 5, no. 4 (April 20, 2016): e003307, https://doi.org/10.1161/JAHA.116.003307.
47 Kapczynski and Morten, "The Big Data Regulator, Rebooted," 516–17.
48 Peter Doshi, Fiona Godlee, and Kamran Abbasi, "Covid-19 Vaccines and Treatments: We Must Have Raw Data, Now," *BMJ* 376, no. 8322 (January 19, 2022): o102, https://doi.org/10.1136/bmj.o102.
49 CDC, "COVID-19 Vaccinations in the United States,Jurisdiction," COVID Data Tracker, May 12, 2023, https://data.cdc.gov/Vaccinations/COVID-19-Vaccinations-in-the-United-States-Jurisdi/unsk-b7fc/data_preview.
50 "Good Pharma Scorecard," Bioethics International, accessed April 22, 2024, https://bioethicsinternational.org/good-pharma-scorecard/; Moe Alsumidaie, "J&J Propels Data Clinical Trial Data Sharing," Applied Clinical Trials, August 4, 2017, https://www.appliedclinicaltrialsonline.com/view/jj-propels-data-clinical-trial-data-sharing.
51 "Johnson & Johnson—Available Data," The YODA Project, accessed April 22, 2024, https://yoda.yale.edu/jj-available-data/.
52 Brandon Novick to YODA Project Representative, "RE: New Submission from Contact Us," April 23, 2024.
53 Abramson, *Sickening*, 173–5; Joseph S. Ross et al., "Overview and Experience of the YODA Project with Clinical Trial Data Sharing after 5 Years," *Scientific Data* 5 (November 27, 2018): Article 180268, https://doi.org/10.1038/sdata.2018.268.
54 Johnson & Johnson, "Johnson & Johnson Announces Clinical Trial Data Sharing Agreement with Yale School of Medicine," PR Newswire, January 30, 2014,

https://www.prnewswire.com/news-releases/johnson--johnson-announces-clinical-trial-data-sharing-agreement-with-yale-school-of-medicine-242694971.html; Office of Public Affairs, "Press Release: Johnson & Johnson to Pay More than $2.2 Billion to Resolve Criminal and Civil Investigations," U.S. Department of Justice, November 4, 2013, https://www.justice.gov/opa/pr/johnson-johnson-pay-more-22-billion-resolve-criminal-and-civil-investigations.

55 "Corporate Integrity Agreement between the Office of Inspector General of the Department of Health and Human Services and Johnson & Johnson," US Department of Justice, October 31, 2013, https://www.justice.gov/sites/default/files/opa/legacy/2013/11/04/corp-integ-agreement.pdf.

56 Holly Fernandez Lynch and I. Glenn Cohen, eds., *FDA in the Twenty-First Century: The Challenges of Regulating Drugs and New Technologies* (New York: Columbia University Press, 2015), 112, https://dokumen.pub/fda-in-the-twenty-first-century-the-challenges-of-regulating-drugs-and-new-technologies-9780231540070.html.

57 Office of Public Affairs, "Press Release: GlaxoSmithKline to Plead Guilty and Pay $3 Billion to Resolve Fraud Allegations and Failure to Report Safety Data," US Department of Justice, July 2, 2012, https://www.justice.gov/opa/pr/glaxosmithkline-plead-guilty-and-pay-3-billion-resolve-fraud-allegations-and-failure-report.

58 "Corporate Integrity Agreement between the Office of Inspector General of the Department of Health and Human Services and Glaxosmithkline LLC," (US Department of Justice, July 2, 2012, https://www.justice.gov/sites/default/files/opa/legacy/2012/07/02/plea-ex-d.pdf.

59 Perry Nisen and Frank Rockhold, "Access to Patient-Level Data from GlaxoSmithKline Clinical Trials," *New England Journal of Medicine* 369, no. 5 (August 1, 2013): 475–8, https://doi.org/10.1056/NEJMsr1302541.

60 "GSK Gives Update on Plans to Share Detailed Clinical Trial Data as Part of Its Commitment to Transparency," GSK, May 7, 2013, https://www.gsk.com/en-gb/media/press-releases/gsk-gives-update-on-plans-to-share-detailed-clinical-trial-data-as-part-of-its-commitment-to-transparency/.

61 "Our Commitment to Data Sharing," GlaxoSmithKline, July 15, 2023, https://www.gsk-studyregister.com/About_GSK_Patient_Level_Data_Sharing_Final_13July2023.pdf.

62 Lynch and Cohen, *FDA in the Twenty-First Century*, 112.

63 Phil B. Fontanarosa, "Reporting Conflicts of Interest, Financial Aspects of Research, and Role of Sponsors in Funded Studies," *JAMA* 294, no. 1 (July 6, 2005): 110–11, https://doi.org/10.1001/jama.294.1.110.

64 Elizabeth Wager et al., "JAMA Published Fewer Industry-Funded Studies after Introducing a Requirement for Independent Statistical Analysis," ed. Erik Von Elm, *PLoS ONE* 5, no. 10 (October 22, 2010): e13591, https://doi.org/10.1371/journal.pone.0013591.

65 Howard Bauchner, "Editorial Policies for Clinical Trials and the Continued Changes in Medical Journalism," *JAMA* 310, no. 2 (July 10, 2013): 149–50, https://doi.org/10.1001/jama.2013.8083.

66 Richard Smith, "Medical Journals Are an Extension of the Marketing Arm of Pharmaceutical Companies," *PLoS Medicine* 2, no. 5 (May 17, 2005): e138, https://doi.org/10.1371/journal.pmed.0020138.

67 Adriane Fugh-Berman and Shahram Ahari, "Following the Script: How Drug Reps Make Friends and Influence Doctors," *PLoS Medicine* 4, no. 4 (April 24, 2007): e150, https://doi.org/10.1371/journal.pmed.0040150.

68 Andreas Lundh et al., "Conflicts of Interest at Medical Journals: The Influence of Industry-Supported Randomised Trials on Journal Impact Factors and Revenue—Cohort Study," *PLoS Medicine* 7, no. 10 (October 26, 2010): e1000354, https://doi.org/10.1371/journal.pmed.1000354.
69 Fiona Godlee, Kamran Abbasi, and Theodora Bloom, "BMJ Declares Its Revenues from Industry," *BMJ* 359, no. 8127 (October 25, 2017): j4930, https://doi.org/10.1136/bmj.j4930.
70 A. E. Handel et al., "High Reprint Orders in Medical Journals and Pharmaceutical Industry Funding: Case-Control Study," *BMJ* 344 (June 28, 2012): e4212, https://doi.org/10.1136/bmj.e4212.
71 Richard Smith, "Richard Smith: The Hypocrisy of Medical Journals over Transparency," *The BMJ Opinion* (blog), January 24, 2018, https://blogs.bmj.com/bmj/2018/01/24/richard-smith-the-hypocrisy-of-medical-journals-over-transparency/.
72 Tim S. Ellison et al., "Open Access Policies of Leading Medical Journals: A Cross-Sectional Study," *BMJ Open* 9, no. 6 (June 20, 2019): e028655, https://doi.org/10.1136/bmjopen-2018-028655.
73 Smith, "The Hypocrisy."
74 S. Scott Graham et al., "Relationships among Commercial Practices and Author Conflicts of Interest in Biomedical Publishing," *PLoS ONE* 15, no. 7 (July 24, 2020): e0236166, https://doi.org/10.1371/journal.pone.0236166.
75 Elizabeth Loder et al., "Mandatory Data and Code Sharing for Research Published by The BMJ," *BMJ* 384, no. 8421 (March 5, 2024): q324, https://doi.org/10.1136/bmj.q324.
76 "About Vivli: Overview," Vivli, accessed April 22, 2024, https://vivli.org/about/overview/.
77 Loder et al., "Mandatory Data and Code Sharing for Research Published by The BMJ."
78 "Data Availability," PLOS Medicine, December 5, 2019, https://journals.plos.org/plosmedicine/s/data-availability.
79 Michael S. Sinha, Aaron S. Kesselheim, and Jonathan J. Darrow, "Pharmaceutical Advertising in Medical Journals," *Chest* 153, no. 1 (2018): 9–11, https://doi.org/10.1016/j.chest.2017.09.048.
80 Lisa M. Schwartz and Steven Woloshin, "Medical Marketing in the United States, 1997–2016," *JAMA* 321, no. 1 (January 1, 2019): 80–96, https://doi.org/10.1001/jama.2018.19320.
81 Jennifer Gettings et al., "Differences in the Volume of Pharmaceutical Advertisements between Print General Medical Journals," ed. Frank Havemann, *PLoS ONE* 9, no. 1 (January 8, 2014): e84790, https://doi.org/10.1371/journal.pone.0084790.
82 Michael J. DiStefano et al., "Association between Drug Characteristics and Manufacturer Spending on Direct-to-Consumer Advertising," *JAMA* 329, no. 5 (February 7, 2023): 386–92, https://doi.org/10.1001/jama.2022.23968.
83 Kim Boesen et al., "Cross-Sectional Study of Medical Advertisements in a National General Medical Journal: Evidence, Cost, and Safe Use of Advertised versus Comparative Drugs," *Research Integrity and Peer Review* 6 (May 10, 2021): Article 8, https://doi.org/10.1186/s41073-021-00111-9.
84 Gary Guenther, "Proposals to Deny a Federal Tax Deduction for Prescription Drug Advertising Expenses," Congressional Research Service, June 10, 2022, https://www.everycrsreport.com/files/2022-06-10_IN11951_27ae87d8e870a6f1def388424fa9562e32baa709.pdf.

85 Virginia State Board of Pharmacy v. Virginia Citizens Consumer Council, Inc., 425 U.S. 748 (US Supreme Court 1976).
86 Schwartz and Woloshin, "Medical Marketing in the United States, 1997–2016."
87 Megan Graham, "Senators to Propose Ban on Drug Advertising to Consumers," *The Wall Street Journal*, June 12, 2025, https://www.wsj.com/articles/senators-to-propose-ban-on-drug-advertising-to-consumers-9ad257c2.
88 Abramson, *Sickening*, 214–15.
89 Richard Durbin and Mike Braun, "Letter from Senators Richard Durbin and Mike Braun to FDA Commissioner Robert Califf," February 14, 2024, https://www.durbin.senate.gov/imo/media/doc/final_durbin-braun_fda_letter_-_rx_promotion_on_social_media.pdf.
90 "Press Release: Early Benefit Assessment—the Whole Range," IQWiG, March 19, 2021, https://www.iqwig.de/en/presse/press-releases/press-releases-detailpage_30784.html.
91 Beate Wieseler, Natalie McGauran, and Thomas Kaiser, "New Drugs: Where Did We Go Wrong and What Can We Do Better?," *BMJ* 366, no. 8207 (July 10, 2019): l4340, https://doi.org/10.1136/bmj.l4340.
92 Leeza Osipenko et al., "Provenance and Clinical Benefit of Medicines Introduced to the French Market, 2008 to 2018," *JAMA Internal Medicine* 184, no. 1 (November 20, 2023): 46–52, https://doi.org/10.1001/jamainternmed.2023.6249.
93 Robin Feldman, "May Your Drug Price Be Evergreen," *Journal of Law and the Biosciences* 5, no. 3 (December 7, 2018): 590–647, https://doi.org/10.1093/jlb/lsy022.
94 Beate Wieseler et al., "Completeness of Reporting of Patient-Relevant Clinical Trial Outcomes: Comparison of Unpublished Clinical Study Reports with Publicly Available Data," ed. Davina Ghersi, *PLoS Med* 10, no. 10 (October 8, 2013): e1001526, https://doi.org/10.1371/journal.pmed.1001526.
95 J. B. Carlisle, "False Individual Patient Data and Zombie Randomised Controlled Trials Submitted to Anaesthesia," *Anaesthesia* 76, no. 4 (October 11, 2020): 472–9, https://doi.org/10.1111/anae.15263.
96 Richard Van Noorden, "Medicine Is Plagued by Untrustworthy Clinical Trials. How Many Studies Are Faked or Flawed?," *Nature* 619, no. 7970 (July 18, 2023): 454–8, https://doi.org/10.1038/d41586-023-02299-w.
97 Carlisle, "False Individual Patient Data and Zombie Randomised Controlled Trials Submitted to Anaesthesia."
98 Van Noorden, "Medicine Is Plagued by Untrustworthy Clinical Trials. How Many Studies Are Faked or Flawed?"
99 Jo Weeks, Anna Cuthbert, and Zarko Alfirevic, "Trustworthiness Assessment as an Inclusion Criterion for Systematic Reviews—What Is the Impact on Results?," *Cochrane Evidence Synthesis and Methods* 1, no. 10 (December 13, 2023): e12037, https://doi.org/10.1002/cesm.12037.
100 Bernhard A. Sabel et al., "Fake Publications in Biomedical Science: Red-Flagging Method Indicates Mass Production," medRxiv, May 8, 2023, https://doi.org/10.1101/2023.05.06.23289563.
101 Ayesha Rascoe, "Fake Studies in Academic Journals May Be More Common than Previously Thought," *NPR*, May 14, 2023, sec. Research News, https://www.npr.org/2023/05/14/1176062276/fake-studies-in-academic-journals-may-be-more-common-than-previously-thought.
102 Richard Van Noorden, "How Big Is Science's Fake-Paper Problem?," *Nature* 623, no. 7987 (November 6, 2023): 466–7, https://doi.org/10.1038/d41586-023-03464-x; Holly Else and Richard Van Noorden, "The Fight against Fake-Paper Factories That

Churn Out Sham Science," *Nature* 591, no. 7851 (March 23, 2021): 516–19, https://doi.org/10.1038/d41586-021-00733-5.

## 4 Poor Instructors and Clinical Practice Guidelines

1 "Clinical Practice Guidelines Development Process," American Academy of Audiology, April 2022, https://www.audiology.org/practice-resources/practice-guidelines-and-standards/clinical-practice-guidelines-development-process/.

2 Prasad and Cifu, *Ending Medical Reversal*, 140–1.

3 M. Hassan Murad, "Clinical Practice Guidelines," *Mayo Clinic Proceedings* 92, no. 3 (March 2017): 423–33, https://doi.org/10.1016/j.mayocp.2017.01.001.

4 Amir Qaseem et al., "The Development of Clinical Guidelines and Guidance Statements by the Clinical Guidelines Committee of the American College of Physicians: Update of Methods," *Annals of Internal Medicine* 170, no. 12 (June 11, 2019): 863–70, https://doi.org/10.7326/M18–3290.

5 George Weisz et al., "The Emergence of Clinical Practice Guidelines," *The Milbank Quarterly* 85, no. 4 (December 7, 2007): 691–727, https://doi.org/10.1111/j.1468-0009.2007.00505.x.

6 Committee on Standards for Developing Trustworthy Clinical Practice Guidelines, Board on Health Care Services, and Institute of Medicine, *Clinical Practice Guidelines We Can Trust*, 2.

7 Weisz et al., "The Emergence of Clinical Practice Guidelines."

8 The agency was initially called the Agency for Health Care Policy and Research (AHCPR).

9 Committee to Advise the Public Health Service on Clinical Practice Guidelines and Institute of Medicine, *Clinical Practice Guidelines: Directions for a New Program*, ed. Marilyn J. Field and Kathleen N. Lohr (Washington, DC: National Academies Press, 1990), 108, https://doi.org/10.17226/1626.

10 Ibid., 6.

11 Ibid., 10–11.

12 Terrence M. Shaneyfelt, Michael F. Mayo-Smith, and Johann Rothwangl, "Are Guidelines Following Guidelines?: The Methodological Quality of Clinical Practice Guidelines in the Peer-Reviewed Medical Literature," *JAMA* 281, no. 20 (May 26, 1999): 1900–5, https://doi.org/10.1001/jama.281.20.1900.

13 The GRADE Working Group et al., "Systems for Grading the Quality of Evidence and the Strength of Recommendations I: Critical Appraisal of Existing Approaches The GRADE Working Group," *BMC Health Services Research* 4 (December 22, 2004): Article 38, https://doi.org/10.1186/1472-6963-4-38.

14 Committee on Standards for Developing Trustworthy Clinical Practice Guidelines, Board on Health Care Services, and Institute of Medicine, *Clinical Practice Guidelines We Can Trust*.

15 Jill Eden et al., *Knowing What Works in Health Care: A Roadmap for the Nation* (Washington, DC: National Academies Press, 2008), 9, https://doi.org/10.17226/12038.

16 Pierluigi Tricoci et al., "Scientific Evidence Underlying the ACC/AHA Clinical Practice Guidelines," *JAMA* 301, no. 8 (February 25, 2009): 831–41, https://doi.org/10.1001/jama.2009.205.

17 Committee on Standards for Developing Trustworthy Clinical Practice Guidelines, Board on Health Care Services, and Institute of Medicine, *Clinical Practice Guidelines We Can Trust*, 53.
18 Ibid., 54.
19 Ibid., 55.
20 Justin Kung, Ram R. Miller, and Philip A. Mackowiak, "Failure of Clinical Practice Guidelines to Meet Institute of Medicine Standards: Two More Decades of Little, If Any, Progress," *Archives of Internal Medicine* 172, no. 21 (November 26, 2012): 1628–33, https://doi.org/10.1001/2013.jamainternmed.56.
21 "The National Guideline Clearinghouse Extent Adherence to Trustworthy Standards (NEATS) Assessments," National Guideline Clearinghouse, October 23, 2017, https://web.archive.org/web/20180609103505/https://www.guideline.gov/help-and-about/summaries/determining-extent-adherence-to-the-iom-standards-in-ngc.
22 Abramson, *Sickening*, 130.
23 Susan Scutti, "Government Shuts Down Website for Doctors," CNN, July 16, 2018, https://www.cnn.com/2018/07/16/health/hhs-website-shuts-down/index.html.
24 Abramson, *Sickening*, 42; National Cholesterol Education Program (NCEP) Expert Panel on Detection, Evaluation, and Treatment of High Blood Cholesterol in Adults (Adult Treatment Panel III), "Third Report of the National Cholesterol Education Program (NCEP) Expert Panel on Detection, Evaluation, and Treatment of High Blood Cholesterol in Adults (Adult Treatment Panel III) Final Report," *Circulation* 106, no. 25 (December 17, 2002): 3143–421, https://doi.org/10.1161/circ.106.25.3143.
25 "Third Report of NCEP," 3351.
26 Expert Panel on Detection, Evaluation, and Treatment of High Blood Cholesterol in Adults, "Executive Summary of the Third Report of the National Cholesterol Education Program (NCEP) Expert Panel on Detection, Evaluation, and Treatment of High Blood Cholesterol in Adults (Adult Treatment Panel III)," *JAMA* 285, no. 19 (May 16, 2001): 2486–97, https://doi.org/10.1001/jama.285.19.2486.
27 Abramson, *Sickening*, 42.
28 John D. Abramson et al., "Should People at Low Risk of Cardiovascular Disease Take a Statin?," *BMJ* 347, no. 7930 (October 22, 2013): f6123, https://doi.org/10.1136/bmj.f6123; James M. Rippe, "Lifestyle Strategies for Risk Factor Reduction, Prevention, and Treatment of Cardiovascular Disease," *American Journal of Lifestyle Medicine* 13, no. 2 (December 2, 2018): 204–12, https://doi.org/10.1177/1559827618812395.
29 Abramson, *Sickening*, 43.
30 Peter S. Sever et al., "Prevention of Coronary and Stroke Events with Atorvastatin in Hypertensive Patients Who Have Average or Lower-than-Average Cholesterol Concentrations, in the Anglo-Scandinavian Cardiac Outcomes Trial—Lipid Lowering Arm (ASCOT-LLA): A Multicentre Randomised Controlled Trial," *The Lancet* 361, no. 9364 (April 5, 2003): 1149–58, https://doi.org/10.1016/S0140-6736(03)12948-0.
31 Kausik K. Ray et al., "Statins and All-Cause Mortality in High-Risk Primary Prevention: A Meta-Analysis of 11 Randomized Controlled Trials Involving 65 229 Participants," *Archives of Internal Medicine* 170, no. 12 (June 28, 2010): 1024–31, https://doi.org/10.1001/archinternmed.2010.182.
32 Abramson, *Sickening*, 45.
33 Cholesterol Treatment Trialists' (Ctt) Collaborators, "The Effects of Lowering LDL Cholesterol with Statin Therapy in People at Low Risk of Vascular

Disease: Meta-Analysis of Individual Data from 27 Randomised Trials," *The Lancet* 380, no. 9841 (May 17, 2012): 581–90, https://doi.org/10.1016/S0140-6736(12)60367-5.
34 Abramson et al., "Should People at Low Risk of Cardiovascular Disease Take a Statin?"
35 Abramson, *Sickening*, 53.
36 I. Heath et al., "Report of the Independent Panel Considering the Retraction of Two Articles in the *BMJ*," *BMJ* 349 (August 15, 2014): g5176, https://doi.org/10.1136/bmj.g5176.
37 Vinay Prasad, "Statins, Primary Prevention, and Overall Mortality," *Annals of Internal Medicine* 160, no. 12 (June 17, 2014): 867–9, https://doi.org/10.7326/M13-2974.
38 Ibid; Abramson, Sickening, 50.
39 Paula Byrne et al., "Evaluating the Association between Low-Density Lipoprotein Cholesterol Reduction and Relative and Absolute Effects of Statin Treatment: A Systematic Review and Meta-Analysis," *JAMA Internal Medicine* 182, no. 5 (March 14, 2022): 474–81, https://doi.org/10.1001/jamainternmed.2022.0134.
40 Ibid.
41 Natalie C. Ward, Gerald F. Watts, and Robert H. Eckel, "Statin Toxicity: Mechanistic Insights and Clinical Implications," *Circulation Research* 124, no. 2 (January 17, 2019): 328–50, https://doi.org/10.1161/CIRCRESAHA.118.312782.
42 Paul D. Thompson et al., "Statin-Associated Side Effects," *Journal of the American College of Cardiology* 67, no. 20 (May 24, 2016): 2395–410, https://doi.org/10.1016/j.jacc.2016.02.071.
43 Beatrice A. Golomb et al., "Effects of Statins on Energy and Fatigue with Exertion: Results from a Randomized Controlled Trial," *Archives of Internal Medicine* 172, no. 15 (August 13, 2012): 1180–2, https://doi.org/10.1001/archinternmed.2012.2171.
44 Abramson et al., "Should People at Low Risk of Cardiovascular Disease Take a Statin?"; Rippe, "Lifestyle Strategies for Risk Factor Reduction, Prevention, and Treatment of Cardiovascular Disease."
45 Maarit J. Korhonen et al., "Lifestyle Changes in Relation to Initiation of Antihypertensive and Lipid-Lowering Medication: A Cohort Study," *Journal of the American Heart Association* 9, no. 4 (February 18, 2020): e014168, https://doi.org/10.1161/JAHA.119.014168.
46 Takehiro Sugiyama et al., "Different Time Trends of Caloric and Fat Intake Between Statin Users and Nonusers among US Adults: Gluttony in the Time of Statins?," *JAMA Internal Medicine* 174, no. 7 (July 2014): 1038–45, https://doi.org/10.1001/jamainternmed.2014.1927.
47 Megan Macfarlane, David Cooper, and Alison Avenell, "Do People Reduce Attempts at Lifestyle Change after Initiating Weight Loss Medication? A Review of Trial Evidence," medRxiv, January 13, 2024, https://doi.org/10.1101/2024.01.12.24301166.
48 Stephen Luther, "Statin Drugs on Trial in Cholesterol's Trillion-Dollar Industry » Symbios Health," Symbios Health, March 23, 2024, https://mysymbios.com/statin-drugs-on-trial-in-cholesterols-trillion-dollar-industry/.
49 "About," CTT Collaboration, accessed June 13, 2024, https://www.cttcollaboration.org/about2; Anand R. Habib, Mitchell H. Katz, and Rita F. Redberg, "Statins for Primary Cardiovascular Disease Prevention: Time to Curb Our Enthusiasm," *JAMA Internal Medicine* 182, no. 10 (August 23, 2022): 1021–4, https://doi.org/10.1001/jamainternmed.2022.3204.

50 Abramson et al., "Should People at Low Risk of Cardiovascular Disease Take a Statin?"
51 "Statins—a Call for Transparent Data," thebmj, accessed June 13, 2024, https://www.bmj.com/campaign/statins-open-data.
52 Catherine Buettner et al., "Prevalence of Musculoskeletal Pain and Statin Use," *Journal of General Internal Medicine* 23, no. 8 (May 1, 2008): 1182–6, https://doi.org/10.1007/s11606-008-0636-7.
53 Ward, Watts, and Eckel, "Statin Toxicity."
54 Cholesterol Treatment Trialists' (CTT) Collaborators, "The Effects of Lowering LDL Cholesterol with Statin Therapy in People at Low Risk of Vascular Disease"; Jane Armitage, "The Safety of Statins in Clinical Practice," *The Lancet* 370, no. 9601 (June 7, 2007): 1781–90, https://doi.org/10.1016/S0140-6736(07)60716-8.
55 Paul D. Thompson, "What to Believe and Do about Statin-Associated Adverse Effects," *JAMA* 316, no. 19 (November 15, 2016): 1969–70, https://doi.org/10.1001/jama.2016.16557.
56 Shuo-yu Lin et al., "Trends in Use and Expenditures for Brand-Name Statins after Introduction of Generic Statins in the US, 2002-2018," *JAMA Network Open* 4, no. 11 (November 22, 2021): e2135371, https://doi.org/10.1001/jamanetworkopen.2021.35371.
57 "Statins," GoodRx, accessed June 16, 2025, https://www.goodrx.com/classes/statins.
58 Patrick J. Skerrett, "Consumers Could Save as Generic Lipitor Hits the Market," Harvard Health Publishing, December 1, 2011, https://www.health.harvard.edu/blog/consumers-could-save-as-generic-lipitor-hits-the-market-201112013884.
59 CDC, "Half of Those Who Need Them Not Taking Cholesterol-Lowering Medications," CDC Archive, April 15, 2024, https://archive.cdc.gov/#/details?url=https://www.cdc.gov/media/releases/2015/p1203-cholesterol-medicine.html.
60 Amro Matyori et al., "Statins Utilization Trends and Expenditures in the U.S. before and after the Implementation of the 2013 ACC/AHA Guidelines," *Saudi Pharmaceutical Journal* 31, no. 6 (June 2023): 795–800, https://doi.org/10.1016/j.jsps.2023.04.002.
61 Casey J. Kim et al., "Trends in Primary Prevention Statin Use by Cardiovascular Risk Score from 1999 to 2018: A Repeated Cross-Sectional Study," *Annals of Internal Medicine* 176, no. 12 (December 5, 2023): 1684–8, https://doi.org/10.7326/M23-1915.
62 Michael J. Pencina et al., "Application of New Cholesterol Guidelines to a Population-Based Sample," *New England Journal of Medicine* 370, no. 15 (April 10, 2014): 1422–31, https://doi.org/10.1056/NEJMoa1315665.
63 Scott M. Grundy et al., "2018 AHA/ACC/AACVPR/AAPA/ABC/ACPM/ADA/AGS/APhA/ASPC/NLA/PCNA Guideline on the Management of Blood Cholesterol: A Report of the American College of Cardiology/American Heart Association Task Force on Clinical Practice Guidelines," *Circulation* 139, no. 25 (November 10, 2018): e1082–143, https://doi.org/10.1161/CIR.0000000000000625; Donna K. Arnett et al., "2019 ACC/AHA Guideline on the Primary Prevention of Cardiovascular Disease: A Report of the American College of Cardiology/American Heart Association Task Force on Clinical Practice Guidelines," *Circulation* 140, no. 11 (March 17, 2019): e596–646, https://doi.org/10.1161/CIR.0000000000000678.
64 USPSTF, "Statin Use for the Primary Prevention of Cardiovascular Disease in Adults: Preventive Medication," US Preventative Servies Task Force, August 23, 2023,

https://www.uspreventiveservicestaskforce.org/uspstf/recommendation/statin-use-in-adults-preventive-medication#fullrecommendationstart.
65 Habib, Katz, and Redberg, "Statins for Primary Cardiovascular Disease Prevention."
66 Lin et al., "Trends in Use and Expenditures for Brand-Name Statins after Introduction of Generic Statins in the US, 2002–2018."
67 Habib, Katz, and Redberg, "Statins for Primary Cardiovascular Disease Prevention."
68 Niteesh K. Choudhry, "Relationships between Authors of Clinical Practice Guidelines and the Pharmaceutical Industry," *JAMA* 287, no. 5 (February 6, 2002): 612–17, https://doi.org/10.1001/jama.287.5.612.
69 "Cholesterol Guidelines Become Morality Play about Conflict of Interest," *The Journal Record*, October 20, 2004, https://journalrecord.com/2004/10/cholesterol-guidelines-become-morality-play-about-conflict-of-interest/.
70 Jerome P. Kassirer, "Conflicted Studies Hard to Swallow," *Tampa Bay Times*, August 6, 2004, https://www.tampabay.com/archive/2004/08/06/conflicted-studies-hard-to-sw.
71 "Cholesterol Guidelines Become Morality Play about Conflict of Interest."
72 John Abramson and Barbara Starfield, "The Effect of Conflict of Interest on Biomedical Research and Clinical Practice Guidelines: Can We Trust the Evidence in Evidence-Based Medicine?," *The Journal of the American Board of Family Medicine* 18, no. 5 (September 1, 2005): 414–18, https://doi.org/10.3122/jabfm.18.5.414; David Willman, "The National Institutes of Health: Public Servant or Private Marketer?," *Los Angeles Times*, December 22, 2004, https://www.latimes.com/news/la-na-nih22dec22-story.html.
73 Prasad and Cifu, *Ending Medical Reversal*, 141.
74 R. Phillip Dellinger et al., "Surviving Sepsis Campaign Guidelines for Management of Severe Sepsis and Septic Shock," *Critical Care Medicine* 32, no. 3 (2004): 858–73, https://doi.org/10.1097/01.CCM.0000117317.18092.E4.
75 Josh Farkas, "Petition to Retire the Surviving Sepsis Campaign Guidelines," PulmCrit (EMCrit), May 2, 2018, https://emcrit.org/pulmcrit/ssc-petition/.
76 "Lilly Announces Withdrawal of Xigris® Following Recent Clinical Trial Results," Lilly, October 24, 2011, https://investor.lilly.com/news-releases/news-release-details/lilly-announces-withdrawal-xigrisr-following-recent-clinical.
77 Lo et al., *Conflict of Interest in Medical Research, Education, and Practice.*
78 Ibid., 2.
79 Ibid., 189.
80 Ibid., 211.
81 Ibid.
82 Committee on Standards for Developing Trustworthy Clinical Practice Guidelines, Board on Health Care Services, and Institute of Medicine, *Clinical Practice Guidelines We Can Trust*, 81.
83 Daylian M. Cain, George Loewenstein, and Don A. Moore, "When Sunlight Fails to Disinfect: Understanding the Perverse Effects of Disclosing Conflicts of Interest," *Journal of Consumer Research* 37, no. 5 (February 1, 2011), 850, https://doi.org/10.1086/656252.
84 Committee on Standards for Developing Trustworthy Clinical Practice Guidelines, Board on Health Care Services, and Institute of Medicine, *Clinical Practice Guidelines We Can Trust*, 83.
85 Kung, Miller, and Mackowiak, "Failure of Clinical Practice Guidelines to Meet Institute of Medicine Standards."

86 Caitlin E. Cox, "Conflicts of Interest in the 2013 Cholesterol Guidelines? New Analysis Revisits the Controversy," tctMD, January 17, 2017, https://www.tctmd.com/news/conflicts-interest-2013-cholesterol-guidelines-new-analysis-revisits-controversy.
87 Unite Here!, "American Heart Association Fails to Disclose $100K in Pharma-Funded Research Led by Vice Chair of Cholesterol Guideline," accessed June 13, 2024, https://unitehere.org/wp-content/uploads/AHA-Vice-Chair-Payments.pdf; Abramson, *Sickening*, 48.
88 Cox, "Conflicts of Interest in the 2013 Cholesterol Guidelines?"
89 Paul Campsall et al., "Financial Relationships between Organizations That Produce Clinical Practice Guidelines and the Biomedical Industry: A Cross-Sectional Study," ed. Hilda Bastian, *PLoS Med* 13, no. 5 (May 31, 2016): e1002029, https://doi.org/10.1371/journal.pmed.1002029.
90 Sahar Tabatabavakili et al., "Financial Conflicts of Interest in Clinical Practice Guidelines: A Systematic Review," *Mayo Clinic Proceedings: Innovations, Quality & Outcomes* 5, no. 2 (January 19, 2021): 466–75, https://doi.org/10.1016/j.mayocpiqo.2020.09.016.
91 "Patient Protection and Affordable Care Act," Pub. L. No. 111–48 (2016), https://www.congress.gov/bill/111th-congress/house-bill/359.
92 Suzanne Murrin, "Open Payments Data: Review of Accuracy, Precision, and Consistency in Reporting," US Department of Health and Human Services Office of Inspector General, August 2018, https://oig.hhs.gov/oei/reports/oei-03-15-00220.pdf.
93 Maryam Mooghali et al., "Financial Conflicts of Interest among US Physician Authors of 2020 Clinical Practice Guidelines: A Cross-Sectional Study," *BMJ Open* 13, no. 1 (January 23, 2023): e069115, https://doi.org/10.1136/bmjopen-2022-069115.
94 "Societies," CMSS, accessed June 13, 2024, https://cmss.org/membership/societies/.
95 Aileen S. Ahiskali, Dimitri M. Drekonja, and Jonathan D. Alpern, "Conflicts of Interest among Infectious Diseases Clinical Practice Guideline Authors and the Pharmaceutical Industry," *JAMA Network Open* 6, no. 4 (April 17, 2023): e238592, https://doi.org/10.1001/jamanetworkopen.2023.8592.
96 Alex Montero et al., "KFF Health Tracking Poll May 2024: The Public's Use and Views of GLP-1 Drugs," KFF, May 10, 2024, https://www.kff.org/health-costs/poll-finding/kff-health-tracking-poll-may-2024-the-publics-use-and-views-of-glp-1-drugs/; "GLP-1 Agonists," Cleveland Clinic, July 3, 2023, https://my.clevelandclinic.org/health/treatments/13901-glp-1-agonists.
97 FDA, "Update on FDA's Ongoing Evaluation of Reports of Suicidal Thoughts or Actions in Patients Taking a Certain Type of Medicines Approved for Type 2 Diabetes and Obesity," US Food & Drug Administration, January 30, 2024, https://www.fda.gov/drugs/drug-safety-and-availability/update-fdas-ongoing-evaluation-reports-suicidal-thoughts-or-actions-patients-taking-certain-type; "Amylin and Lilly Announce FDA Approval of BYETTA(TM) (Exenatide) Injection," Lilly, April 29, 2005, https://investor.lilly.com/news-releases/news-release-details/amylin-and-lilly-announce-fda-approval-byettatm-exenatide.
98 Sanjula Jain, "2023 Trends Shaping the Health Economy: Value for Money," Trilliant Health, 2023, https://www.trillianthealth.com/hubfs/TH_Annual%20Report_2

023.10.25%20(2).pdf?hsCtaTracking=e0a5d398-f873-4e1f-b574-54c459b40597%7C64ca9886-cf47-4a6f-9a43-814418eb9864.

99 John W. Ostrominski et al., "Trends in Utilization of Glucose- and Weight-Lowering Medications after Tirzepatide Approval in the United States: A Population-Based Cohort Study," *Annals of Internal Medicine* 178, no. 5 (April 15, 2025): 620–33, https://doi.org/10.7326/ANNALS-24-02870.

100 "Drug Label: Tamiflu (Oseltamivir Phosphate) Capsules and Oral Suspension," US Food & Drug Administration, December 2017, https://www.accessdata.fda.gov/drugsatfda_docs/label/2011/021087s056_021246s039lbl.pdf.

101 Christopher Sorli et al., "Efficacy and Safety of Once-Weekly Semaglutide Monotherapy versus Placebo in Patients with Type 2 Diabetes (SUSTAIN 1): A Double-Blind, Randomised, Placebo-Controlled, Parallel-Group, Multinational, Multicentre Phase 3a Trial," *The Lancet Diabetes & Endocrinology* 5, no. 4 (2017): 251–60, https://doi.org/10.1016/S2213-8587(17)30013-X.

102 Peter Wehrwein, "For Weight Loss, Off-Label GLP-1s Are Increasingly the Chosen Ones | AMCP 2023," Managed Healthcare Executive, March 23, 2024, https://www.managedhealthcareexecutive.com/view/for-weight-loss-the-glp-1s-are-the-ones-amcp-2023.

103 Berkeley Lovelace Jr., Lauren Dunn, and Kristen Dahlgren, "People with Diabetes Struggle to Find Ozempic as It Soars in Popularity as a Weight Loss Aid," NBC News, January 12, 2023, https://www.nbcnews.com/health/health-news/people-diabetes-struggle-find-ozempic-soars-popularity-weight-loss-aid-rcna64916; Lisa Rozner, "Diabetes Patients Frustrated as Popularity of Ozempic and Trulicity Limits Supply," CBS News, January 23, 2024, https://www.cbsnews.com/newyork/news/diabetes-patients-frustrated-as-popularity-of-ozempic-and-trulicity-limits-supply/; Monique Ming Laven, "Crippling Consequences over Shortage of Diabetes Drug Used for Weight Loss," KIRO 7, February 15, 2024, https://www.kiro7.com/news/local/crippling-consequences-over-shortage-diabetes-drug-used-weight-loss/HT4QSMPQVBDBZJENQPQRC6CTNI/.

104 FDA, "Update on FDA's Ongoing Evaluation of Reports of Suicidal Thoughts or Actions in Patients Taking a Certain Type of Medicines Approved for Type 2 Diabetes and Obesity."

105 Dani Blum, "The Wegovy Shortage Drags on, Leaving Patients in Limbo," *The New York Times*, October 5, 2023, https://www.nytimes.com/2023/10/05/well/live/wegovy-shortage-ozempic-fda.html.

106 Eduardo Grunvald et al., "AGA Clinical Practice Guideline on Pharmacological Interventions for Adults with Obesity," *Gastroenterology* 163, no. 5 (2022): 1198–225, https://doi.org/10.1053/j.gastro.2022.08.045.

107 Sarah E. Hampl et al., "Clinical Practice Guideline for the Evaluation and Treatment of Children and Adolescents with Obesity," *Pediatrics* 151, no. 2 (January 9, 2023): e2022060640, https://doi.org/10.1542/peds.2022-060640.

108 Olivia Gilbert et al., "2025 Concise Clinical Guidance: An ACC Expert Consensus Statement on Medical Weight Management for Optimization of Cardiovascular Health," *Journal of the American College of Cardiology*, June 20, 2025, https://doi.org/10.1016/j.jacc.2025.05.024.

109 USPSTF, "High Body Mass Index in Children and Adolescents: Interventions," US Preventative Services Task Force, June 18, 2024, https://www.uspreventiveservicesta

skforce.org/uspstf/document/RecommendationStatementFinal/obesity-in-children-and-adolescents-screening.

110 USPSTF, "Weight Loss to Prevent Obesity-Related Morbidity and Mortality in Adults: Behavioral Interventions," US Preventative Services Task Force, September 18, 2018, https://www.uspreventiveservicestaskforce.org/uspstf/recommendation/obesity-in-adults-interventions.

111 Kaitlin Sullivan, "Weight Loss Drugs Can Lead to Muscle Loss, Too. Is That a Bad Thing?," NBC News, May 20, 2023, https://www.nbcnews.com/health/health-news/weight-loss-drugs-muscle-loss-rcna84936.

112 John P. H. Wilding et al., "Once-Weekly Semaglutide in Adults with Overweight or Obesity," *New England Journal of Medicine* 384, no. 11 (February 10, 2021): Supplementary Appendix, https://doi.org/10.1056/NEJMoa2032183.

113 George Moschonis and Gina Louise Trakman, "Overweight and Obesity: The Interplay of Eating Habits and Physical Activity," *Nutrients* 15, no. 13 (June 27, 2023): 2896, https://doi.org/10.3390/nu15132896.

114 Christiaan G. Abildso et al., "Prevalence of Meeting Aerobic, Muscle-Strengthening, and Combined Physical Activity Guidelines During Leisure Time among Adults, by Rural-Urban Classification and Region—United States, 2020," *MMWR Morbidity and Mortality Weekly Report* 72, no. 4 (January 27, 2023): 85–9, https://doi.org/10.15585/mmwr.mm7204a1.

115 Seung Hee Lee et al., "Adults Meeting Fruit and Vegetable Intake Recommendations—United States, 2019," *MMWR Morbidity and Mortality Weekly Report* 71, no. 1 (January 7, 2022): 1–9, https://doi.org/10.15585/mmwr.mm7101a1.

116 Adam Collins and The Conversation US, "Why You Don't Just Lose Fat When You're on a Diet," *Scientific American*, July 13, 2023, https://www.scientificamerican.com/article/weight-loss-why-you-dont-just-lose-fat-when-youre-on-a-diet/; Gary R. Hunter et al., "Resistance Training Conserves Fat-free Mass and Resting Energy Expenditure Following Weight Loss," *Obesity* 16, no. 5 (2008): 1045–51, https://doi.org/10.1038/oby.2008.38; Edda Cava, Nai Chien Yeat, and Bettina Mittendorfer, "Preserving Healthy Muscle during Weight Loss," *Advances in Nutrition* 8, no. 3 (2017): 511–19, https://doi.org/10.3945/an.116.014506; Moschonis and Trakman, "Overweight and Obesity."

117 The Associated Press, "Weight-Loss Drugs like Wegovy Are Meant for Long-Term Use. What Happens If You Stop?," NBC News, March 7, 2024, https://www.nbcnews.com/health/health-news/weight-loss-drugs-wegovy-are-meant-long-term-use-happens-stop-rcna142291.

118 Tina Reed, "The Big Question about Obesity Drugs: Can People Ever Stop Taking Them?," Axios, November 27, 2023, https://www.axios.com/2023/11/27/obesity-weight-loss-drugs-lifetime-ozempic-wegovy.

119 John P. H. Wilding et al., "Weight Regain and Cardiometabolic Effects after Withdrawal of Semaglutide: The STEP 1 Trial Extension," *Diabetes, Obesity and Metabolism* 24, no. 8 (April 19, 2022): 1553–64, https://doi.org/10.1111/dom.14725.

120 Jack Alistair Sargeant et al., "A Review of the Effects of Glucagon-Like Peptide-1 Receptor Agonists and Sodium-Glucose Cotransporter 2 Inhibitors on Lean Body Mass in Humans," *Endocrinology and Metabolism* 34, no. 3 (September 26, 2019): 247–62, https://doi.org/10.3803/EnM.2019.34.3.247; Satoshi Ida et al., "Effects of Antidiabetic Drugs on Muscle Mass in Type 2 Diabetes Mellitus," *Current Diabetes*

*Reviews* 17, no. 3 (July 5, 2020): 293–303, https://doi.org/10.2174/1573399816666200705210006.

121 "Age and Muscle Loss," Harvard Health Publishing, February 14, 2023, https://www.health.harvard.edu/exercise-and-fitness/age-and-muscle-loss.

122 Sara Y. Oikawa, Tanya M. Holloway, and Stuart M. Phillips, "The Impact of Step Reduction on Muscle Health in Aging: Protein and Exercise as Countermeasures," *Frontiers in Nutrition* 6 (May 24, 2019): Article 75, https://doi.org/10.3389/fnut.2019.00075.

123 Dani Blum, "The Race Is on to Stop Ozempic Muscle Loss," *The New York Times*, February 8, 2024, https://www.nytimes.com/2024/02/08/well/live/ozempic-muscle-loss-exercise.html.

124 Marc-André Cornier, "A Review of Current Guidelines for the Treatment of Obesity," *The American Journal of Managed Care* 28, no. suppl. 15 (December 14, 2022): S288–96, https://doi.org/10.37765/ajmc.2022.89292.

125 Montero et al., "KFF Health Tracking Poll May 2024."

126 Shawn Radcliffe, "How Common Are GLP-1 Drugs Like Ozempic? 13% of U.S. Adults Have Used Them," Healthline, May 13, 2024, https://www.healthline.com/health-news/how-common-are-glp-1-drugs-like-ozempic-13-of-u-s-adults-have-used-them; "Executive Clinical Leadership," Options Medical Weight Loss, accessed July 5, 2024, https://optionsmedicalweightloss.com/our-people/.

127 Amjad Kanj and Diane Levine, "Overcoming Obesity: Weight-Loss Drugs Are Underused," *Cleveland Clinic Journal of Medicine* 87, no. 10 (2020): 602–4, https://doi.org/10.3949/ccjm.87a.19102.

128 CDC, "About the Division of Nutrition, Physical Activity, and Obesity," National Center for Chronic Disease Prevention and Health Promotion (NCCDPHP), May 15, 2024, https://www.cdc.gov/nccdphp/divisions-offices/about-the-division-of-nutrition-physical-activity-and-obesity.html#:~:text=Poor%20nutrition%20and%20inadequate%20physical,%2C%20certain%20cancers%2C%20and%20depression; "Causes: Obesity," NHS, February 15, 2023, https://www.nhs.uk/conditions/obesity/causes/#:~:text=Obesity%20is%20a%20complex%20issue,in%20the%20body%20as%20fat.

129 "Ozempic," GoodRx, accessed July 13, 2025, https://www.goodrx.com/ozempic; "Wegovy," GoodRx, accessed July 13, 2025, https://www.goodrx.com/wegovy.

130 Samuel D. Emmerich et al., "Obesity and Severe Obesity Prevalence in Adults: United States, August 2021–August 2023," National Center for Health Statistics, September 2024, https://static.foxnews.com/foxnews.com/content/uploads/2024/09/db508.pdf; Forrest et al., "Trends in US Children's Mortality, Chronic Conditions, Obesity, Functional Status, and Symptoms"; Cheryl D. Fryar et al., "Prevalence of Overweight, Obesity, and Severe Obesity among Adults Aged 20 and Over: United States, 1960–1962 through 2017–2018," National Center for Health Statistics, January 29, 2021, https://www.cdc.gov/nchs/data/hestat/obesity-adult-17-18/overweight-obesity-adults-H.pdf.

131 Thomas S. Roukis, "White Papers, Position Papers, Clinical Consensus Statements, and Clinical Practice Guidelines: Future Directions for ACFAS," *The Journal of Foot and Ankle Surgery* 54, no. 2 (January 21, 2015): 151–2, https://doi.org/10.1053/j.jfas.2015.01.003; Carmel Jacobs et al., "Clinical Practice Guidelines and Consensus Statements in Oncology—An Assessment of Their Methodological Quality,"

ed. Eugenio Paci, *PLoS ONE* 9, no. 10 (October 17, 2014): e110469, https://doi.org/10.1371/journal.pone.0110469.

132 Richard M. Rosenfeld, Lorraine C. Nnacheta, and Maureen D. Corrigan, "Clinical Consensus Statement Development Manual," *Otolaryngology—Head and Neck Surgery* 153, no. S2 (November 2, 2015): S1–14, https://doi.org/10.1177/0194599815601394.

133 "Creating Sound Clinical Consensus Statements," American Medical Writers Association, May 20, 2024, https://blog.amwa.org/creating-sound-clinical-consensus-statements.

134 Kasper P. Kepp et al., "Panel Stacking Is a Threat to Consensus Statement Validity," *Journal of Clinical Epidemiology* 173 (June 17, 2024): 111428, https://doi.org/10.1016/j.jclinepi.2024.111428.

135 Guideline Production Group of the European Academy of Neurology et al., "Guidelines Should Be Guidelines: Time to Leave the Terms 'Consensus' and 'Position' for Other Purposes," *European Journal of Neurology* 28, no. 8 (May 22, 2021): 2461–6, https://doi.org/10.1111/ene.14933.

136 Roukis, "White Papers, Position Papers, Clinical Consensus Statements, and Clinical Practice Guidelines."

137 Jacobs et al., "Clinical Practice Guidelines and Consensus Statements in Oncology—An Assessment of Their Methodological Quality."

138 Liang Yao et al., "Discordant and Inappropriate Discordant Recommendations in Consensus and Evidence Based Guidelines: Empirical Analysis," *BMJ* 375, no. 8316 (November 25, 2021): e066045, https://doi.org/10.1136/bmj-2021-066045.

139 Jacobs et al., "Clinical Practice Guidelines and Consensus Statements in Oncology—an Assessment of Their Methodological Quality."

140 "2023 AACE Consensus Statement: Comprehensive Type 2 Diabetes Management Algorithm," AACE, accessed June 22, 2024, https://pro.aace.com/clinical-guidance/2023-aace-consensus-statement-comprehensive-type-2-diabetes-management-algorithm.

141 "About AACE: Corporate AACE Partnership (CAP)," AACE, accessed July 13, 2024, https://pro.aace.com/about/corporate-aace-partnership-cap.

142 Susan L. Samson et al., "American Association of Clinical Endocrinology Consensus Statement: Comprehensive Type 2 Diabetes Management Algorithm—2023 Update," *Endocrine Practice* 29, no. 5 (2023): 305–40, https://doi.org/10.1016/j.eprac.2023.02.001.

143 "Weight Loss," Medizen Institute, accessed June 22, 2024, https://medizeninstitute.com/weight-loss/.

144 Alan J. Garber et al., "Consensus Statement by the American Association of Clinical Endocrinologists and American College of Endocrinology on the Comprehensive Type 2 Diabetes Management Algorithm—2018 Executive Summary," *Endocrine Practice* 24, no. 1 (2018): 91–121, https://doi.org/10.4158/CS-2017-0153.

145 Abramson, *Sickening*, chap. 4.

146 Andrea Siebenhofer et al., "Short Acting Insulin Analogues versus Regular Human Insulin in Patients with Diabetes Mellitus," *Cochrane Database of Systematic Reviews* 2006, no. 2 (April 19, 2006): Article CD003287, https://doi.org/10.1002/14651858.CD003287.pub4; Karl Horvath et al., "Long-Acting Insulin Analogues versus NPH Insulin (Human Isophane Insulin) for Type 2 Diabetes Mellitus," ed. Cochrane Metabolic and Endocrine Disorders Group, *Cochrane Database of Systematic Reviews*

2007, no. 2 (April 18, 2007): Article CD005613, https://doi.org/10.1002/14651858.CD005613.pub3; Moshe Vardi et al., "Intermediate Acting versus Long Acting Insulin for Type 1 Diabetes Mellitus," *Cochrane Database of Systematic Reviews* 2008, no. 3 (July 16, 2008): Article CD006297, https://doi.org/10.1002/14651858.CD006297.pub2.

147 Abramson, *Sickening*, Chapter 4.

148 Ibid., 65.

149 Kasia J. Lipska et al., "Use and Out-of-Pocket Costs of Insulin for Type 2 Diabetes Mellitus from 2000 Through 2010," *JAMA* 311, no. 22 (June 11, 2014): 2331–3, https://doi.org/10.1001/jama.2014.6316.

150 Alan J. Garber et al., "Consensus Statement by the American Association of Clinical Endocrinologists and American College of Endocrinology on the Comprehensive Type 2 Diabetes Management Algorithm—2016 EXECUTIVE SUMMARY," *Endocrine Practice* 22, no. 1 (2016): 84–113, https://doi.org/10.4158/EP151126.CS.

151 Garber et al., "Consensus Statement by the American Association of Clinical Endocrinologists and American College of Endocrinology on the Comprehensive Type 2 Diabetes Management Algorithm—2018 Executive Summary," 99.

152 Samson et al., "American Association of Clinical Endocrinology Consensus Statement."

153 Kepp et al., "Panel Stacking Is a Threat to Consensus Statement Validity."

154 Jeffrey V. Lazarus et al., "A Multinational Delphi Consensus to End the COVID-19 Public Health Threat," *Nature* 611, no. 7935 (November 3, 2022): 332–45, https://doi.org/10.1038/s41586-022-05398-2.

155 Jennifer Rigby, Josephine Mason, and Jennifer Rigby, "WHO Chief Says China's Zero-COVID Policy Not 'Sustainable,'" *Reuters*, May 10, 2022, sec. China, https://www.reuters.com/world/china/who-chief-says-chinas-zero-covid-policy-not-sustainable-2022-05-10/.

156 Yao et al., "Discordant and Inappropriate Discordant Recommendations in Consensus and Evidence Based Guidelines."

157 Liang Yao, Gordon H Guyatt, and Benjamin Djulbegovic, "Can We Trust Strong Recommendations Based on Low Quality Evidence?," *BMJ* 375, no. 8316 (November 25, 2021): n2833, https://doi.org/10.1136/bmj.n2833.

## 5 Faster Approvals and Weaker Evidence

1 Sydney Lupkin, "FDA Approves Drugs Faster than Ever but Relies on Weaker Evidence, Researchers Find," *NPR*, January 14, 2020, sec. Health Inc., https://www.npr.org/sections/health-shots/2020/01/14/796227083/fda-approves-drugs-faster-than-ever-but-relies-on-weaker-evidence-researchers-fi.

2 Jonathan J. Darrow, Jerry Avorn, and Aaron S. Kesselheim, "FDA Approval and Regulation of Pharmaceuticals, 1983–2018," *JAMA* 323, no. 2 (January 14, 2020): 164–76, https://doi.org/10.1001/jama.2019.20288.

3 FDA, "FDA at a Glance October 2024," US Food & Drug Administration, October 2024, https://www.fda.gov/media/182749/download.

4 To Amend the Federal Food, Drug, and Cosmetic Act to Authorize Human Drug Application, Prescription Drug Establishment, and Prescription Drug Product Fees and for Other Purposes," Pub. L. No. 102–571 (1992), https://www.congress.gov/bill/102nd-congress/house-bill/6181/text?q=%7B%22search%22%3A%5B%22prescription+drug+user+fee+act%22%5D%7D&r=2&s=7; Susan Thaul, "The Prescription Drug User Fee Act: History through the 2007 PDUFA IV Reauthorization," Congressional Research Service, June 27, 2008, https://www.congress.gov/crs_external_products/RL/PDF/RL33914/RL33914.10.pdf.

5 Judith A. Johnson et al., "The Food and Drug Administration: Budget and Statutory History, FY1980–FY2007," Congressional Research Service, January 29, 2008, https://crsreports.congress.gov/product/pdf/RL/RL34334/11.

6 Ibid.

7 Thaul, "The Prescription Drug User Fee Act: History through the 2007 PDUFA IV Reauthorization."

8 Janet Woodcock and Suzanne Junod, "PDUFA Lays the Foundation: Launching into the Era of User Fee Acts," Food & Drug Administration, accessed June 21, 2025, https://www.fda.gov/files/about%20fda/published/PDUFA-Lays-the-Foundation--Launching-Into-the-Era-of-User-Fee-Acts.pdf.

9 Joanne S. Eglovitch, "Industry Experts Peel Back the Curtain on User Fee Negotiations," Regulatory Focus, June 7, 2024, https://www.raps.org/News-and-Articles/News-Articles/2024/6/Industry-experts-peel-back-the-curtain-on-user-fee.

10 Donna U. Vogt and Blanchard I. Randall IV, "The Prescription Drug User Fee Act: Structure and Reauthorization Issues," Congressional Research Service, October 7, 2002, https://crsreports.congress.gov/product/pdf/RL/RL31453/3.

11 John Schwartz, "FDA Graded Highly on Relative Speed of Review Process," *The Washington Post*, November 7, 1995, https://www.washingtonpost.com/archive/politics/1995/11/08/fda-graded-highly-on-relative-speed-of-review-process/1eeb463d-5cc6-4106-be45-9592025fd637/.

12 Prescription Drug User Fee Act of 1992, Pub. L. Nos. 102–571 (1992), https://www.congress.gov/102/statute/STATUTE-106/STATUTE-106-Pg4491.pdf; Susan Thaul, "The Prescription Drug User Fee Act (PDUFA): Background and Issues for PDUFA IV Reauthorization" (Congressional Research Service, March 13, 2007), https://www.everycrsreport.com/files/20070313_RL33914_f473f0cb5dec3ba97a38b3ed46b6590c6e0b7dac.pdf.

13 Thaul, "The Prescription Drug User Fee Act: History through the 2007 PDUFA IV Reauthorization."

14 Ibid.; FDA, "Drugs@FDA Glossary of Terms," US Food & Drug Administration, November 14, 2017, https://www.fda.gov/drugs/drug-approvals-and-databases/drugsfda-glossary-terms.

15 Food and Drug Administration, "21 CFR Part 314 Subpart H—Accelerated Approval of New Drugs for Serious or Life-Threatening Illnesses," Code of Federal Regulations, June 7, 2024, https://www.ecfr.gov/current/title-21/part-314/subpart-H.

16 FDA, "Accelerated Approval Program," US Food & Drug Administration, December 24, 2024, https://web.archive.org/web/20250709030313/https://www.fda.gov/drugs/nda-and-bla-approvals/accelerated-approval-program.

17 Vogt and Randall IV, "The Prescription Drug User Fee Act: Structure and Reauthorization Issues."

18 Food and Drug Administration Modernization Act of 1997.
19 Erin H. Ward, "COVID-19: Legal Considerations for Bringing a New Vaccine to Market," Congressional Research Service, March 24, 2020, https://crsreports.congress.gov/product/pdf/LSB/LSB10427.
20 Food and Drug Administration Modernization Act of 1997.
21 Michael Malinowski and Grant Gautreaux, "Drug Development—Stuck in a State of Puberty?: Regulatory Reform of Human Clinical Research to Raise Responsiveness to the Reality of Human Variability," *Saint Louis University Law Journal* 56, no. 2 (2012): 399, https://scholarship.law.slu.edu/lj/vol56/iss2/3.
22 James L. Zelenay, "The Prescription Drug User Fee Act: Is a Faster Food and Drug Administration Always a Better Food and Drug Administration?," *Food and Drug Law Journal* 60, no. 2 (2005): 261–338, https://www.jstor.org/stable/26660831.
23 Food and Drug Administration Modernization Act of 1997.
24 Ibid.
25 "Public Health Security and Bioterrorism Preparedness and Response Act of 2002," Pub. L. No. 107–88 (2002), https://www.congress.gov/bill/107th-congress/house-bill/3448?q=%7B%22search%22%3A%5B%22cite%3APL 107-188%22%5D%7D&s=3&r=1.
26 Ibid.
27 Lisa A. Bero and Lisa Parker, "Risky Business? Pharmaceutical Industry Sponsorship of Health Consumer Groups," *Australian Prescriber* 44, no. 3 (June 1, 2021): 74–6, https://doi.org/10.18773/austprescr.2021.017; Rachana Pradhan, "Millions of Dollars Flow from Pharma to Patient Advocacy Groups," *KFF Health News* (blog), December 15, 2023, https://kffhealthnews.org/news/article/health-202-pharma-money-patient-advocacy-groups-public-citizen/.
28 Mike Tanglis, "Mapping the PhRMA Grant Universe," Public Citizen, December 14, 2023, https://www.citizen.org/article/mapping-the-phrma-grant-universe/.
29 Susannah L. Rose et al., "Patient Advocacy Organizations, Industry Funding, and Conflicts of Interest," *JAMA Internal Medicine* 177, no. 3 (March 2017): 344–50, https://doi.org/10.1001/jamainternmed.2016.8443.
30 Food and Drug Administration Amendments Act of 2007.
31 Susan Thaul, "Drug Safety: A Side-by-Side Comparison of Bills in the 110th Congress," Congressional Research Service, March 13, 2007, https://file.wikileaks.org/file/crs/RL33925.pdf.
32 Alicia Baciu et al., *The Future of Drug Safety: Promoting and Protecting the Health of the Public* (Washington, DC: National Academies Press, 2007), 4, https://doi.org/10.17226/11750.
33 FDA, "Risk Evaluation and Mitigation Strategies | REMS," US Food & Drug Administration, May 16, 2023, https://www.fda.gov/drugs/drug-safety-and-availability/risk-evaluation-and-mitigation-strategies-rems; Office of Inspector General, "FDA's Risk Evaluation and Mitigation Strategies: Uncertain Effectiveness in Addressing the Opioid Crisis," U.S. Department of Health and Human Services, September 2020, https://oig.hhs.gov/oei/reports/OEI-01-17-00510.pdf.
34 Food and Drug Administration Amendments Act of 2007.
35 "Food and Drug Administration Safety and Innovation Act," Pub. L. No. 112–44 (2012), https://www.congress.gov/bill/112th-congress/senate-bill/3187?q=%7B%22search%22%3A%5B%22Public+Law+112-144%22%5D%7D&resultIndex=1.
36 Ibid.

37 Ibid.
38 Ibid.
39 FDA, "Breakthrough Therapy," US Food & Drug Administration, January 4, 2018, https://www.fda.gov/patients/fast-track-breakthrough-therapy-accelerated-approval-priority-review/breakthrough-therapy.
40 Hassan Z. Sheikh, "How FDA Approves Drugs and Regulates Their Safety and Effectiveness," Congressional Research Service, May 8, 2018, https://crsreports.congress.gov/product/pdf/R/R41983.
41 "An Act to Amend the Federal Food, Drug, and Cosmetic Act to Revise and Extend the User-Fee Programs for Prescription Drugs, Medical Devices, Generic Drugs, and Biosimilar Biological Products, and for Other Purposes," Pub. L. No. 115–52 (2017), https://www.congress.gov/bill/115th-congress/house-bill/2430/text.
42 Ibid.
43 Center for Drug Evaluation and Research, "Competitive Generic Therapies Guidance for Industry," Food and Drug Administration, October 2022, https://www.fda.gov/media/136063/download.
44 "21st Century Cures Act," Pub. L. No. 114–255 (2016), https://www.congress.gov/bill/114th-congress/house-bill/34.
45 Ibid.
46 Ibid.
47 Ibid.
48 Ibid.
49 Ibid.
50 "An Act to Authorize the Use of Unapproved Medical Products by Patients Diagnosed with a Terminal Illness in Accordance with State Law, and for Other Purposes," Pub. L. No. 115–76 (2018), https://www.congress.gov/bill/115th-congress/senate-bill/204.
51 A legally authorized representative of a patient can also provide such written consent.
52 FDA, "FDA Fact Sheet: Right to Try," accessed June 21, 2025, https://www.fda.gov/media/133864/download.
53 FDA, "Expanded Access," US Food & Drug Administration, February 28, 2024, https://www.fda.gov/news-events/public-health-focus/expanded-access.
54 American Cancer Society Cancer Action Network et al., "Right to Try Coalition Letter," February 6, 2018, https://www.facingourrisk.org/uploads/advocacy/Right%20to%20Try%20Coalition%20Letter_Feb2018.pdf; Scot Walker, "Expanded Access versus Right-to-Try," *Hospital Pharmacy* 55, no. 2 (October 25, 2019): 79–81, https://doi.org/10.1177/0018578719883801.
55 "Continuing Appropriations and Ukraine Supplemental Appropriations Act, 2023," Pub. L. No. 117–38 (2022), https://www.congress.gov/bill/117th-congress/house-bill/6833.
56 Gregory H. Levine et al., "Congress Enacts Clean Reauthorization of FDA User Fees, Leaving Uncertain Future for Important Policy Reforms," Ropes & Gray, September 30, 2022, https://www.ropesgray.com/en/insights/alerts/2022/09/congress-enacts-clean-reauthorization-of-fda-user-fees-leaving-uncertain-future.
57 Amanda K. Sarata, "The Food and Drug Administration (FDA) Budget: Fact Sheet," Congressional Research Service, December 9, 2022, https://crsreports.congress.gov/product/pdf/R/R44576.

58 FDA, "FDA at a Glance October 2024."

59 Woodcock and Junod, "PDUFA Lays the Foundation: Launching into the Era of User Fee Acts."

60 Enrique Seoane-Vazquez, Rosa Rodriguez-Monguio, and John H. Powers, "Analysis of US Food and Drug Administration New Drug and Biologic Approvals, Regulatory Pathways, and Review Times, 1980–2022," *Scientific Reports* 14 (February 9, 2024): Article 3325, https://doi.org/10.1038/s41598-024-53554-7.

61 Center for Drug Evaluation and Research, "Advancing Health through Innovation: New Drug Therapy Approvals 2024," US Food & Drug Administration, January 2025, https://www.fda.gov/media/184967/download?attachment.

62 Center for Drug Evaluation and Research, "Advancing Health through Innovation: New Drug Therapy Approvals," US Food & Drug Administration, 2018–2024; each report available at: 2023: https://www.fda.gov/media/175253/download?attachment; 2022: https://www.fda.gov/drugs/novel-drug-approvals-fda/new-drug-therapy-approvals-2022#innovation; 2021: https://www.fda.gov/media/155227/download?attachment; 2020: https://www.fda.gov/media/144982/download?attachment; 2019: https://www.fda.gov/media/134493/download?attachment; 2018: https://www.fda.gov/files/drugs/published/New-Drug-Therapy-Approvals-2018_3.pdf; 2017: https://www.fda.gov/files/about%20fda/published/2017-New-Drug-Therapy-Approvals-Report.pdf; Center for Drug Evaluation and Research, "Novel Drugs Summary," US Food & Drug Administration, 2016–17; each report available at: 2016: https://www.fda.gov/media/102618/download; 2015: https://web.archive.org/web/20240118205118/https://www.fda.gov/media/95661/download.

63 S. Murphy and R. Roberts, "'Black Box' 101: How the Food and Drug Administration Evaluates, Communicates, and Manages Drug Benefit/Risk," *Journal of Allergy and Clinical Immunology* 117, no. 1 (2006): 34–9, https://doi.org/10.1016/j.jaci.2005.10.031; "Black Box Warnings," Drugwatch, September 5, 2023, https://www.drugwatch.com/fda/black-box-warnings/.

64 Daniel Carpenter, Evan James Zucker, and Jerry Avorn, "Drug-Review Deadlines and Safety Problems," *New England Journal of Medicine* 358, no. 13 (March 27, 2008): 1354–61, https://doi.org/10.1056/NEJMsa0706341.

65 Downing et al., "Postmarket Safety Events among Novel Therapeutics Approved by the US Food and Drug Administration between 2001 and 2010."

66 Andreas Schick et al., "Evaluation of Pre-marketing Factors to Predict Post-marketing Boxed Warnings and Safety Withdrawals," *Drug Safety* 40, no. 6 (March 24, 2017): 497–503, https://doi.org/10.1007/s40264-017-0526-1.

67 Sana R. Mostaghim, Joshua J. Gagne, and Aaron S. Kesselheim, "Safety Related Label Changes for New Drugs after Approval in the US through Expedited Regulatory Pathways: Retrospective Cohort Study," *BMJ* 358, no. 8120 (September 7, 2017): j3837, https://doi.org/10.1136/bmj.j3837.

68 Cassie Frank et al., "Era of Faster FDA Drug Approval Has Also Seen Increased Black-Box Warnings and Market Withdrawals," *Health Affairs* 33, no. 8 (2014): 1453–9, https://doi.org/10.1377/hlthaff.2014.0122.

69 The Lever and McGraw Center for Business Journalism, "Do Your Drugs Work? A Searchable Database," The Lever, accessed June 13, 2025, https://www.levernews.com/do-your-drugs-work-a-searchable-database/.

70 "FDA Approved—And Ineffective: Database Explainer," The Lever, accessed June 19, 2025, https://www.levernews.com/fda-approved-and-ineffective-database-explainer/.
71 Zhang et al., "Assessment of Clinical Trials Supporting US Food and Drug Administration Approval of Novel Therapeutic Agents, 1995–2017."
72 Mayookha Mitra-Majumdar et al., "Analysis of Supportive Evidence for US Food and Drug Administration Approvals of Novel Drugs in 2020," *JAMA Network Open* 5, no. 5 (May 17, 2022): e2212454, https://doi.org/10.1001/jamanetworkopen.2022.12454; The analysis excludes the FDA-approved four diagnostic agents in 2020.
73 Joshua D. Wallach et al., "Associations between Surrogate Markers and Clinical Outcomes for Nononcologic Chronic Disease Treatments," *JAMA* 331, no. 19 (April 22, 2024): 1646–54, https://doi.org/10.1001/jama.2024.4175.
74 FDA, "Table of Surrogate Endpoints That Were the Basis of Drug Approval or Licensure," US Food & Drug Administration, February 28, 2022, https://www.fda.gov/drugs/development-resources/table-surrogate-endpoints-were-basis-drug-approval-or-licensure; 21st Century Cures Act.
75 Chul Kim and Vinay Prasad, "Strength of Validation for Surrogate End Points Used in the US Food and Drug Administration's Approval of Oncology Drugs," *Mayo Clinic Proceedings* 91, no. 6 (May 25, 2016): 713–25, https://doi.org/10.1016/j.mayocp.2016.02.012.
76 Emerson Y. Chen, Alyson Haslam, and Vinay Prasad, "FDA Acceptance of Surrogate End Points for Cancer Drug Approval: 1992–2019," *JAMA Internal Medicine* 180, no. 6 (April 27, 2020): 912–14, https://doi.org/10.1001/jamainternmed.2020.1097.
77 Anushka Walia, Alyson Haslam, and Vinay Prasad, "FDA Validation of Surrogate Endpoints in Oncology: 2005–2022," *Journal of Cancer Policy* 34 (September 26, 2022): 100364, https://doi.org/10.1016/j.jcpo.2022.100364.
78 Chul Kim and Vinay Prasad, "Cancer Drugs Approved on the Basis of a Surrogate End Point and Subsequent Overall Survival: An Analysis of 5 Years of US Food and Drug Administration Approvals," *JAMA Internal Medicine* 175, no. 12 (December 2015): 1992–4, https://doi.org/10.1001/jamainternmed.2015.5868.
79 FDA, "FDA Expands Approval of Gene Therapy for Patients with Duchenne Muscular Dystrophy," US Food & Drug Administration, June 20, 2024, https://www.fda.gov/news-events/press-announcements/fda-expands-approval-gene-therapy-patients-duchenne-muscular-dystrophy.
80 Reshma Ramachandran and Holly Fernandez Lynch, "Should FDA Grant Accelerated Approval to Duchenne Muscular Dystrophy Gene Therapy?," MedPage Today, May 18, 2023, https://www.medpagetoday.com/opinion/second-opinions/104574.
81 Judy George, "Duchenne Muscular Dystrophy Treatment Narrowly Captures Support of FDA Advisors," MedPage Today, May 13, 2023, https://www.medpagetoday.com/neurology/generalneurology/104492.
82 Jason Mast and Adam Feuerstein, "Sarepta's Duchenne Gene Therapy Fails to Meet Primary Endpoint in Pivotal Trial," *STAT* (blog), October 30, 2023, https://www.statnews.com/2023/10/30/sareptas-duchenne-gene-therapy-fails-to-meet-primary-endpoint-in-pivotal-trial/.
83 Mike Singer and Xiaofei Wang, "BLA Integrated Clinical and Clinical Pharmacology Review Memorandum," US Food & Drug Administration, June 18, 2024, https://www.fda.gov/media/179486/download?attachment.
84 Jason Mast and Matthew Herper, "Top FDA Official Peter Marks Overruled Staff, Review Team to Approve Sarepta Gene Therapy," *STAT* (blog), June 20, 2024,

https://www.statnews.com/2024/06/20/sarepta-duchenne-elevidys-fda-approval-peter-marks-overruled-staff/; Derek Lowe, "Sarepta. Why?," Science, June 21, 2024, https://www.science.org/content/blog-post/sarepta-why.

85 Beth Mole, "Top FDA Official Overrules Staff to Approve Gene Therapy That Failed Trial," Ars Technica, June 21, 2024, https://arstechnica.com/science/2024/06/top-fda-official-overrules-staff-to-approve-gene-therapy-that-failed-trial/.

86 Lola A. Fashoyin-Aje and Nicole Verdun, "Office Director Memorandum: Summary of Regulatory Decision on Biologics License Application," Office of Clinical Evaluation, June 18, 2024, https://www.fda.gov/media/179487/download?attachment.

87 Angus Liu, "Sarepta Reports 2nd Death after DMD Gene Therapy Elevidys, Stops Dosing in Half of Patients," Fierce Pharma, June 16, 2025, https://www.fiercepharma.com/pharma/sarepta-records-second-death-after-dmd-gene-therapy-elevidys-stops-dosing-half-patients; Angus Liu, "Sarepta Reports One Death after Patient Received DMD Gene Therapy Elevidys," Fierce Pharma, March 18, 2025, https://www.fiercepharma.com/pharma/sarepta-reports-1-death-after-dmd-patient-received-gene-therapy-elevidys.

88 "Orphan Drug Act," Pub. L. No. 97–114 (1983), https://www.congress.gov/bill/97th-congress/house-bill/5238#:~:text=Orphan%20Drug%20Act%20%2D%20Amends%20the,be%20conducted%20with%20the%20drug; Matthew Herder, "What Is the Purpose of the Orphan Drug Act?," *PLoS Med* 14, no. 1 (January 3, 2017): e1002191, https://doi.org/10.1371/journal.pmed.1002191.

89 John Swann, "The Story Behind the Orphan Drug Act," US Food & Drug Administration, February 23, 2018, https://web.archive.org/web/20240915141737/https://www.fda.gov/industry/fdas-rare-disease-day/story-behind-orphan-drug-act.

90 FDA, "Designating an Orphan Product: Drugs and Biological Products," US Food & Drug Administration, July 8, 2022, https://www.fda.gov/industry/medical-products-rare-diseases-and-conditions/designating-orphan-product-drugs-and-biologicalproducts; M. Angeles Villarreal, "Orphan Drug Act: Background and Proposed Legislation in the 107th Congress," Congressional Research Service, July 25, 2001, https://digital.library.unt.edu/ark:/67531/metadc805930/m1/1/.

91 Orphan Drug Act.

92 "Health Promotion and Disease Prevention Amendments of 1984," Pub. L. No. 98–551 (1983), https://www.congress.gov/bill/98th-congress/senate-bill/771/text.

93 Herder, "What Is the Purpose of the Orphan Drug Act?"

94 Hana Althobaiti et al., "Disentangling the Cost of Orphan Drugs Marketed in the United States," *Healthcare* 11, no. 4 (February 13, 2023): 558, https://doi.org/10.3390/healthcare11040558.

95 Hannah-Alise Rogers and Hassan Z. Sheikh, "The Orphan Drug Act: Legal Overview and Policy," Congressional Research Service, March 5, 2024: 2, https://crsreports.congress.gov/product/pdf/IF/IF12605/2.

96 These calculations were made from published numbers in annual FDA new/novel drug therapy reports (see notes 61–2).

97 Thomas Michaeli, Hendrik Jürges, and Daniel Tobias Michaeli, "FDA Approval, Clinical Trial Evidence, Efficacy, Epidemiology, and Price for Non-orphan and Ultra-rare, Rare, and Common Orphan Cancer Drug Indications: Cross Sectional Analysis," *BMJ* 381, no. 8382 (May 9, 2023): e073242, https://doi.org/10.1136/bmj-2022-073242.

98 Aaron S. Kesselheim, "Characteristics of Clinical Trials to Support Approval of Orphan vs Nonorphan Drugs for Cancer," *JAMA* 305, no. 22 (June 8, 2011): 2320–6, https://doi.org/10.1001/jama.2011.769.
99 Palvi Kudyar et al., "Evaluation of Clinical Trials Done for Orphan Drugs versus Nonorphan Drugs in Infectious Diseasesan Eleven Year Analysis [2010–2020]," *Perspectives in Clinical Research* 14, no. 2 (June 2023): 56–60, https://doi.org/10.4103/picr.picr_137_21.
100 Min Fan et al., "Postmarketing Safety of Orphan Drugs: A Longitudinal Analysis of the US Food and Drug Administration Database between 1999 and 2018," *Orphanet Journal of Rare Diseases* 17 (January 4, 2022): Article 3, https://doi.org/10.1186/s13023-021-02166-9.
101 Matthew Herder, "Pharmaceutical Drugs of Uncertain Value, Lifecycle Regulation at the US Food and Drug Administration, and Institutional Incumbency," *The Milbank Quarterly* 97, no. 3 (August 12, 2019): 820–57, https://doi.org/10.1111/1468-0009.12413.
102 FDA, "Postmarketing Requirements and Commitments: Introduction," US Food & Drug Administration, January 12, 2016, https://www.fda.gov/drugs/guidance-compliance-regulatory-information/postmarket-requirements-and-commitments.
103 Food and Drug Administration, "21 CFR Part 314 Subpart H—Accelerated Approval of New Drugs for Serious or Life-Threatening Illnesses"; Food and Drug Administration, "21 CFR Part 601 Subpart E—Accelerated Approval of Biological Products for Serious or Life-Threatening Illnesses," Code of Federal Regulations, June 7, 2024, https://www.ecfr.gov/current/title-21/chapter-I/subchapter-F/part-601/subpart-E; Food and Drug Administration, "21 CFR Part 314.55 Pediatric Use Information," Code of Federal Regulations, June 7, 2024, https://www.ecfr.gov/current/title-21/chapter-I/subchapter-D/part-314/subpart-B/section-314.55; Food and Drug Administration, "21 CFR Part 601.27 Pediatric Studies," Code of Federal Regulations, June 7, 2024, https://www.ecfr.gov/current/title-21/chapter-I/subchapter-F/part-601#601.27; Food and Drug Administration, "21 CFR Part 314 Subpart I—Approval of New Drugs When Human Efficacy Studies Are Not Ethical or Feasible," Code of Federal Regulations, June 7, 2024, https://www.ecfr.gov/current/title-21/chapter-I/subchapter-D/part-314/subpart-I; Food and Drug Administration, "21 CFR Part 601 Subpart H—Approval of Biological Products When Human Efficacy Studies Are Not Ethical or Feasible," Code of Federal Regulations, June 7, 2024, https://www.ecfr.gov/current/title-21/chapter-I/subchapter-F/part-601/subpart-H.
104 Food and Drug Administration Amendments Act of 2007.
105 Herder, "Pharmaceutical Drugs of Uncertain Value, Lifecycle Regulation at the US Food and Drug Administration, and Institutional Incumbency."
106 Sarah Ridge et al., "US FDA Postmarketing Requirements and Commitments: A Systematic Assessment of Clinical Pharmacology Studies and Their Impact on US FDA Prescribing Information," *The Journal of Clinical Pharmacology* 63, no. 6 (February 2, 2023): 695–703, https://doi.org/10.1002/jcph.2208.
107 Joshua D Wallach et al., "Postmarket Studies Required by the US Food and Drug Administration for New Drugs and Biologics Approved between 2009 and 2012: Cross Sectional Analysis," *BMJ* 361, no. 8155 (May 24, 2018): k2031, https://doi.org/10.1136/bmj.k2031.

108 Huseyin Naci, Katelyn R. Smalley, and Aaron S. Kesselheim, "Characteristics of Preapproval and Postapproval Studies for Drugs Granted Accelerated Approval by the US Food and Drug Administration," *JAMA* 318, no. 7 (August 15, 2017): 626–36, https://doi.org/10.1001/jama.2017.9415.

109 Thomas J. Hwang et al., "Completion Rate and Reporting of Mandatory Pediatric Postmarketing Studies under the US Pediatric Research Equity Act," *JAMA Pediatrics* 173, no. 1 (January 2019): 68–74, https://doi.org/10.1001/jamapediatrics.2018.3416.

110 Garth T. Whiteside and Jeffrey D. Kennedy, "Chapter 16: Consideration of Pharmacokinetic Pharmacodynamic Relationships in the Discovery of New Pain Drugs," in *Translational Pain Research: From Mouse to Man*, ed. Lawrence Kruger and Alan R. Light, Frontiers in Neuroscience (Boca Raton, FL: CRC Press, 2010), http://www.ncbi.nlm.nih.gov/books/NBK57267/.

111 HHS Office of Inspector General, "Delays in Confirmatory Trials for Drug Applications Granted FDA's Accelerated Approval Raise Concerns," US Department of Health & Human Services, September 2022, https://oig.hhs.gov/oei/reports/OEI-01-21-00401.pdf.

112 FDA, "FDA Commissioner and Chief Scientist Announce Decision to Withdraw Approval of Makena," US Food & Drug Administration, April 6, 2023, https://www.fda.gov/news-events/press-announcements/fda-commissioner-and-chief-scientist-announce-decision-withdraw-approval-makena.

113 Angus Liu, "Viatris Pulls Decades-Old Accelerated Approval Thanks to 'Unfeasible' Confirmatory Trial Demand," Fierce Pharma, November 30, 2022, https://www.fiercepharma.com/pharma/accelerated-approval-withdrawn-after-25-years-viatris-pulls-antibiotic-powder-thanks.

114 Yale Collaboration for Research Integrity and Transparency, "What's in Your Medicine Cabinet?: Ensuring the Safety and Efficacy of Prescription Drugs, Biologics and Medical Devices in the United States," February 2018, https://law.yale.edu/sites/default/files/area/center/crit/document/crit_policy_paper_february_2018_3rd_edition.pdf.

115 Joshua D. Wallach et al., "Postmarketing Commitments for Novel Drugs and Biologics Approved by the US Food and Drug Administration: A Cross-Sectional Analysis," *BMC Medicine* 17 (June 17, 2019): Article 117, https://doi.org/10.1186/s12916-019-1344-3.

116 Beatrice L. Brown et al., "Fulfillment of Postmarket Commitments and Requirements for New Drugs Approved by the FDA, 2013–2016," *JAMA Internal Medicine* 182, no. 11 (October 3, 2022): 1223–6, https://doi.org/10.1001/jamainternmed.2022.4226.

117 Herder, "Pharmaceutical Drugs of Uncertain Value, Lifecycle Regulation at the US Food and Drug Administration, and Institutional Incumbency."

118 Government Accountability Office, "Drug Safety: FDA Expedites Many Applications, But Data for Postapproval Oversight Need Improvement," December 2015, 22, https://www.gao.gov/assets/gao-16-192.pdf.

119 FDA, "Guidance for Industry: Postmarketing Studies and Clinical Trials—Implementation of Section 505(o)(3) of the Federal Food, Drug, and Cosmetic Act," US Food and Drug Administration, April 2011, https://www.fda.gov/media/131980/download.

120 FDA, "Notice to Industry: Postmarketing Requirements—Postmarket Studies and Clinical Trials," US Food & Drug Administration, February 12, 2016, https://www.fda.gov/drugs/guidance-compliance-regulatory-information/notice-industry-postma

rketing-requirements-postmarket-studies-and-clinical-trials#:~:text=If%20a%20company%20fails%20to,and%20assessing%20civil%20monetary%20penalties.

121 Steven Woloshin et al., "The Fate of FDA Postapproval Studies," *New England Journal of Medicine* 377, no. 12 (September 21, 2017): 1114–17, https://doi.org/10.1056/NEJMp1705800.

122 Office of Inspector General, "FDA's Risk Evaluation and Mitigation Strategies: Uncertain Effectiveness in Addressing the Opioid Crisis."

123 Ibid., 2.

124 Ibid., 17.

125 Mary K. Olson and Nina Yin, "New Clinical Information and Physician Prescribing: How Do Pediatric Labeling Changes Affect Prescribing to Children?," *Health Economics* 30, no. 1 (November 2, 2020): 144–64, https://doi.org/10.1002/hec.4182.

126 HHS Office of Inspector General, "Delays in Confirmatory Trials for Drug Applications Granted FDA's Accelerated Approval Raise Concerns."

127 Staffs of the Committee on Oversight and Reform and Committee on Energy and Commerce, "The High Price of Aduhelm's Approval: An Investigation into FDA's Atypical Review Process and Biogen's Aggressive Launch Plans," US House of Representatives, December 2022, https://democrats-energycommerce.house.gov/sites/evo-subsites/democrats-energycommerce.house.gov/files/documents/Final%20Aduhelm%20Report_12.29.22.pdf; Abramson, Sickening, 233.

128 Abramson, *Sickening*, 232.

129 Kathy Y. Liu, Lon S. Schneider, and Robert Howard, "The Need to Show Minimum Clinically Important Differences in Alzheimer's Disease Trials," *The Lancet Psychiatry* 8, no. 11 (June 1, 2021): 1013–16, https://doi.org/10.1016/S2215-0366(21)00197-8.

130 Stephen Salloway et al., "Amyloid-Related Imaging Abnormalities in 2 Phase 3 Studies Evaluating Aducanumab in Patients with Early Alzheimer Disease," *JAMA Neurology* 79, no. 1 (November 22, 2021): 13–21, https://doi.org/10.1001/jamaneurol.2021.4161.

131 Pam Belluck and Rebecca Robbins, "Three F.D.A. Advisers Resign over Agency's Approval of Alzheimer's Drug," *The New York Times*, June 10, 2021, sec. Health, https://www.nytimes.com/2021/06/10/health/aduhelm-fda-resign-alzheimers.html.

132 Aaron S. Kesselheim and Jerry Avorn, "The F.D.A. Has Reached a New Low," *The New York Times*, June 15, 2021, sec. Opinion, https://www.nytimes.com/2021/06/15/opinion/alzheimers-drug-aducanumab-fda.html.

133 CMS, "CMS Finalizes Medicare Coverage Policy for Monoclonal Antibodies Directed against Amyloid for the Treatment of Alzheimer's Disease," CMS.gov, April 7, 2022, https://www.cms.gov/newsroom/press-releases/cms-finalizes-medicare-coverage-policy-monoclonal-antibodies-directed-against-amyloid-treatment.

134 Staffs of the Committee on Oversight and Reform and Committee on Energy and Commerce, "The High Price of Aduhelm's Approval: An Investigation into FDA's Atypical Review Process and Biogen's Aggressive Launch Plans"; Carma Hassan and Jen Christensen, "Biogen Discontinues Alzheimer's Medication Aduhelm," CNN, January 31, 2024, https://www.cnn.com/2024/01/31/health/aduhelm-alzheimers-biogen/index.html.

135 "Biogen Drops Alzheimer's Drug Aduhelm, Ending a 17-Year Chapter," *Reuters*, January 31, 2024, sec. Healthcare & Pharmaceuticals, https://www.reuters.com/busin

ess/healthcare-pharmaceuticals/biogen-discontinue-development-older-alzheimers-drug-aduhelm-2024-01-31/.

136 Staffs of the Committee on Oversight and Reform and Committee on Energy and Commerce, "The High Price of Aduhelm's Approval: An Investigation into FDA's Atypical Review Process and Biogen's Aggressive Launch Plans."

137 Ibid., 17.

138 Ibid., 4.

139 Ibid., 22.

140 Ibid., 41–3.

141 Ibid., 42.

142 Ibid., 43; This includes Alaska Natives.

143 Ibid., 44.

144 DiStefano et al., "Association between Drug Characteristics and Manufacturer Spending on Direct-to-Consumer Advertising."

145 Staffs of the Committee on Oversight and Reform and Committee on Energy and Commerce, "The High Price of Aduhelm's Approval: An Investigation into FDA's Atypical Review Process and Biogen's Aggressive Launch Plans," 22.

146 Loper Bright Enterprises et al. v. Raimondo, Secretary of Commerce, et al., 603 U.S. (US Supreme Court 2024); Chevron U.S.A. Inc. v. Natural Resources Defense Council, Inc., 467 U.S. 837 (US Supreme Court 1984).

147 "21 U.S. Code § 355—New Drugs," Legal Information Institute, accessed June 30, 2024, https://www.law.cornell.edu/uscode/text/21/355.

148 "The Potential Implications of Loper Bright for FDA and FDA-Regulated Industries," Sidley, June 28, 2024, https://www.sidley.com/en/insights/newsupdates/2024/06/the-potential-implications-of-loper-bright-for-fda-and-fda-regulated-industries; Michelle Campbell, "Measuring How Patients Feel and Function," Silver Spring, MD, May 12, 2017, https://www.fda.gov/media/104969/download.

149 Loper Bright Enterprises et al. v. Raimondo, Secretary of Commerce, et al., 603 U.S.

150 Meghan Bartels, "A Supreme Court Ruling May Make It Harder for Government Agencies to Use Good Science," *Scientific American*, June 25, 2024, https://www.scientificamerican.com/article/supreme-courts-chevron-deference-decision-could-make-science-based/.

151 "FDA's Laboratory-Developed Test Rule Struck Down in Major Test of Loper Bright," Sidley, April 3, 2025, https://www.sidley.com/en/insights/newsupdates/2025/04/fdas-laboratory-developed-tests-ldt-rule-struck-down-in-major-test-of-loper-bright.

152 Lev Facher, "More than Two-Thirds of Congress Cashed a Pharma Campaign Check in 2020, New STAT Analysis Shows," STAT, June 9, 2021, https://www.statnews.com/feature/prescription-politics/federal-full-data-set/.

## 6 It Gets Worse: Medical Devices

1 FDA, "Medical Device User Fee Amendments (MDUFA)," US Food & Drug Administration, October 3, 2024, https://www.fda.gov/industry/fda-user-fee-programs/medical-device-user-fee-amendments-mdufa.

2 FDA, "FDA At a Glance October 2024."

3 FDA, "Biosimilar User Fee Amendments," US Food & Drug Administration, June 10, 2024, https://www.fda.gov/industry/fda-user-fee-programs/biosimilar-user-fee-amendments#:~:text=The%20Federal%20Food%2C%20Drug%2C%20and,October%202022%20through%20September%202027; FDA, "FDA: User Fees Explained," US Food & Drug Administration, May 22, 2024, https://www.fda.gov/industry/fda-user-fee-programs/fda-user-fees-explained.

4 FDA, "A History of Medical Device Regulation & Oversight in the United States," US Food & Drug Administration, August 21, 2023, https://www.fda.gov/medical-devices/overview-device-regulation/history-medical-device-regulation-oversight-united-states.

5 Amanda K. Sarata, "FDA Regulation of Medical Devices," Congressional Research Service, January 4, 2023, https://crsreports.congress.gov/product/pdf/R/R47374.

6 FDA, "Classification of Products as Drugs and Devices & Additional Product Classification Issues: Guidance for Industry and FDA Staff," US Food and Drug Administration, September 2017: 5, https://www.fda.gov/media/80384/download.

7 FDA, "A History of Medical Device Regulation & Oversight in the United States."

8 FDA, "Learn if a Medical Device Has Been Cleared by FDA for Marketing," US Food & Drug Administration, December 29, 2021, https://www.fda.gov/medical-devices/consumers-medical-devices/learn-if-medical-device-has-been-cleared-fda-marketing.

9 FDA, "General Controls for Medical Devices," US Food & Drug Administration, December 15, 2023, https://www.fda.gov/medical-devices/regulatory-controls/general-controls-medical-devices; Sumatha Kondabolu, "The 3 FDA Medical Device Classes: Differences and Examples Explained," Qualio, January 25, 2023, https://www.qualio.com/blog/fda-medical-device-classes-differences.

10 FDA, "Learn if a Medical Device Has Been Cleared by FDA for Marketing."

11 "21 U.S. Code § 360c—Classification of Devices Intended for Human Use," Legal Information Institute, accessed June 13, 2024, https://www.law.cornell.edu/uscode/text/21/360c.

12 Ibid.; Sarata, "FDA Regulation of Medical Devices," 4.

13 Jonathan J. Darrow, Jerry Avorn, and Aaron S. Kesselheim, "FDA Regulation and Approval of Medical Devices: 1976–2020," *JAMA* 326, no. 5 (August 3, 2021): 420–32, https://doi.org/10.1001/jama.2021.11171.

14 Sarata, "FDA Regulation of Medical Devices," 9.

15 Mateo Aboy, Cristina Crespo, and Ariel Stern, "Beyond the 510(k): The Regulation of Novel Moderate-Risk Medical Devices, Intellectual Property Considerations, and Innovation Incentives in the FDA's De Novo Pathway," *Npj Digital Medicine* 7 (February 8, 2024): Article 29, https://doi.org/10.1038/s41746-024-01021-y; Alexander O. Everhart et al., "Association between Regulatory Submission Characteristics and Recalls of Medical Devices Receiving 510(k) Clearance," *JAMA* 329, no. 2 (January 10, 2023): 144–56, https://doi.org/10.1001/jama.2022.22974.

16 Robert Seiple and Sarah Fitzgerald, "Clinical Data in Support of U.S. FDA 510(k) Submissions," Emergo, November 2022, https://www.emergobyul.com/sites/default/files/2023-04/Clinical%20Data-%20whitepaper%20Emergo-Final.pdf.

17 FDA, "The Least Burdensome Provisions: Concept and Principles Guidance for Industry and Food and Drug Administration Staff," US Food and Drug Administration, February 5, 2019, https://www.fda.gov/media/73188/download.

18 FDA, "FDA Fact Sheet: What's Involved in Reviewing and Approving Generic Drug Applications?," US Food & Drug Administration, accessed June 19, 2024, https://www.fda.gov/media/99163/download; FDA, "Evaluation of Therapeutic Equivalence: Guidance for Industry" (US Food and Drug Administration, July 2022), https://www.fda.gov/media/160054/download.
19 Committee on the Public Health Effectiveness of the FDA 510(k) Clearance Process, Board on Population Health and Public Health Practice, and Institute of Medicine, *Medical Devices and the Public's Health: The FDA 510(k) Clearance Process at 35 Years* (Washington, DC: National Academies Press, 2011), https://doi.org/10.17226/13150; FDA, "The 510(k) Program: Evaluating Substantial Equivalence in Premarket Notifications [510(k)]: Guidance for Industry and Food and Drug Administration Staff," US Food & Drug Administration, July 28, 2014, https://www.fda.gov/media/82395/download.
20 FDA, "Medical Device User Fee Amendments (MDUFA)."
21 "Premarket Approval (PMA)," Drugwatch, September 5, 2023, https://www.drugwatch.com/fda/premarket-approval/.
22 Kushal T. Kadakia et al., "Renewing the Call for Reforms to Medical Device Safety—The Case of Penumbra," *JAMA Internal Medicine* 182, no. 1 (November 29, 2021): 59–65, https://doi.org/10.1001/jamainternmed.2021.6626.
23 Kushal T. Kadakia and Harlan M. Krumholz, "Reforms Needed for FDA's Regulation of Medical Devices," STAT, December 3, 2021, https://www.statnews.com/2021/12/03/reforms-needed-for-fdas-regulation-of-medical-devices/.
24 Xiaolin Zheng to Micaela Victoria, "K190010," June 16, 2019, https://www.accessdata.fda.gov/cdrh_docs/pdf19/K190010.pdf.
25 Mary Ellen Schneider, "Experts: Penumbra Recall Highlights 'Device Creep,' Makes Case for Regulatory Reform," Regulatory Focus, November 30, 2021, https://www.raps.org/News-and-Articles/News-Articles/2021/11/Experts-Penumbra-recall-highlights-device-creep-ma.
26 Kadakia et al., "Renewing the Call for Reforms to Medical Device Safety—The Case of Penumbra"; The Penumbra Pivotal Stroke Trial Investigators, "The Penumbra Pivotal Stroke Trial: Safety and Effectiveness of a New Generation of Mechanical Devices for Clot Removal in Intracranial Large Vessel Occlusive Disease," *Stroke* 40, no. 8 (July 6, 2009): 2761–8, https://doi.org/10.1161/STROKEAHA.108.544957.
27 Quintessential Capital Management, "Penumbra and Its 'Killer Catheter,' " https://www.qcmfunds.com/wp-content/uploads/2020/11/QCM-on-Penumbra-presentation-Final-.pdf.
28 "Penumbra Aspiration System Jet7 Xtra Flex Precuations For Use," Medicos Hirata Safety Measure Team, June 2020, https://www.dropbox.com/scl/fi/4lzepbocl5yb5ouz7qd3v/Japan%20Letter%20Translated%20to%20English.jpg?rlkey=mgkizuyj96sstkwtoaoe8nrc7&e=2&dl=0.
29 Greg Farrell and Josh Fineman, "Catheter-Linked Death Jolts Penumbra, a Target of Short Sellers," Bloomberg, December 4, 2020, https://www.bloomberg.com/tosv2.html?vid=&uuid=6b436746-29c3-11ef-8575-ad74e7bc797b&url=L25ld3MvYXJ0aWNsZXMvMjAyMC0xMi0wNC9jYXRoZXRlci1saW5rZWQtZGVhdGgtam9sdHMtcGVudW1icmEtYS10YXJnZXQtb2Ytc2hvcnQtc2VsbGVycw==.
30 Kadakia et al., "Renewing the Call for Reforms to Medical Device Safety—The Case of Penumbra."

31 Claudia See et al., "Class I Recalls of Cardiovascular Devices between 2013 and 2022: A Cross-Sectional Analysis," *Annals of Internal Medicine* 177, no. 11 (September 17, 2024): 1499–508, https://doi.org/10.7326/ANNALS-24-00724.
32 Everhart et al., "Association between Regulatory Submission Characteristics and Recalls of Medical Devices Receiving 510(k) Clearance."
33 Jonathan R. Dubin et al., "Risk of Recall among Medical Devices Undergoing US Food and Drug Administration 510(k) Clearance and Premarket Approval, 2008–2017," *JAMA Network Open* 4, no. 5 (May 6, 2021): e217274, https://doi.org/10.1001/jamanetworkopen.2021.7274.
34 Committee on the Public Health Effectiveness of the FDA 510(k) Clearance Process, Board on Population Health and Public Health Practice, and Institute of Medicine, *Medical Devices and the Public's Health*, 5.
35 Kushal T. Kadakia et al., "Use of Recalled Devices in New Device Authorizations under the US Food and Drug Administration's 510(k) Pathway and Risk of Subsequent Recalls," *JAMA* 329, no. 2 (January 10, 2023): 136–43, https://doi.org/10.1001/jama.2022.23279.
36 Committee on the Public Health Effectiveness of the FDA 510(k) Clearance Process, Board on Population Health and Public Health Practice, and Institute of Medicine, *Medical Devices and the Public's Health*, 143.
37 Ibid., 9–10.
38 Office of Inspector General, "Hospital Incident Reporting Systems Do Not Capture Most Patient Harm," U.S. Department of Health and Human Services, January 2012, https://oig.hhs.gov/oei/reports/oei-06-09-00091.pdf.
39 Government Accountability Office, "Medical Devices: FDA Has Begun Building an Active Postmarket Surveillance System," July 2024, https://www.gao.gov/assets/gao-24-106699.pdf.
40 FDA, "Recalls, Corrections and Removals (Devices)," US Food & Drug Administration, January 13, 2025, https://www.fda.gov/medical-devices/postmarket-requirements-devices/recalls-corrections-and-removals-devices.
41 Food and Drug Administration, "21 CFR Part 806—Medical Devices; Reports of Corrections and Removals," Code of Federal Regulations, August 22, 2024, https://www.ecfr.gov/current/title-21/chapter-I/subchapter-H/part-806.
42 David Hilzenrath, "The FDA Calls Them 'Recalls,' yet the Targeted Medical Devices Often Remain in Use," CBS News, August 13, 2024, https://www.cbsnews.com/news/fda-medical-device-recalls-stay-in-use/.
43 Darrow, Avorn, and Kesselheim, "FDA Regulation and Approval of Medical Devices."
44 Government Accountability Office, "Medical Devices: FDA Should Take Steps to Ensure That High-Risk Device Types Are Approved through the Most Stringent Premarket Review Process," January 2009, https://www.gao.gov/assets/gao-09-190.pdf.
45 Ibid., 18.
46 "Safe Medical Devices Act of 1990," Pub. L. No. 101–629 (1990), https://www.congress.gov/bill/101st-congress/house-bill/3095#:~:text=Safe%20Medical%20Devices%20Act%20of%201990%20%2D%20Amends%20the%20Federal%20Food,or%20contributed%20to%20a%20death%2C.
47 Government Accountability Office, "Medical Devices: FDA Should Take Steps to Ensure That High-Risk Device Types Are Approved through the Most Stringent Premarket Review Process."

48 Office of Inspector General, "FDA's Clearance of Medical Devices through the 510(k) Process," US Department of Health and Human Services, September 2013, https://oig.hhs.gov/documents/evaluation/2843/OEI-04-10-00480-Complete%20Report.pdf.
49 Maryam Mooghali et al., "Medical Device Risk (Re)Classification: Lessons from the FDA's 515 Program Initiative," *BMJ Surgery, Interventions, & Health Technologies* 5, no. 1 (September 27, 2023): e000186, https://doi.org/10.1136/bmjsit-2023-000186.
50 Elaine Silvestrini and Kevin Connolly, "Report: Medical Device Modifications Approved with Poor Data," Drugwatch, September 14, 2017, https://www.drugwatch.com/news/2017/09/14/medical-device-approval-process-flaws/.
51 Sanket S. Dhruva, "Strength of Study Evidence Examined by the FDA in Premarket Approval of Cardiovascular Devices," *JAMA* 302, no. 24 (December 23, 2009): 2679–85, https://doi.org/10.1001/jama.2009.1899.
52 Rita Redberg, "FDA Medical Device Approval: Is There a Better Way?," Congressional Hearing Testimony, June 2, 2011, https://oversight.house.gov/wp-content/uploads/2012/01/6-2-11_Redberg_FDA_testimony.pdf.
53 Connie E. Chen, Sanket S. Dhruva, and Rita F. Redberg, "Inclusion of Comparative Effectiveness Data in High-Risk Cardiovascular Device Studies at the Time of Premarket Approval," *JAMA* 308, no. 17 (November 7, 2012): 1740–2, https://doi.org/10.1001/jama.2012.14491.
54 Sarah Y. Zheng, Sanket S. Dhruva, and Rita F. Redberg, "Characteristics of Clinical Studies Used for US Food and Drug Administration Approval of High-Risk Medical Device Supplements," *JAMA* 318, no. 7 (August 15, 2017): 619–25, https://doi.org/10.1001/jama.2017.9414.
55 21st Century Cures Act.
56 FDA, "Breakthrough Devices Program: Guidance for Industry and Food and Drug Administration Staff," US Food and Drug Administration, September 15, 2023: 7, https://www.fda.gov/media/162413/download.
57 Ibid., 8.
58 Kushal T. Kadakia et al., "FDA Authorization of Therapeutic Devices under the Breakthrough Devices Program," *JAMA Internal Medicine*, June 30, 2025, https://doi.org/10.1001/jamainternmed.2025.2235.
59 L. Camille Jones, Sanket S. Dhruva, and Rita F. Redberg, "Assessment of Clinical Trial Evidence for High-Risk Cardiovascular Devices Approved under the Food and Drug Administration Priority Review Program," *JAMA Internal Medicine* 178, no. 10 (October 2018): 1418–20, https://doi.org/10.1001/jamainternmed.2018.3649.
60 Caroline Ong, Vy K. Ly, and Rita F. Redberg, "Comparison of Priority vs Standard US Food and Drug Administration Premarket Approval Review for High-Risk Medical Devices," *JAMA Internal Medicine* 180, no. 5 (March 30, 2020): 801–3, https://doi.org/10.1001/jamainternmed.2020.0297.
61 FDA, "Recalls, Corrections and Removals (Devices)," US Food & Drug Administration, September 29, 2020, https://www.fda.gov/medical-devices/postmarket-requirements-devices/recalls-corrections-and-removals-devices.
62 "Internal Emails Show FDA, Industry Jointly Framed 'Cures' Device Language," InsideHealthPolicy, December 10, 2015, https://insidehealthpolicy.com/share/87113.
63 Ibid.; "Diana Zuckerman," LinkedIn, accessed June 23, 2024, https://www.linkedin.com/in/diana-zuckerman-3126b95/details/experience/.
64 Vinay K. Rathi et al., "Characteristics of Clinical Studies Conducted over the Total Product Life Cycle of High-Risk Therapeutic Medical Devices Receiving FDA

Premarket Approval in 2010 and 2011," *JAMA* 314, no. 6 (August 11, 2015): 604–12, https://doi.org/10.1001/jama.2015.8761.
65 Vinay K. Rathi et al., "Postmarket Clinical Evidence for High-Risk Therapeutic Medical Devices Receiving Food and Drug Administration Premarket Approval in 2010 and 2011," *JAMA Network Open* 3, no. 8 (August 28, 2020): e2014496, https://doi.org/10.1001/jamanetworkopen.2020.14496.
66 Safe Medical Devices Act of 1990.
67 FDA, "Humanitarian Device Exemption," US Food & Drug Administration, October 3, 2022, https://www.fda.gov/medical-devices/premarket-submissions-selecting-and-preparing-correct-submission/humanitarian-device-exemption.
68 FDA, "Humanitarian Device Exemption (HDE) Program: Guidance for Industry and Food and Drug Administration Staff," US Food and Drug Administration, September 6, 2019, https://www.fda.gov/media/74307/download.
69 "21 U.S. Code § 360j—General Provisions Respecting Control of Devices Intended for Human Use," Legal Information Institute, accessed June 23, 2024, https://www.law.cornell.edu/uscode/text/21/360j.
70 A. J. Gartenberg et al., "Presumed Safe No More: Lessons from the Wingspan Saga on Regulation of Devices," *BMJ* 348, no. 7942 (January 22, 2014): g93, https://doi.org/10.1136/bmj.g93.
71 FDA, "Humanitarian Device Exemption (HDE): Wingspan Stent System with Gateway PTA Balloon Catheter," 522 Postmarket Surveillance Studies Database, June 17, 2024, https://www.accessdata.fda.gov/scripts/cdrh/cfdocs/cfhde/hde.cfm?id=375531.
72 Arani Bose et al., "A Novel, Self-Expanding, Nitinol Stent in Medically Refractory Intracranial Atherosclerotic Stenoses: The Wingspan Study," *Stroke* 38, no. 5 (March 29, 2007): 1531–7, https://doi.org/10.1161/STROKEAHA.106.477711.
73 FDA, "Summary of Safety and Probable Benefit: Intracranial Stent," US Food & Drug Administration, accessed June 22, 2024, https://www.accessdata.fda.gov/cdrh_docs/pdf5/h050001b.pdf; Gartenberg et al., "Presumed Safe No More."
74 Marc I. Chimowitz et al., "Stenting versus Aggressive Medical Therapy for Intracranial Arterial Stenosis," *New England Journal of Medicine* 365, no. 11 (September 15, 2011): 993–1003, https://doi.org/10.1056/NEJMoa1105335.
75 Gartenberg et al., "Presumed Safe No More."
76 Safe Medical Devices Act of 1990.
77 Center for Devices and Radiological Health, "Medical Devices Advisory Committee: Neurological Devices Panel," US Food & Drug Administration, March 23, 2012): 296, https://web.archive.org/web/20161023135552/https://www.fda.gov/downloads/AdvisoryCommittees/CommitteesMeetingMaterials/MedicalDevices/MedicalDevicesAdvisoryCommittee/NeurologicalDevicesPanel/UCM300900.pdf.
78 Gartenberg et al., "Presumed Safe No More."
79 Michael J. Alexander et al., "WEAVE Trial: Final Results in 152 On-Label Patients," *Stroke* 50, no. 4 (February 28, 2019): 889–94, https://doi.org/10.1161/STROKEAHA.118.023996.
80 FDA, "522 Postmarket Surveillance Studies Database: Rates of Stroke and Death," 522 Postmarket Surveillance Studies Database, June 17, 2024, https://www.accessdata.fda.gov/scripts/cdrh/cfdocs/cfPMA/pss.cfm?t_id=297&c_id=762.
81 Peng Gao et al., "Effect of Stenting Plus Medical Therapy vs Medical Therapy Alone on Risk of Stroke and Death in Patients with Symptomatic Intracranial Stenosis: The

CASSISS Randomized Clinical Trial," *JAMA* 328, no. 6 (August 9, 2022): 534–42, https://doi.org/10.1001/jama.2022.12000.

82 Tanya N. Turan and Marios-Nikos Psychogios, "The CASSISS Randomized Clinical Trial," *Stroke* 54, no. 1 (November 11, 2022): 286–9, https://doi.org/10.1161/STROKEAHA.122.041096.

83 Darrow, Avorn, and Kesselheim, "FDA Regulation and Approval of Medical Devices."

84 David A. Simon, Michael K. Paasche-Orlow, and Hooman Noorchashm, "Establishing Medical Device Transparency at the FDA—a Public Database for Device Labels," *JAMA* 334, no. 2 (June 2, 2025): 109–10, https://doi.org/10.1001/jama.2025.7407.

## 7 Regulatory Capture and Corruption of the FDA

1 Daniel P. Carpenter and David A. Moss, eds., *Preventing Regulatory Capture: Special Interest Influence and How to Limit It* (New York: Cambridge University Press, 2014).

2 Jed Handelsman Shugerman, "The Dependent Origins of Independent Agencies: The Interstate Commerce Commission, the Tenure of Office Act, and the Rise of Modern Campaign Finance," *Journal of Law and Politics* 31, no. 2 (Fall 2015): 139–86, https://scholarship.law.bu.edu/cgi/viewcontent.cgi?article=4570&context=faculty_scholarship.

3 Paul Stephen Dempsey, "The Rise and Fall of the Interstate Commerce Commission: The Tortuous Path from Regulation to Deregulation of America's Infrastructure," *Marquette Law Review* 95, no. 4 (Summer 2012): 1151–89, https://scholarship.law.marquette.edu/mulr/vol95/iss4/7.

4 Daniel Carpenter and David A. Moss, eds., *Preventing Regulatory Capture: Special Interest Influence and How to Limit It* (New York City: Cambridge University Press, 2014), 6.

5 Jeffrey Lazarus, Amy McKay, and Lindsey Herbel, "Who Walks through the Revolving Door? Examining the Lobbying Activity of Former Members of Congress," *Interest Groups & Advocacy* 5, no. 1 (January 14, 2016): 82–100, https://doi.org/10.1057/iga.2015.16.

6 Alan Zibel, "Revolving Congress: The Revolving Door Class of 2019 Flocks to K Street," Public Citizen, May 30, 2019, https://www.citizen.org/article/revolving-congress/.

7 Chris Macke, "Ex-Rep. Is Still Costing Taxpayers Billions in Prescription Fees," *The Hill*, February 15, 2018, https://thehill.com/opinion/healthcare/374035-ex-congressman-still-costing-taxpayers-billions-in-prescription-fees/.

8 Common Cause, "The Medicare/Prescription Drug Bill: A Study in How Government Shouldn't Work," June 3, 2004, https://www.govinfo.gov/content/pkg/CREC-2004-06-04/html/CREC-2004-06-04-pt1-PgE1038-4.htm.

9 Mike Stuckey, "Tauzin Aided Drug Firms, Then They Hired Him," NBC News, March 22, 2006, https://www.nbcnews.com/id/wbna11714763.

10 Alex Wayne and Drew Armstrong, "Tauzin's $11.6 Million Made Him Highest-Paid Health-Law Lobbyist," Bloomberg, November 29, 2011, https://www.bloomberg.com/news/articles/2011-11-29/tauzin-s-11-6-million-made-him-highest-paid-health-law-lobbyist.

11 "Federal Agencies," OpenSecrets, accessed June 13, 2024, https://www.opensecrets.org/revolving-door/federal-agencies.

12 "Agency Search: Food & Drug Administration," OpenSecrets, accessed July 1, 2024, https://www.opensecrets.org/revolving-door/search_result?agency_code=EAHHS09&name=Food+%26+Drug+Administration+&agency=G; "Methodology," OpenSecrets, accessed July 1, 2024, https://www.opensecrets.org/revolving-door/methodology.

13 Genevieve P. Kanter and Daniel Carpenter, "The Revolving Door in Health Care Regulation," *Health Affairs* 42, no. 9 (September 2023): 1298–303, https://doi.org/10.1377/hlthaff.2023.00418.

14 Katherine Ellen Foley, "Trust Issues Deepen as yet Another FDA Commissioner Joins the Pharmaceutical Industry," Quartz, July 1, 2019, https://qz.com/1656529/yet-another-fda-commissioner-joins-the-pharmaceutical-industry.

15 "Ellodi Pharmaceuticals Welcomes Dr. David Kessler and John Fraher to Its Board of Directors," *Ellodi Pharmaceuticals* (blog), October 21, 2020, https://ellodipharma.com/ellodi-pharmaceuticals-welcomes-dr-david-kessler-and-john-fraher-to-its-board-of-directors/.

16 "G1 Therapeutics Announces Addition of Norman E. Sharpless to Board of Directors," G1 Therapeutics, July 25, 2022, https://investor.g1therapeutics.com/news-releases/news-release-details/g1-therapeut ics-announces-addition-norman-e-sharpless-board; "Altesa BioSciences, Inc., Launches Operations to Develop, Commercialize Drugs for Respiratory Viruses and Global Viral Threats," Altesa BioSciences, February 10, 2022, https://altesabio.com/wp-content/uplo ads/2022/05/NR_ALTESA_LAUNCHES_OPS_02.10.2022.pdf.

17 Graham et al., "Risk of Acute Myocardial Infarction"; Graham, "Testimony of David J. Graham, MD, MPH"; Gøtzsche, *Deadly Medicines and Organised Crime*, 108.

18 Janice Hopkins Tanne, "Former FDA Commissioner Is Fined $90 000 for Failing to Disclose Conflicts of Interest," *BMJ* 334, no. 7592 (March 8, 2007): 492, https://doi.org/10.1136/bmj.39142.592130.DB.

19 FDA, "Lester M. Crawford," US Food & Drug Administration, February 21, 2020, https://www.fda.gov/about-fda/fda-leadership-1907-today/lester-crawford; Stephanie Saul, "Former F.D.A. Chief Is Charged with Conflict," *The New York Times*, October 17, 2006, https://www.nytimes.com/2006/10/17/washington/former-fda-chief-is-charged-with-conflict.html.

20 Peter Doshi, "Revolving Doors: Board Memberships, Hedge Funds, and the FDA Chiefs Responsible for Regulating Industry," *BMJ* 385 (May 8, 2024): q975, https://doi.org/10.1136/bmj.q975.

21 OGE, "OGE Agency Profile 2024," US Office of Government Ethics, October 31, 2024, https://www.oge.gov/web/OGE.nsf/0/2523C11C3F34E38885258BC8004788D1/$FILE/US%20Office%20of%20Government%20Ethics_2024%20Agency%20Profile.pdf.

22 Foley, "Trust Issues Deepen as yet Another FDA Commissioner Joins the Pharmaceutical Industry"; "Our Leadership," Alnylam, accessed July 9, 2025, https://www.alnylam.com/about-alnylam/alnylam-leadership.

23 Jeffrey Bien and Vinay Prasad, "Future Jobs of FDA's Haematology-Oncology Reviewers," *BMJ* 354 (September 27, 2016): i5055, https://doi.org/10.1136/bmj.i5055.

24 Charles Piller, "FDA's Revolving Door: Companies Often Hire Agency Staffers Who Managed Their Successful Drug Reviews," Science, July 5, 2018, https://www.science.

org/content/article/fda-s-revolving-door-companies-often-hire-agency-staffers-who-managed-their-successful.
25 Wayne A. Ray et al., "Atypical Antipsychotic Drugs and the Risk of Sudden Cardiac Death," *New England Journal of Medicine* 360, no. 3 (January 15, 2009): 225–35, https://doi.org/10.1056/NEJMoa0806994.
26 Piller, "FDA's Revolving Door: Companies Often Hire Agency Staffers Who Managed Their Successful Drug Reviews."
27 "FDA Panel Snubs Seroquel as 1st Choice Depression Treatment," ABC News, April 8, 2009, https://abcnews.go.com/Health/Healthday/story?id=7294641&page=1; James Floyd and Sidney Wolfe to Thomas Laughren, "Letter Urging FDA to Reject Use of Quetiapine Fumarate (Seroquel) in Depression," April 9, 2009, https://www.citizen.org/article/letter-urging-fda-to-reject-use-of-quetiapine-fumarate-seroquel-in-depression/.
28 Piller, "FDA's Revolving Door: Companies Often Hire Agency Staffers Who Managed Their Successful Drug Reviews."
29 "Thomas Laughren," LinkedIn, accessed July 13, 2025, https://www.linkedin.com/in/thomas-laughren-1b568364/.
30 "Advisory Board," Vistagen, accessed July 13, 2025, https://www.vistagen.com/about/advisory-board.
31 Peter Doshi, "The FDA and Moderna's Cosy Relationship: How Lax Rules Enable a Revolving Door Culture," *BMJ* 383 (November 1, 2023): p2486, https://doi.org/10.1136/bmj.p2486.
32 "Doran Fink, MD, PhD," LinkedIn, accessed June 13, 2024, https://www.linkedin.com/in/doran-fink-md-phd-473a20a3/.
33 "Jaya Goswami, M.D., M.A.," LinkedIn, accessed June 13, 2024, https://www.linkedin.com/in/jaya-goswami-m-d-m-a-81b678b9/.
34 Doshi, "The FDA and Moderna's Cosy Relationship."
35 "Moderna Receives U.S. FDA Approval for RSV Vaccine MRESVIA(R)," Moderna, May 31, 2024, https://investors.modernatx.com/news/news-details/2024/Moderna-Receives-U.S.-FDA-Approval-for-RSV-Vaccine-mRESVIAR/default.aspx.
36 Isaac Arnsdorf, "Trump's Vaccine Czar Refuses to Give Up Stock in Drug Company Involved in His Government Role," ProPublica, September 23, 2020, https://www.propublica.org/article/trumps-vaccine-czar-refuses-to-give-up-stock-in-drug-company-involved-in-his-government-role.
37 "Sanofi and GSK Selected for Operation Warp Speed to Supply United States Government with 100 Million Doses of COVID-19 Vaccine," GSK, July 31, 2020, https://www.gsk.com/en-gb/media/press-releases/sanofi-and-gsk-selected-for-operation-warp-speed-to-supply-united-states-government-with-100-million-doses-of-covid-19-vaccine/.
38 Kyle LaHucik, "He Authorized Moderna's Vaccine 6 Months Ago. Now, Ex-FDA Chief Hahn Joins Biotech's Backer," Fierce Biotech, June 14, 2021, https://www.fiercebiotech.com/biotech/six-months-after-granting-moderna-covid-19-eua-ex-fda-commish-joins-biotech-s-founding.
39 "Stephen M. Hahn," Flagship Pioneering, accessed June 14, 2024, https://web.archive.org/web/20240710200022/https://www.flagshippioneering.com/people/stephen-m-hahn-2.
40 "18 USC 207: Restrictions on Former Officers, Employees, and Elected Officials of the Executive and Legislative Branches," Office of the Law Revision Counsel United

States Code, accessed June 13, 2024, https://uscode.house.gov/view.xhtml?req=granuleid:USC-prelim-title18-section207&num=0&edition=prelim.

41 "Summary of Post-Employment Restrictions of 18 U.S.C. § 207," US Department of Justice, July 29, 2004: 3, https://www.justice.gov/sites/default/files/jmd/legacy/2014/05/01/oge-summ-of-207-2004.pdf.

42 Ibid., 5.

43 "18 U.S.C. § 207: Applicability Chart," United States Office of Government Ethics, accessed June 13, 2024, https://www.oge.gov/Web/oge.nsf/0/6F0B33C29C0E772E852585B6005A1BB7/$FILE/Combined%20Senior%20Employees.pdf.

44 "5 USC 5315: Positions at Level IV," Office of the Law Revision Counsel United States Code, accessed June 13, 2024, https://uscode.house.gov/view.xhtml?req=(title:5%20section:5315%20edition:prelim).

45 "Salary Table No. 2024-EX," US Office of Personnel Management, accessed June 21, 2025, https://www.opm.gov/policy-data-oversight/pay-leave/salaries-wages/salary-tables/pdf/2024/EX.pdf.

46 "Employment—Current Month—IBM Cognos PowerPlay Studio," FedScope, accessed May 29, 2025, https://www.fedscope.opm.gov/ibmcognos/bi/v1/disp?b_action=powerPlayService&m_encoding=UTF-8&BZ=1AAABnsT72MN42oVOsW6DQAz9mTNph0Y_wyVhYIDjUBiANLBXlFzSqsBFcB3y9xUwpFWGvidL9vN7lp2yWJdVcVRpHIzWDDqNn4DocyNI4jZU6PncQ0%7EtfIHRZiO5UKREtAWiZ2fKqvAo94ew2gdASWN6q3sLlJxNe9IDiAg87OtOgxuvDnXzVV%7E0_Ka6a2tune7tCkQMlFyXzV%7E73QWEL0Aov4dhmTLT248p68SlXMsiz5Ws0iLPw0wF%7E_Wc6DU4IzKOiJwjYwyZQEbIJjIWXnTf3IAQ6ASEYdsC_pkZ7eMpQJ8B7YBcBNIc6B3IXwR_F9gMIHey%7EwKfOXfLO3MtTyz4AbZLbJc%3D.

47 "Food and Drug Administration (FDA) Highest Paid Employees," OpenPayrolls, accessed June 13, 2024, https://openpayrolls.com/rank/highest-paid-employees/food-and-drug-administration.

48 Daniel L. Koffsky, "Who Qualifies as a 'Very Senior' Employee Under 18 U.S.C. § 207(d)(1)(B)," US Department of Justice, January 19, 2017, https://www.justice.gov/olc/file/1078066/dl.

49 "3 USC Ch. 2: Chapter 2—Office and Compensation of President," Office of the Law Revision Counsel United States Code, accessed June 13, 2024, https://uscode.house.gov/view.xhtml?path=/prelim@title3/chapter2&edition=prelim.

50 Angelica Peebles, "Former FDA Commissioner Scott Gottlieb Joins Pfizer's Board of Directors," CNBC, June 27, 2019, https://www.cnbc.com/2019/06/27/former-fda-commissioner-scott-gottlieb-joins-pfizers-board.html.

51 "18 USC 207: Restrictions on Former Officers, Employees, and Elected Officials of the Executive and Legislative Branches."

52 Joseph R. Biden Jr., "Executive Order 13989: Ethics Commitments by Executive Branch Personnel," Federal Register, January 20, 2021, https://www.oge.gov/Web/OGE.nsf/0/16D49D01588276F985258668004F1094/$FILE/Exec.%20Order%2013989.pdf.

53 Ibid., 7029–30.

54 "Covered Executive Branch Official," Legal Information Institute, accessed June 13, 2024, https://www.law.cornell.edu/definitions/uscode.php?width=840&height=800&iframe=true&def_id=26-USC-1052080537-1976857055&term_occur=999&term_src=title:26:subtitle:A:chapter:1:subchapter:B:part:VI:section:162.

55 Donald J. Trump, "Executive Order 13770: Ethics Commitments by Executive Branch Personnel," Federal Register, January 28, 2017, https://www.federalregister.gov/documents/2017/02/03/2017-02450/ethics-commitments-by-executive-branch-appointees.
56 Biden Jr., "Executive Order 13989: Ethics Commitments by Executive Branch Personnel," 7030.
57 Melissa L. Laurenza, Kenneth A. Gross, and Kevin M. Paulsen, "Ethics Changes for Trump Administration Appointees," Akin, February 10, 2025, https://www.akingump.com/en/insights/alerts/ethics-changes-for-trump-administration-appointees.
58 Jacob R. Straus, "Ethics Pledges and Other Executive Branch Restrictions Since 1993: Historical, Current Practices, and Options For," Congressional Research Service, February 23, 2021, https://sgp.fas.org/crs/misc/R44974.pdf.
59 "Summary of Post-Employment Restrictions of 18 U.S.C. § 207," 4.
60 Craig Holman and Caralyn Esser, "Slowing the Federal Revolving Door," Public Citizen, July 22, 2019, https://www.citizen.org/article/slowing-the-federal-revolving-door/.
61 John P. Sarbanes, "For the People Act of 2021," H.R. 1 (2021), https://www.congress.gov/bill/117th-congress/house-bill/1#:~:text=Shown%20Here%3A&text=This%20bill%20addresses%20voter%20access,%2Dmail%20and%20early%20voting); "2 U.S. Code § 1602 - Definitions," Legal Information Institute, accessed July 12, 2025, https://www.law.cornell.edu/uscode/text/2/1602.
62 Biden Jr., "Executive Order 13989: Ethics Commitments by Executive Branch Personnel."
63 CBO, "Comparing the Compensation of Federal and Private-Sector Employees in 2022," Congressional Budget Office, April 2024, https://www.cbo.gov/publication/60235.
64 Scott Gottlieb, "FDA 21st Century Cures Workforce Planning Report to Congress," US Food & Drug Administration, June 2018, https://web.archive.org/web/20250118162321/https://www.fda.gov/media/114163/download.
65 Robert E. Mutch, *Buying the Vote: A History of Campaign Finance Reform* (Oxford; New York: Oxford University Press, 2014).
66 Ibid., 40.
67 Jordi Blanes I Vidal, Mirko Draca, and Christian Fons-Rosen, "Revolving Door Lobbyists," *American Economic Review* 102, no. 7 (December 2012): 3731–48, https://doi.org/10.1257/aer.102.7.3731.
68 Jason W. Ridge, Amy Ingram, and Aaron D. Hill, "Beyond Lobbying Expenditures: How Lobbying Breadth and Political Connectedness Affect Firm Outcomes," *Academy of Management Journal* 60, no. 3 (March 15, 2016): 1147, 1156, https://doi.org/10.5465/amj.2015.0584.
69 Gottlieb, "FDA 21st Century Cures Workforce Planning Report to Congress," 10.
70 C. Joseph Ross Daval et al., "Association of Advisory Committee Votes with US Food and Drug Administration Decision-Making on Prescription Drugs, 2010–2021," *JAMA Health Forum* 4, no. 7 (July 7, 2023): e231718, https://doi.org/10.1001/jamahealthforum.2023.1718.
71 Food and Drug Administration Modernization Act of 1997.
72 18 USC 208: Acts Affecting a Personal Financial Interest," Office of the Law Revision Counsel United States Code, accessed June 13, 2024, https://uscode.house.gov/view.xhtml?req=granuleid:USC-prelim-title18-section208&num=0&edition=prelim.

73 Public Health Service, "42 CFR 50.603—Definitions," Code of Federal Regulations, May 28, 2025, https://www.ecfr.gov/current/title-42/chapter-I/subchapter-D/part-50/subpart-F/section-50.603.
74 Advisory Committee Oversight and Management Staff, "FDA Advisory Committees: Financial Conflicts of Interest Overview," accessed June 13, 2024, https://www.fda.gov/media/87421/download#:~:text=What%20is%20a%20%E2%80%9Cconflict%20of%20interest%E2%80%9D%3F&text=A%20conflict%20of%20interest%2C%20for,work%20on%20the%20advisory%20committee.&text=18%20U.S.C; "A Bit More about Financial Interests," National Institutes of Health, accessed June 13, 2024, https://ethics.od.nih.gov/bit-more-about-financial-interests.
75 FDA, "Special Government Employee (SGE) Resources," US Food & Drug Administration, February 18, 2022, https://www.fda.gov/about-fda/ethics/special-government-employee-sge-resources.
76 "FDA-3410: Confidential Financial Disclosure Report for Special Government Employees," US Food & Drug Administration, accessed June 13, 2024: 3 https://www.fda.gov/about-fda/ethics/special-government-employee-sge-resources.
77 FDA, "Guidance for the Public, FDA Advisory Committee Members, and FDA Staff: Public Availability of Advisory Committee Members' Financial Interest Information and Waivers," US Food and Drug Administration, March 2014, https://www.fda.gov/media/83188/download.
78 Ibid., 10; Food and Drug Administration, "73 FR 45458 - Guidance for the Public, FDA Advisory Committee Members, and FDA Staff on Procedures for Determining Conflict of Interest and Eligibility for Participation in FDA Advisory Committees; Availability," Code of Federal Regulations, August 5, 2008, https://www.federalregister.gov/documents/2008/08/05/E8-17998/guidance-for-the-public-fda-advisory-committee-members-and-fda-staff-on-procedures-for-determining.
79 Food and Drug Administration, "73 FR 45458"; FDA, *Guidance for the Public, FDA Advisory Committee Members*, 7.
80 Food and Drug Administration Amendments Act of 2007; Susan F. Wood and Jillian K. Mador, "Uncapping Conflict of Interest?," *Science* 340, no. 6137 (June 7, 2013): 1172–3, https://doi.org/10.1126/science.1231955.
81 Food and Drug Administration Safety and Innovation Act; Wood and Mador, "Uncapping Conflict of Interest?"
82 Janet Woodcock, "PDUFA V: Medical Innovation, Jobs, and Patients," Congressional Hearing Testimony, July 7, 2011, https://www.govinfo.gov/content/pkg/CHRG-112hhrg72917/pdf/CHRG-112hhrg72917.pdf.
83 Ned Feder, "POGO Letter Urges FDA Not to Weaken Conflict of Interest Standards at Center for Drug Evaluation and Research," POGO, August 11, 2011, https://www.pogo.org/policy-letters/pogo-letter-urges-fda-not-to-weaken-conflict-of-interest-standards-at-center-for-drug-evaluation-and-research.
84 Darren E. Zinner et al., "Participation of Academic Scientists in Relationships with Industry," *Health Affairs* 28, no. 6 (December 2009): 1814–25, https://doi.org/10.1377/hlthaff.28.6.1814.
85 Todd B. Mendelson et al., "Conflicts of Interest in Cardiovascular Clinical Practice Guidelines," *Archives of Internal Medicine* 171, no. 6 (March 28, 2011): 577–84, https://doi.org/10.1001/archinternmed.2011.96.
86 Wood and Mador, "Uncapping Conflict of Interest?"

87 "Susan F. Wood," Milken Institute School of Public Health, accessed June 13, 2024, https://publichealth.gwu.edu/departments/health-policy-and-management/susan-wood; "Conflict-of-Interest Restrictions Needed to Ensure Strong FDA Review," ScienceDaily, June 6, 2013, https://www.sciencedaily.com/releases/2013/06/130606154706.htm.

88 Wood and Mador, "Uncapping Conflict of Interest?"

89 Colleen O. Davis, "Red Tape Tightrope: Regulating Financial Conflicts of Interest in FDA Advisory Committees," *Washington University Law Review* 91, no. 6 (2014): 1591–632, https://openscholarship.wustl.edu/law_lawreview/vol91/iss6/8.

90 O. Lidegaard et al., "Risk of Venous Thromboembolism from Use of Oral Contraceptives Containing Different Progestogens and Oestrogen Doses: Danish Cohort Study, 2001–9," *BMJ* 343 (October 25, 2011): d6423, https://doi.org/10.1136/bmj.d6423.

91 Jeanne Lenzer and Keith Epstein, "The Yaz Men: Members of FDA Panel Reviewing the Risks of Popular Bayer Contraceptive Had Industry Ties," *Washington Monthly*, January 9, 2012, http://washingtonmonthly.com/2012/01/09/the-yaz-men-members-of-fda-panel-reviewing-the-risks-of-popular-bayer-contraceptive-had-industry-ties/.

92 "20050223 Conflicts of Committee on Cox-2 Inhibitors," Center for Science in the Public Interest, February 23, 2005, https://www.cspinet.org/sites/default/files/media/documents/resource/cox2_conflicts_of_committee.pdf.

93 The Associated Press, "10 on FDA Vioxx Panel Had Ties to Companies," NBC News, February 25, 2005, http://www.nbcnews.com/health/health-news/10-fda-vioxx-panel-had-ties-companies-flna1C9440119.

94 Gardiner Harris and Alex Berenson, "10 Voters on Panel Backing Pain Pills Had Industry Ties," *The New York Times*, February 25, 2005, sec. U.S., https://www.nytimes.com/2005/02/25/politics/10-voters-on-panel-backing-pain-pills-had-industry-ties.html.

95 The Associated Press, "Painkiller Bextrapulled [sic] from Market," NBC News, April 7, 2005, https://www.nbcnews.com/health/health-news/painkiller-bextrapulled-market-flna1c9443740; John K. Jenkins and Paul J. Seligman, "Analysis and Recommendations for Agency Action Regarding Non Anti-Inflammatory Drugs and Cardiovascular Risk," Memorandum, US Food & Drug Administration, April 6, 2005, https://www.fda.gov/media/74279/download.

96 The Associated Press, "10 on FDA Vioxx Panel Had Ties to Companies"; Snigdha Prakash and Vikki Valentine, "Timeline: The Rise and Fall of Vioxx," *NPR*, November 10, 2007, sec. Vioxx: The Downfall of a Drug, https://www.npr.org/2007/11/10/5470430/timeline-the-rise-and-fall-of-vioxx; Graham et al., "Risk of Acute Myocardial Infarction"; Graham, "Testimony of David J. Graham, MD, MPH."

97 Peter Lurie et al., "Financial Conflict of Interest Disclosure and Voting Patterns at Food and Drug Administration Drug Advisory Committee Meetings," *JAMA* 295, no. 16 (April 26, 2006): 1921–8, https://doi.org/10.1001/jama.295.16.1921.

98 Rishad Khan et al., "Characteristics and Conflicts of Interest at Food and Drug Administration Gastrointestinal Drug Advisory Committee Meetings," *PLoS ONE* 16, no. 5 (2021): e0252155, https://doi.org/10.1371/journal.pone.0252155.

99 Matthew V. Abola and Vinay Prasad, "Characteristics and Conflicts of Public Speakers at Meetings of the Oncologic Drugs Advisory Committee to the US Food

and Drug Administration," *JAMA Internal Medicine* 176, no. 3 (March 2016): 389–91, https://doi.org/10.1001/jamainternmed.2015.7805.
100 Matthew S. McCoy et al., "Conflicts of Interest of Public Speakers at Meetings of the Anesthetic and Analgesic Drug Products Advisory Committee," *JAMA Internal Medicine* 178, no. 7 (July 2018): 996–7, https://doi.org/10.1001/jamainternmed.2018.1325.
101 Sharon Batt and Adriane Fugh-Berman, "What Needs to Change at the FDA?," PharmedOut, September 20, 2022, https://georgetown.app.box.com/s/u1gtp59iy4as18px53rcvh44n3aneu2y.
102 Aaron Glickman, "Conflict of Interest among Public Speakers at FDA Advisory Committees," Penn LDI, April 23, 2018, https://ldi.upenn.edu/our-work/research-updates/conflict-of-interest-among-public-speakers-at-fda-advisory-committees/.
103 Genevieve Pham-Kanter, "Revisiting Financial Conflicts of Interest in FDA Advisory Committees," *The Milbank Quarterly* 92, no. 3 (September 9, 2014): 446–70, https://doi.org/10.1111/1468-0009.12073.
104 Charles Piller, "Hidden Conflicts? Pharma Payments to FDA Advisers after Drug Approvals Spark Ethical Concerns," Science, July 5, 2018, https://www.science.org/content/article/hidden-conflicts-pharma-payments-fda-advisers-after-drug-approvals-spark-ethical.
105 "FDA Advisory Committee Votes in Favor of Abbott's First-of-Its-Kind Triclip System to Treat People with a Leaky Tricuspid Heart Valve," Abbott, February 13, 2024, https://abbott.mediaroom.com/2024-02-13-FDA-Advisory-Committee-Votes-in-Favor-of-Abbotts-First-of-Its-Kind-TriClip-TM-System-to-Treat-People-With-a-Leaky-Tricuspid-Heart-Valve.
106 Holly K. Hacker and David Hilzenrath, "Ten Doctors on FDA Panel Reviewing Abbott Heart Device Had Financial Ties with Company," *KFF Health News* (blog), April 8, 2024, https://kffhealthnews.org/news/article/abbott-triclip-fda-advisory-panel-payments-funding-conflict-of-interest/.
107 FDA, "FDA Commissioner Makary Announces New Policy on Individuals Serving on FDA Advisory Committees," US Food & Drug Administration, April 17, 2025, https://www.fda.gov/news-events/press-announcements/fda-commissioner-makary-announces-new-policy-individuals-serving-fda-advisory-committees.
108 FDA, "FDA at a Glance October 2024."
109 Public Health Security and Bioterrorism Preparedness and Response Act of 2002.
110 Food and Drug Administration Amendments Act of 2007.
111 Christina Jewett, "F.D.A.'s Drug Industry Fees Fuel Concerns Over Influence," *The New York Times*, September 15, 2022, sec. Health, https://www.nytimes.com/2022/09/15/health/fda-drug-industry-fees.html.
112 "Industry Influence on Drug and Medical Device Safety at FDA: $700 Million in Lobbying Buys Significant Access," Union of Concerned Scientists, March 29, 2012, https://www.ucsusa.org/sites/default/files/legacy/assets/documents/scientific_integrity/industry-influence-drug-medical-device-safety-FDA.pdf.
113 "Industry Profile: Pharmaceuticals/Health Products," OpenSecrets, April 24, 2025, https://www.opensecrets.org/federal-lobbying/industries/summary?id=H04.
114 Mutch, *Buying the Vote*.

115 "Contribution Limits," Federal Election Commission, accessed June 13, 2024, https://www.fec.gov/help-candidates-and-committees/candidate-taking-receipts/contribution-limits/.
116 R. Sam Garrett, "The State of Campaign Finance Policy: Recent Developments and Issues for Congress," Congressional Research Service, July 29, 2025, https://www.congress.gov/crs-product/R41542.
117 "Pharmaceuticals / Health Products Summary," OpenSecrets, accessed May 30, 2025, https://www.opensecrets.org/industries/totals?cycle=2022&ind=H04.
118 Mutch, *Buying the Vote*.
119 "Pharmaceuticals / Health Products Summary."
120 FDA, "Performance Report to Congress: Prescription Drug User Fee Act FY 2023," US Food and Drug Administration, accessed June 13, 2024: 10, https://www.fda.gov/media/177976/download?attachment.
121 FDA, "PDUFA Reauthorization Performance Goals and Procedures Fiscal Years 2023 through 2027," US Food & Drug Administration, August 23, 2021, https://www.fda.gov/media/151712/download.
122 Zelenay, "The Prescription Drug User Fee Act."
123 David E. Wheadon, "FDA User Fees 2012: How Innovation Helps Patients and Jobs," Congressional Hearing Testimony, April 18, 2012, https://www.congress.gov/112/chrg/CHRG-112hhrg78635/CHRG-112hhrg78635.pdf.
124 Ferdous Al-Faruque, "MDUFA V: We Have a Deal," Regulatory Focus, March 8, 2022, https://www.raps.org/news-and-articles/news-articles/2022/3/mdufa-v-we-have-a-deal.
125 FDA, "Total Product Life Cycle Advisory Program (TAP)," US Food & Drug Administration, July 1, 2024, https://www.fda.gov/medical-devices/how-study-and-market-your-device/total-product-life-cycle-advisory-program-tap.
126 Staffs of the Committee on Oversight and Reform and Committee on Energy and Commerce, "The High Price of Aduhelm's Approval: An Investigation into FDA's Atypical Review Process and Biogen's Aggressive Launch Plans."
127 Woodcock, "PDUFA V: Medical Innovation, Jobs, and Patients," 37–8.
128 Andrew von Eschenbach, "Toward a 21st-Century FDA," Manhattan Institute, April 15, 2012, https://manhattan.institute/article/toward-a-21st-century-fda/.
129 Andrew von Eschenbach, "Medical Innovation: How the U.S. Can Retain Its Lead," *The Wall Street Journal*, February 14, 2012, https://www.wsj.com/articles/SB10001424052970203646004577215403399350874.
130 Richard Horton, "Vioxx, the Implosion of Merck, and Aftershocks at the FDA," *The Lancet* 364, no. 9450 (November 5, 2004): 1995, https://doi.org/10.1016/S0140-6736(04)17523-5.
131 Annalee Armstrong, "For Every Million-Dollar Gene Therapy, Peter Marks Gets an Email from FDA Chief Robert Califf," Fierce Pharma, May 8, 2024, https://www.fiercepharma.com/pharma/every-million-dollar-gene-therapy-peter-marks-gets-email-fda-chief-robert-califf.
132 Kesselheim and Avorn, "The F.D.A. Has Reached a New Low."
133 Ellen Nakashima and Lisa Rein, "FDA Staffers Sue Agency over Surveillance of Personal E-mail," *The Washington Post*, January 29, 2012, https://www.washingtonpost.com/world/national-security/fda-staffers-sue-agency-over-surveillance-of-personal-e-mail/2012/01/23/gIQAj34DbQ_story.html.

134 Ibid; Eric Lichtblau and Scott Shane, "Vast F.D.A. Effort Tracked E-mails of Its Scientists," *The New York Times*, July 14, 2012, sec. U.S., https://www.nytimes.com/2012/07/15/us/fda-surveillance-of-scientists-spread-to-outside-critics.html.
135 Jonathan H. Marks, *The Perils of Partnership: Industry Influence, Institutional Integrity, and Public Health* (New York City: Oxford University Press, 2019), 67.

## 8 Why Do Doctors Accept This?

1 Zuger, "A Doctor's Guide to What to Read on the Opioid Crisis."
2 Thomas S. Kuhn, *The Structure of Scientific Revolutions*, 3rd Edition (Chicago, IL: University of Chicago Press, 1996).
3 Ibid., 5–6.
4 Ibid., 5.
5 Ibid.
6 "Table A-17: MCAT and GPAs for Applicants and Matriculants to U.S. MD-Granting Medical Schools by Primary Undergraduate Major, 2023–2024," Association of American Medical Colleges, October 25, 2023, https://www.aamc.org/media/6061/download; "What Is Pre-med? Exploring the Path from College to Medical School," Berry College, April 4, 2022, https://www.berry.edu/articles/blog/2022/pre-med-path-from-college-to-medical-school.
7 "What's on the MCAT® Exam?," Association of American Medical Colleges, 2020, https://students-residents.aamc.org/media/9261/download.
8 "What to Expect in Medical School," The Princeton Review, accessed June 26, 2024, https://www.princetonreview.com/med-school-advice/what-to-expect-in-medical-school.
9 Kevin Jubbal, "Medical School Timeline (All 4 Years Explained)," Med School Insiders, March 1, 2022, https://medschoolinsiders.com/pre-med/4-years-of-medical-school-timeline/.
10 "What to Expect in Medical School."
11 Jubbal, "Medical School Timeline (All 4 Years Explained)."
12 Brendan Murphy, "Key Data Trends Applicants Should Keep Tabs on before Match Day," AMA, March 1, 2024, https://www.ama-assn.org/medical-students/preparing-residency/key-data-trends-applicants-should-keep-tabs-match-day; "What Is Residency?," AMA, May 20, 2024, https://www.ama-assn.org/medical-students/preparing-residency/what-residency#:~:text=It%20is%20a%20supervised%20clinical,guidance%20of%20experienced%20attending%20physicians.
13 "About Physician Licensure," Federation of State Medical Boards, accessed June 26, 2024, https://www.fsmb.org/u.s.-medical-regulatory-trends-and-actions/guide-to-medical-regulation-in-the-united-states/about-physician-licensure/.
14 "What Is a Fellow Doctor? Understanding Medical Fellowships," Med School Insiders, October 26, 2022, https://medschoolinsiders.com/lifestyle/medical-fellowship-what-is-a-fellow-doctor/.
15 "Fellowship Programs," Johns Hopkins Medicine, accessed June 26, 2024, https://www.hopkinsmedicine.org/medicine/education/fellows.
16 John Abramson, *Overdosed America: The Broken Promise of American Medicine*, 1st Edition (New York City: HarperCollins, 2004), 119.

17 Kuhn, *The Structure of Scientific Revolutions*, 177.
18 Adam Cifu, Vinay Prasad, and D. Rani Nandiwada, "Reforming Medical Education," *Sensible Medicine* (blog), September 20, 2022, https://www.sensible-med.com/p/our-new-analysis-of-myocarditis-after.
19 Abramson, *Overdosed America*, xiv; Abramson, *Sickening*, xx.
20 Garret A. FitzGerald and Carlo Patrono, "The Coxibs, Selective Inhibitors of Cyclooxygenase-2," *New England Journal of Medicine* 345, no. 6 (August 9, 2001): 433–42, https://doi.org/10.1056/NEJM200108093450607; Abramson, *Overdosed America*, 33.
21 Graham et al., "Risk of Acute Myocardial Infarction"; Graham, "Testimony of David J. Graham, MD, MPH."
22 Claire Bombardier et al., "Comparison of Upper Gastrointestinal Toxicity of Rofecoxib and Naproxen in Patients with Rheumatoid Arthritis," *New England Journal of Medicine* 343, no. 21 (November 23, 2000): 1520–8, https://doi.org/10.1056/NEJM200011233432103.
23 FitzGerald and Patrono, "The Coxibs, Selective Inhibitors of Cyclooxygenase-2."
24 Abramson, *Sickening*, 5.
25 FitzGerald and Patrono, "The Coxibs, Selective Inhibitors of Cyclooxygenase-2."
26 Abramson, *Overdosed America*, 34.
27 Abramson, *Sickening*, 5–6.
28 Abramson, *Overdosed America*, 36.
29 Joe Neel, "Medical Journal: Vioxx Paper Flawed," NPR, December 8, 2005, https://www.npr.org/2005/12/08/5045087/medical-journal-vioxx-paper-flawed; Gregory D. Curfman, Stephen Morrissey, and Jeffrey M. Drazen, "Expression of Concern: Bombardier et al., 'Comparison of Upper Gastrointestinal Toxicity of Rofecoxib and Naproxen in Patients with Rheumatoid Arthritis,' N Engl J Med 2000;343:1520–8," *New England Journal of Medicine* 353, no. 26 (December 29, 2005): 2813–14, https://doi.org/10.1056/NEJMe058314.
30 Abramson, *Overdosed America*, 35.
31 David Armstrong, "How the New England Journal Missed Warning Signs on Vioxx," *The Wall Street Journal*, May 15, 2006, https://www.wsj.com/amp/articles/SB114765430315252591.
32 NIHCM Foundation, "Prescription Drug Expenditures in 2001: Another Year of Escalating Costs," National Institute for Health Care Management Research and Educational Foundation, May 6, 2002, https://web.archive.org/web/20030625210039/https://www.nihcm.org/spending2001.pdf.
33 Krumholz et al., "What Have We Learnt from Vioxx?"
34 "Evaluating Health Information," UCSF Health, accessed May 30, 2025, https://www.ucsfhealth.org/education/evaluating-health-information; Laura Kurtzman, "US News Ranks Medical and Nursing Schools in Top 10," UCSF, May 10, 2023, https://www.ucsf.edu/news/2023/05/425331/us-news-ranks-medical-and-nursing-schools-top-10.
35 Djulbegovic and Guyatt, "Progress in Evidence-Based Medicine."
36 Graham et al., "Risk of Acute Myocardial Infarction"; Graham, "Testimony of David J. Graham, MD, MPH"
37 Jeanne Lenzer, "Crisis Deepens at the US Food and Drug Administration," *BMJ* 329, no. 7478 (December 2, 2004): 1308, https://doi.org/10.1136/bmj.329.7478.1308; Gøtzsche, *Deadly Medicines and Organised Crime*, 239.

38 "Steven Galson, MD, MPH," LinkedIn, accessed July 4, 2025, https://www.linkedin.com/in/steven-galson-md-mph-4414bb108/details/experience/.
39 Gøtzsche, *Deadly Medicines and Organised Crime*, 239–40.
40 Lenzer, "Crisis Deepens at the US Food and Drug Administration"; Jeanne Lenzer, "Public Interest Group Accuses FDA of Trying to Discredit Whistleblower," *BMJ* 329, no. 7477 (November 25, 2004): 1255, https://doi.org/10.1136/bmj.329.7477.1255-a.
41 Charles E. Grassley to Raymond V. Gilmartin, "Chairman Grassley Questions Merck about Communication with the FDA on Vioxx," October 14, 2004, https://www.finance.senate.gov/chairmans-news/chairman-grassley-questions-merck-about-communication-with-the-fda-on-vioxx.
42 "U.S. Physicians: Medical Misinformation Is Harming Patients' Health," de Beaumont Foundation, March 29, 2023, https://debeaumont.org/wp-content/uploads/2023/03/misinformation-poll-brief-FINAL.pdf.
43 Bashar Qumseya et al., "Barriers to Clinical Practice Guideline Implementation among Physicians: A Physician Survey," *International Journal of General Medicine* 2021, no. 14 (November 2, 2021): 7591–8, https://doi.org/10.2147/IJGM.S333501.
44 Susan R. Bailey, "Words and Actions That Erode Trust in the CDC Hurt Us All," AMA, September 15, 2020, https://www.ama-assn.org/about/leadership/words-and-actions-erode-trust-cdc-hurt-us-all.
45 "Surveys of Trust in the U.S. Health Care System: Physician Survey," National Opinion Research Center and American Board of Internal Medicine Foundation, May 21, 2021, https://buildingtrust.org/wp-content/uploads/2021/05/20210518_ABIM_Foundation_Topline1_Physician-Survey.pdf.
46 Spherix Global Insights, "Specialty Physicians Weigh in with Opinions about the US Food and Drug Administration," PR Newswire, July 27, 2021, https://www.prnewswire.com/news-releases/specialty-physicians-weigh-in-with-opinions-about-the-us-food-and-drug-administration-301342509.html.
47 Staffs of the Committee on Oversight and Reform and Committee on Energy and Commerce, "The High Price of Aduhelm's Approval: An Investigation into FDA's Atypical Review Process and Biogen's Aggressive Launch Plans."
48 Kirsten E. Austad, Jerry Avorn, and Aaron S. Kesselheim, "Medical Students' Exposure to and Attitudes about the Pharmaceutical Industry: A Systematic Review," ed. Joel Lexchin, *PLoS Med* 8, no. 5 (May 24, 2011): e1001037, https://doi.org/10.1371/journal.pmed.1001037.
49 Frederick S. Sierles et al., "Medical Students' Exposure to and Attitudes about Drug Company Interactions: A National Survey," *JAMA* 294, no. 9 (September 7, 2005): 1034–42, https://doi.org/10.1001/jama.294.9.1034.
50 Colette DeJong et al., "Pharmaceutical Industry–Sponsored Meals and Physician Prescribing Patterns for Medicare Beneficiaries," *JAMA Internal Medicine* 176, no. 8 (August 2016): 1114–22, https://doi.org/10.1001/jamainternmed.2016.2765.
51 Taeho Greg Rhee and Joseph S. Ross, "Association Between industry Payments to Physicians and Gabapentinoid Prescribing," *JAMA Internal Medicine* 179, no. 10 (July 8, 2019): 1425–8, https://doi.org/10.1001/jamainternmed.2019.1082.
52 Shahram Ahari, "Under the Influence: Can We Provide Doctors an Alternative to Biased Drug Reviews," Congressional Hearing Testimony, March 12, 2008, https://www.aging.senate.gov/imo/media/doc/hr190sa.pdf.

53 Aaron P. Mitchell et al., "Are Financial Payments from the Pharmaceutical Industry Associated with Physician Prescribing?: A Systematic Review," *Annals of Internal Medicine* 174, no. 3 (November 24, 2020): 353–61, https://doi.org/10.7326/M20-5665.
54 Scott E. Hadland et al., "Association of Pharmaceutical Industry Marketing of Opioid Products with Mortality from Opioid-Related Overdoses," *JAMA Network Open* 2, no. 1 (January 18, 2019): e186007, https://doi.org/10.1001/jamanetworkopen.2018.6007.
55 Yavar Moghimi, "The 'PharmFree' Campaign: Educating Medical Students about Industry Influence," *PLoS Med* 3, no. 1 (January 31, 2006): e30, https://doi.org/10.1371/journal.pmed.0030030.
56 "AMSA's PharmFree Campaign," AMSA.org, June 15, 2002, https://web.archive.org/web/20020615171709/https://www.amsa.org/prof/pharmfree.cfm.
57 "Step 1. Educate Yourself," AMSA.org, May 29, 2002, https://web.archive.org/web/20020529051119/http://www.amsa.org/prof/step1.cfm; "An Overview of the Literature: 'Does That One Slice of Pizza Matter?,'" American Medical Students Association, accessed June 26, 2024, https://web.archive.org/web/20050903051949/http://www.amsa.org/prof/nofreelunch.pdf.
58 "AMSA PharmFree Medical Student Pledge," American Medical Students Association, accessed June 26, 2024, https://web.archive.org/web/20040411153801/http://www.amsa.org/prof/pharmfreepledge.pdf.
59 "Students Tell Pharma: 'Take Back Your Pens,'" AMSA, May 2005, https://web.archive.org/web/20050907030702/https:/www.amsa.org/news/focus/0305news.cfm.
60 Daniel J. Carlat et al., "The Updated AMSA Scorecard of Conflict-of-Interest Policies: A Survey of U.S. Medical Schools," *BMC Medical Education* 16 (August 12, 2016): Article 202, https://doi.org/10.1186/s12909-016-0725-y.
61 Duff Wilson, "Harvard Medical School in Ethics Quandary," *The New York Times*, March 2, 2009, sec. Business, https://www.nytimes.com/2009/03/03/business/03medschool.html; "Conflict of Interest Policies at Academic Medical Centers: Harvard Medical School," AMSA, 2008, https://web.archive.org/web/20080606102709/http://amsascorecard.org/institutions/112.
62 Charles E. Grassley to Jeffrey B. Kindler, March 3, 2009, https://graphics8.nytimes.com/packages/pdf/business/2009_03_03_Pfizer_letter.pdf.
63 "Industry Funding of Medical Education: Report of an AAMC Task Force," Association of American Medical Colleges, June 2008, https://www.aamc.org/media/24271/download.
64 Carlat et al., "The Updated AMSA Scorecard of Conflict-of-Interest Policies."
65 "AMSA PharmaFree Scorecard 2013: Executive Summary," AMSA, April 9, 2013, https://web.archive.org/web/20140114213846/http://www.amsascorecard.org/executive-summary.
66 Carlat et al., "The Updated AMSA Scorecard of Conflict-of-Interest Policies."
67 Kirsten E. Austad et al., "Changing Interactions between Physician Trainees and the Pharmaceutical Industry: A National Survey," *Journal of General Internal Medicine* 28, no. 8 (2013): 1064–71, https://doi.org/10.1007/s11606-013-2361-0.
68 Thomas Sullivan, "Medical Students Eating Lunches but Feeling Guilty," Policy & Medicine, May 6, 2018, https://web.archive.org/web/20210520173504/https://www.policymed.com/2013/03/medical-students-eating-lunches-but-feeling-guilty.html.
69 Tracy Weber Ornstein Charles, "Med Schools Flunk at Keeping Faculty off Pharma Speaking Circuit," ProPublica, December 19, 2010, https://www.propublica.org/article/medical-schools-policies-on-faculty-and-drug-company-speaking-circuit.

70 Robert Preidt, "Med School Students Still Get Gifts from Drug Companies: Survey," HealthDay, March 6, 2013, https://www.healthday.com/health-news/public-health/med-school-students-still-get-gifts-from-drug-companies-survey-673902.html.
71 Toby Keys et al., "Premedical Student Exposure to Pharmaceutical Marketing: Too Much, Too Soon?," *Family Medicine* 51, no. 9 (2019): 722–7, https://doi.org/10.22454/FamMed.2019.360469.
72 Sean O. Hogan et al., "Industry Payments Received by Residents During Training," *JAMA Network Open* 6, no. 10 (October 16, 2023): e2337904, https://doi.org/10.1001/jamanetworkopen.2023.37904.
73 Misop Han et al., "Trends in Industry Payments to Physicians in the First 6 Years after Graduate Medical Training," *JAMA Network Open* 5, no. 10 (October 19, 2022): e2237574, https://doi.org/10.1001/jamanetworkopen.2022.37574.
74 Waqas Haque, Magdalena Espinoza, and David Hsiehchen, "Industry Payments Are Prevalent and Contagious in Subspecialty Medical Education," *Journal of General Internal Medicine* 36, no. 10 (January 27, 2021): 3257–60, https://doi.org/10.1007/s11606-021-06612-z.
75 "AMSA Takes a Deeper Look into Conflicts of Interest as It Relates to Health Policy," AMSA, accessed June 26, 2024, https://www.amsa.org/advocate/activism-resources/amsa-scorecard/.
76 Ed Silverman, "Student Group That Ranked Med Schools over Industry Conflicts Votes to Accept Pharma Funding," *STAT* (blog), June 5, 2024, https://www.statnews.com/pharmalot/2024/06/05/conflicts-pharmaceuticals-universities/.
77 "A–1 Clarification of Relationships with Industry," AMSA, 2024, https://web.archive.org/web/20240607151549/https://www.amsa.org/current_resolutions/a-1-principles-regarding-membership-classifications/.
78 "Industry Funding of Medical Education: Report of an AAMC Task Force," iii.
79 Dan Bowman, "Stanford: Pfizer Will Fund Our Med School Curriculum with 'No Strings Attached,'" Fierce Healthcare, January 12, 2010, https://www.fiercehealthcare.com/healthcare/stanford-pfizer-will-fund-our-med-school-curriculum-no-strings-attached.
80 Kara Nyberg, "Pharma and Academia Partner for Better Health," Yale School of Medicine, Spring 2013, https://medicine.yale.edu/news/yale-medicine-magazine/article/pharma-and-academia-partner-for-better-health/.
81 Veronica Paulus and Akshaya Ravi, "'Deal with the Devil': Harvard Medical School Faculty Grapple with Increased Industry Research Funding," *The Harvard Crimson*, April 23, 2024, https://www.thecrimson.com/article/2024/4/23/hms-biopharma-funding/.
82 Sadiq K. Soofi and Claire Yuan, "Harvard Inks $30M Deal with Pharmaceutical Company for Therapeutic Research," *The Harvard Crimson*, October 19, 2021, https://www.thecrimson.com/article/2021/10/19/harvard-alliance-therapeutic-tech/; Ariel H. Kim and Meimei Xu, "HMS Dean Outlines Financial, Institutional Goals in State of the School Address," The Harvard Crimson, October 6, 2021, https://www.thecrimson.com/article/2021/10/6/hms-state-of-the-school/.
83 Dorcas Y. Gadras and Krishi Kishore, "Harvard Medical School Dean Says HMS Has Improved Financial Stability at State of the School Address," *The Harvard Crimson*, October 3, 2022, https://www.thecrimson.com/article/2022/10/3/hms-financial-stability-address-2022/.
84 Paulus and Ravi, "'Deal with the Devil.'"

85 "UCSF Funding Opportunities," UCSF Innovation Ventures, accessed June 26, 2024, https://innovation.ucsf.edu/UCSF_Funding_Opportunities.
86 "Funding," Johns Hopkins Drug Discovery, accessed May 30, 2025, https://drugdiscovery.jhu.edu/about-us/funding/.
87 "Browse by U.S. State Requirements," AMA Ed Hub, accessed July 14, 2025, https://edhub.ama-assn.org/state-cme.
88 "Online Courses for Indiana CME Requirements," AMA Ed Hub, accessed July 14, 2025, https://edhub.ama-assn.org/state-cme/Indiana.
89 "Earning CME Requirements: Different Types of CME Credits," BoardVitals, January 5, 2023, https://www.boardvitals.com/blog/types-of-cme-credits/.
90 "Committee Staff Report to the Chairman and Ranking Member: Use of Educational Grants by Pharmaceutical Manufacturers," United States Senate Committee on Finance, April 2007, https://www.finance.senate.gov/imo/media/doc/prb042507a.pdf.
91 Ibid., 2.
92 Ibid., 1.
93 Ibid., 16.
94 John Gever, "U of Michigan to Reject Industry Sponsors for CME," MedPage Today, June 25, 2010, https://www.medpagetoday.com/publichealthpolicy/medicaleducation/20897.
95 John Fauber and Coulter Jones, "Risk/Reward: Wary of Conflicts, Universities Taking Less Money from Drug Companies," *Milwaukee Journal Sentinel*, August 22, 2021, https://www.jsonline.com/story/archives/2021/08/22/wary-conflicts-universities-taking-less-money-drug-companies/7713996002/.
96 "ACCME Annual Report Data 2006," Accreditation Council for Continuing Medical Education, 2007, https://web.archive.org/web/20150906184749/https://www.accme.org/sites/default/files/null/395_2006_Annual_report_2006_20070706.pdf.
97 "Commercial Promotion Guidelines," ACS, accessed June 26, 2024, https://www.facs.org/for-medical-professionals/education/cme-resources/commercial-promotion-guidelines/.
98 "ACCME Data Report: Thriving Through Growth and Innovation—2023," Accreditation Council for Continuing Medical Education, August 15, 2024, https://accme.org/wp-content/uploads/2024/08/2023-ACCME-Annual-Data-Report-1045_20240815.pdf.
99 Michael C. Dalsing, "Industry Working with Physicians through Professional Medical Associations," *Journal of Vascular Surgery* 54, no. 3 (2011): 41S–46S, https://doi.org/10.1016/j.jvs.2011.04.068.
100 "ACCME Data Report: Thriving Through Growth and Innovation—2023."
101 Adriane Fugh-Berman, "Industry-Funded Medical Education Is Always Promotion—an Essay by Adriane Fugh-Berman," *BMJ* 373, no. 8296 (June 4, 2021): n1273, https://doi.org/10.1136/bmj.n1273.
102 Lo et al., *Conflict of Interest in Medical Research, Education, and Practice*, 145.
103 Joseph S. Ross, Peter Lurie, and Sidney M. Wolfe, "Medical Education Services Suppliers: A Threat to Physician Education," Public Citizen, July 19, 2000, https://www.citizen.org/article/medical-education-services-suppliers-a-threat-to-physician-education/.
104 "Who We Are," CPE Communications, accessed May 30, 2025, https://www.cpeducate.com/who-we-are/.

105 "How We're Different," CPE Communications, accessed May 30, 2025, https://www.cpeducate.com/how-we-are-different/.
106 Antonie Meixel, Elena Yanchar, and Adriane Fugh-Berman, "Hypoactive Sexual Desire Disorder: Inventing a Disease to Sell Low Libido," *Journal of Medical Ethics* 41, no. 10 (June 29, 2015): 859–62, https://doi.org/10.1136/medethics-2014-102596; Hylton V. Joffe et al., "FDA Approval of Flibanserin—Treating Hypoactive Sexual Desire Disorder," *New England Journal of Medicine* 374, no. 2 (January 14, 2016): 101–4, https://doi.org/10.1056/NEJMp1513686.
107 Jinhyun Jung and Adriane Fugh-Berman, "Marketing Messages in Continuing Medical Education (CME) Modules on Binge-Eating Disorder (BED)," *The Journal of the American Board of Family Medicine* 33, no. 2 (2020): 240–51, https://doi.org/10.3122/jabfm.2020.02.190129.
108 Abramson, *Overdosed America*, 119.
109 Jose U. Scher and Georg Schett, "Key Opinion Leaders—a Critical Perspective," *Nature Reviews Rheumatology* 17 (November 30, 2020): 119–24, https://doi.org/10.1038/s41584-020-00539-1.
110 "KOL Mapping," H1, accessed August 6, 2025, https://web.archive.org/web/20250806092958/https://h1.co/use-case/kol-mapping-and-engagement/.
111 Ray Moynihan et al., "Financial Ties between Leaders of Influential US Professional Medical Associations and Industry: Cross Sectional Study," *BMJ* 369, no. 8247 (May 27, 2020): m1505, https://doi.org/10.1136/bmj.m1505.
112 Kristin Wright et al., "Industry Relationships with Medical Oncologists: Who Are the High-Payment Physicians?," *JCO Oncology Practice* 18, no. 7 (June 13, 2022): e1164–9, https://doi.org/10.1200/OP.21.00756.
113 Jeffrey J. Meffert, "Key Opinion Leaders: Where They Come from and How That Affects the Drugs You Prescribe," *Dermatologic Therapy* 22, no. 3 (May 6, 2009): 262–8, https://doi.org/10.1111/j.1529-8019.2009.01240.x.
114 Ray Moynihan, "Key Opinion Leaders: Independent Experts or Drug Representatives in Disguise?," *BMJ* 336, no. 7658 (June 19, 2008): 1402–3, https://doi.org/10.1136/bmj.39575.675787.651.
115 Shahram Ahari, "I Was a Drug Rep. I Know How Pharma Companies Pushed Opioids," *The Washington Post*, November 26, 2019, https://www.washingtonpost.com/outlook/i-was-a-drug-rep-i-know-how-pharma-companies-pushed-opioids/2019/11/25/82b1da88-beb9-11e9-9b73-fd3c65ef8f9c_story.html.
116 Arthur Gale, "Sacklers Sacked But Purdue Still Caused Opioid Epidemic," *Missouri Medicine* 119, no. 2 (April 2022): 109, https://www.ncbi.nlm.nih.gov/pmc/articles/PMC9339402/.
117 Office of Inspector General, "Special Fraud Alert: Speaker Programs," Department of Health and Human Services, November 16, 2020, https://oig.hhs.gov/documents/special-fraud-alerts/865/SpecialFraudAlertSpeakerPrograms.pdf.
118 US Attorney's Office for the Southern District of New York, "Acting Manhattan U.S. Attorney Announces $678 Million Settlement Of Fraud Lawsuit Against Novartis Pharmaceuticals For Operating Sham Speaker Programs Through Which It Paid Over $100 Million To Doctors To Unlawfully Induce Them To Prescribe Novartis Drugs," US Department of Justice, July 1, 2020, https://www.justice.gov/usao-sdny/pr/acting-manhattan-us-attorney-announces-678-million-settlement-fraud-lawsuit-against; Office of Public Affairs, "Press Release: Novartis Pays over $642 Million to Settle Allegations of Improper Payments to Patients and Physicians," US Department

of Justice, July 1, 2020, https://www.justice.gov/archives/opa/pr/novartis-pays-over-642-million-settle-allegations-improper-payments-patients-and-physicians.
119 Office of Inspector General, "Special Fraud Alert: Speaker Programs."
120 Douglas Alan Greene and Barry J. Gertz, "RE: William Harvey Research Conference," October 15, 2001, https://www.industrydocuments.ucsf.edu/drug/docs/#id=khpd0217.
121 "List of Doctors—Neutralize/Discredit" (UCSF), accessed July 4, 2024, https://www.industrydocuments.ucsf.edu/drug/docs/#id=pmhw0217.
122 Ray Moynihan, "Court Hears How Drug Giant Merck Tried to 'Neutralise' and 'Discredit' Doctors Critical of Vioxx," *BMJ* 338 (April 6, 2009): b1432, https://doi.org/10.1136/bmj.b1432.
123 "The Art of Detailing to Doctors: Building Strong Pharmaceutical Relationships," Platforce, April 24, 2024, https://platforce.io/detailing-to-doctors-building-strong-pharmaceutical-relationships/.
124 Institute for Health Policy, "Drug Policy 101: Kaiser Permanente's Approach to Pharmaceutical Detailing," Kaiser Permanente, February 2022, https://www.kpihp.org/wp-content/uploads/2022/02/0186_IHP_DrugPolicy101_flyr_021822-1.pdf.
125 "A Day in the Life of a Pharmaceutical Sales Representative," MedReps, June 15, 2022, https://www.medreps.com/medical-sales-careers/what-do-pharmaceutical-sales-reps-do/.
126 "Exploring Pharmaceutical Sales Reps Salaries: A Deep Dive," Rep-Lite, February 24, 2024, https://rep-lite.com/how-much-do-pharmaceutical-sales-reps-make/.
127 Ahari, "I Was a Drug Rep. I Know How Pharma Companies Pushed Opioids."
128 Ahari, "Under the Influence: Can We Provide Doctors an Alternative to Biased Drug Reviews," March 12, 2008.
129 Carl Elliott, "The Drug Pushers," *The Atlantic*, April 2006, https://www.theatlantic.com/magazine/archive/2006/04/the-drug-pushers/304714/.
130 "National Survey of Physicians II: Doctors and Prescription Drugs," Kaiser Family Foundation, March 2002, https://www.kff.org/wp-content/uploads/2002/03/nhp022-physician-survey-part-ii-rx-drugs-final-4-15-02.pdf.
131 "Pharmaceutical Sales Representative Demographics and Statistics in the US," Zippia, accessed June 26, 2024, https://www.zippia.com/pharmaceutical-sales-representative-jobs/demographics/.
132 Schwartz and Woloshin, "Medical Marketing in the United States, 1997–2016."
133 Ashleigh C. King, Lisa M. Schwartz, and Steven Woloshin, "A National Survey of the Frequency of Drug Company Detailing Visits and Free Sample Closets in Practices Delivering Primary Care," *JAMA Internal Medicine* 180, no. 4 (January 27, 2020): 592–5, https://doi.org/10.1001/jamainternmed.2019.6770.
134 Joanne Finnegan, "Physicians Increasingly Too Busy to See Pharma Sales Reps, Report Finds," Fierce Healthcare, September 17, 2019, https://www.fiercehealthcare.com/practices/physicians-increasingly-too-busy-to-see-pharma-sales-reps-report-finds.
135 Dave Melville, "Post-Pandemic Physician Engagement: 4 Areas to Consider When Rethinking Your Sales Talent and Their Approach," PharmExec.com, April 20, 2021, https://www.pharmexec.com/view/post-pandemic-physician-engagement-4-areas-to-consider-when-rethinking-your-sales-talent-and-their-approach.
136 Matthew Arnold, "Remote and In-Person, Sales Reps Continue to Inform Patient Care, but Physician Needs Vary," Clarivate, July 27, 2022, https://clarivate.com/

blog/remote-and-in-person-sales-reps-continue-to-inform-patient-care-but-physic ian-needs-vary/.

137 "How Much Do Medical Device Sales Reps Make in 2024?," David Bagga Company, 2024, https://www.davidbagga.com/how-much-do-medical-device-sales-reps-mak e-in-2024/.

138 Bonnie O'Connor, Fran Pollner, and Adriane Fugh-Berman, "Salespeople in the Surgical Suite: Relationships between Surgeons and Medical Device Representatives," ed. Chunfeng Zhao, *PLoS ONE* 11, no. 8 (August 3, 2016): e0158510, https://doi.org/10.1371/journal.pone.0158510.

139 Kristin Huntoon et al., "Sales Representatives in the Operating Room: Conflict of Interest or Clinical Support?," *World Neurosurgery* 155 (2021): e480–3, https://doi.org/10.1016/j.wneu.2021.08.088.

140 "National Survey of Physicians II: Doctors and Prescription Drugs."

141 Eric G. Campbell et al., "A National Survey of Physician–Industry Relationships," *New England Journal of Medicine* 356, no. 17 (April 26, 2007): 1742–50, https://doi.org/10.1056/NEJMsa064508.

142 Schwartz and Woloshin, "Medical Marketing in the United States, 1997–2016."

143 CMS, "Facts about Open Payments Data," OpenPaymentsData.CMS.gov, accessed May 30, 2025, https://openpaymentsdata.cms.gov/summary.

144 AAMC, "U.S. Physician Workforce Data Dashboard," Association of American Medical Colleges, May 30, 2025, https://www.aamc.org/data-reports/report/us-physician-workforce-data-dashboard.

145 Ahmed Sayed et al., "Industry Payments to US Physicians by Specialty and Product Type," *JAMA* 331, no. 15 (March 28, 2024): 1325–7, https://doi.org/10.1001/jama.2024.1989.

146 Amarnath R. Annapureddy et al., "Association between Industry Payments to Physicians and Device Selection in ICD Implantation," *JAMA* 324, no. 17 (November 3, 2020): 1755–64, https://doi.org/10.1001/jama.2020.17436.

147 Michael A. Steinman et al., "Narrative Review: The Promotion of Gabapentin: An Analysis of Internal Industry Documents," *Annals of Internal Medicine* 145, no. 4 (August 15, 2006): 284–93, https://doi.org/10.7326/0003-4819-145-4-200608150-00008.

148 "Neurontin 1996 SE CBU Plan, Goal: 12% N Rx by December 1996," Parke-Davis, 1996, https://www.industrydocuments.ucsf.edu/drug/docs/#id=mtyd0217.

149 Natasha Giordano et al., "Business Strategies to Penetrate the Hospital Segment of the Northeast Customer Business Unit," Parke-Davis, accessed June 27, 2024, https://www.industrydocuments.ucsf.edu/drug/docs/#id=nsyd0217.

150 Steinman et al., "Narrative Review."

151 "1998 Strategic Plan and A&P Allocation Grid, Neurontin," Parke-Davis, August 27, 1997, https://www.industrydocuments.ucsf.edu/drug/docs/#id=lmyd0217.

152 Giordano et al., "Business Strategies to Penetrate the Hospital Segment of the Northeast Customer Business Unit."

153 Steinman et al., "Narrative Review."

154 "Physician Compensation Report 2024," Doximity and Curative, 2024, https://web.archive.org/web/20260112065110/https://www.assets.doxcdn.com/image/upload/pdfs/doximity-physician-compensation-report-2024.pdf.

155 Leslie Kane, "Medscape Physician Compensation Report 2023: Your Income vs Your Peers,'" Medscape, April 14, 2023, https://www.medscape.com/slides

how/2023-compensation-overview-6016341#:~:text=Medscape%20Physician%20Compensation%20Report%202023%3A%20Your%20Income%20vs%20Your%20Peers',-Leslie%20Kane%2C%20MA&text=Physician%20compensation%20is%20still%20on,%24352%2C000%20in%20this%20year's%20report; "BLS Data Viewer: Average Weekly Hours of All Employees, Total Private, Seasonally Adjusted," US Bureau of Labor Statistics, accessed June 26, 2024, https://data.bls.gov/dataViewer/view/timeseries/CES0500000002;jsessionid=161CAB7B12C6B14583A56F500DE4A028.

156 Bradley M. Gray et al., "Clinical Knowledge and Trends in Physicians' Prescribing of Opioids for New Onset Back Pain, 2009–2017," *JAMA Network Open* 4, no. 7 (July 1, 2021): e2115328, https://doi.org/10.1001/jamanetworkopen.2021.15328.

## 9 The Root Incentive: Patents

1 CBO, "Research and Development in the Pharmaceutical Industry," Congressional Budget Office, April 2021, https://www.cbo.gov/publication/57126.

2 Stephanie Rennane, Lawrence Baker, and Andrew Mulcahy, "Estimating the Cost of Industry Investment in Drug Research and Development: A Review of Methods and Results," *INQUIRY: The Journal of Health Care Organization, Provision, and Financing* 58 (February 16, 2022): 469580211059731, https://doi.org/10.1177/00469580211059731.

3 CoinNews Media Group, US Inflation Calculator, accessed May 31, 2025, https://www.usinflationcalculator.com/.

4 Economic and Statistics Administration and United States Patent and Trademark Office, "Intellectual Property and the U.S. Economy: Industries in Focus," US Department of Commerce, March 2012, https://www.uspto.gov/sites/default/files/news/publications/IP_Report_March_2012.pdf.

5 Ibid.

6 Juliette Cubanski et al., "How Does Prescription Drug Spending and Use Compare Across Large Employer Plans, Medicare Part D, and Medicaid?," *KFF* (blog), May 20, 2019, https://www.kff.org/medicare/issue-brief/how-does-prescription-drug-spending-and-use-compare-across-large-employer-plans-medicare-part-d-and-medicaid/.

7 Jeanne S. Ringel et al., *The Elasticity of Demand for Health Care: A Review of the Literature and Its Application to the Military Health System* (Santa Monica, CA: RAND, 2002), https://www.rand.org/content/dam/rand/pubs/monograph_reports/2005/MR1355.pdf.

8 John Abramson, "Fixing American Health Care: Session 2: Corporate Capture of Medical 'Knowledge,'" Pelican Cove University, February 27, 2024; Abramson, *Sickening*, 167–77.

9 "The United States Constitution," National Constitution Center, accessed June 14, 2024, https://constitutioncenter.org/the-constitution/full-text; "A Brief History of the Patent Law of the United States," Ladas & Parry, May 7, 2014, https://ladas.com/education-center/a-brief-history-of-the-patent-law-of-the-united-states-2/.

10 "ArtI.S8.C8.1 Overview of Congress's Power over Intellectual Property," Constitution Annotated, accessed June 13, 2024, https://constitution.congress.gov/browse/essay/

artI-S8-C8-1/ALDE_00013060/#:~:text=Article%20I%2C%20Section%208%2C%20Clause,their%20respective%20Writings%20and%20Discoveries.

11 "Intellectual Property Clause," Legal Information Institute, June 2023, https://www.law.cornell.edu/wex/intellectual_property_clause.

12 "A Brief History of the Patent Law of the United States"; Idaho State Bar, "A Brief History of the U.S. Patent System," https://isb.idaho.gov/wp-content/uploads/IPL-Section-Meeting-Material-Apr.-15-2021.pdf.

13 Taylar-Simone McCants, "The U.S. Patent and Trademark Office," FindLaw, May 22, 2024, https://www.findlaw.com/smallbusiness/intellectual-property/the-u-s-patent-and-trademark-office.html; "A Brief History of the Patent Law of the United States."

14 United States Patent and Trademark Office, "General Information Concerning Patents," US Department of Commerce, 2014, https://www.uspto.gov/sites/default/files/inventors/edu-inf/BasicPatentGuide.pdf.

15 Kara W. Swanson, "Food and Drug Law as Intellectual Property Law: Historical Reflections.," *Wisconsin Law Review* 2011, no. 2 (April 25, 2011): 331–98, https://papers.ssrn.com/sol3/papers.cfm?abstract_id=1822223.

16 Joseph M. Gabriel, *Medical Monopoly: Intellectual Property Rights and the Origins of the Modern Pharmaceutical Industry*, Paperback edition., Synthesis (Chicago: The University of Chicago Press, 2020).

17 Swanson, "Food and Drug Law as Intellectual Property Law," 352.

18 Joseph M. Gabriel, "The US Drug Industry Used to Oppose Patents—What Changed?," The Conversation, June 29, 2021, http://theconversation.com/the-us-drug-industry-used-to-oppose-patents-what-changed-161319.

19 Swanson, "Food and Drug Law as Intellectual Property Law."

20 "Principles of Medical Ethics," American Medical Association, 1903, https://global.oup.com/us/companion.websites/9780199774111/doc/IXa.doc.

21 Gabriel, "The US Drug Industry Used to Oppose Patents—What Changed?"

22 Swanson, "Food and Drug Law as Intellectual Property Law."

23 Morris Fishbein, "Are Patents on Medicinal Discoveries and on Foods in the Public Interest—Medical Patents," *Industrial & Engineering Chemistry* 29, no. 11 (November 1, 1937): 1315–18, https://doi.org/10.1021/ie50335a026.

24 Gabriel, "The US Drug Industry Used to Oppose Patents—What Changed?"

25 "A Brief History of the Patent Law of the United States."

26 "An Act to Revise and Codify the Laws Relating to Patents and the Patent Office, and to Enact into Law Title 35 of the United States Code Entitled 'Patents,'" Pub. L. No. 82–593 (1952), https://www.congress.gov/bill/82nd-congress/house-bill/7794/text.

27 Halliburton Oil Well Cementing Co. v. Walker, 329 U.S. 1 (US Supreme Court 1946).

28 An Act to revise and codify the laws relating to patents and the Patent Office, and to enact into law title 35 of the United States Code entitled "Patents."

29 Wanli (Lily) Tang, "Revitalizing the Patent System to Incentivize Pharmaceutical Innovation: The Potential of Claims with Means-Plus-Function Clauses," *Duke Law Journal* 62, no. 5 (2013): 1069–108, https://scholarship.law.duke.edu/dlj/vol62/iss5/3.

30 Gabrielle Athanasia, "The Legacy of Bayh-Dole's Success on U.S. Global Competitiveness Today," Center for Strategic & International Studies, January 12, 2022, https://www.csis.org/blogs/perspectives-innovation/legacy-bayh-doles-success-us-global-competitiveness-today.

31 "An Act to Amend the Patent and Trademark Laws.," Pub. L. No. 96–517 (1980), https://www.congress.gov/bill/96th-congress/house-bill/693; Andrei Iancu and Cooper Godfrey, "The Bayh-Dole Act and the Debate over 'Reasonable Price' March-In Rights," The Federalist Society, April 18, 2024, https://fedsoc.org/commentary/fedsoc-blog/the-bayh-dole-act-and-the-debate-over-reasonable-price-march-in-rights#:~:text=Realizing%20that%20%E2%80%9C%5Bg%5Dovernment,licenses%20to%20federally%20funded%20patents.
32 "35 U.S. Code § 203—March-in Rights," Legal Information Institute, accessed June 14, 2024, https://www.law.cornell.edu/uscode/text/35/203.
33 "A Brief History of the Patent Law of the United States."
34 "Uruguay Round Agreements Act," Pub. L. No. 103–465 (1994), https://www.congress.gov/bill/103rd-congress/house-bill/5110.
35 Jan Berger et al., "How Drug Life-Cycle Management Patent Strategies May Impact Formulary Management," *The American Journal of Managed Care* 22, no. 16 Suppl (August 6, 2020): S487–95, https://www.ajmc.com/view/a636-article; Chie Hoon Song and Jeung-Whan Han, "Patent Cliff and Strategic Switch: Exploring Strategic Design Possibilities in the Pharmaceutical Industry," *SpringerPlus* 5 (May 23, 2016): Article 692, https://doi.org/10.1186/s40064-016-2323-1.
36 WTO, "The Uruguay Round," World Trade Organization, accessed June 14, 2024, https://www.wto.org/english/thewto_e/whatis_e/tif_e/fact5_e.htm; WTO, "Members and Observers," World Trade Organization, accessed May 31, 2025, https://www.wto.org/english/thewto_e/whatis_e/tif_e/org6_e.htm.
37 Dean Baker, *Rigged: How Globalization and the Rules of the Modern Economy Were Structured to Make the Rich Richer* (Washington, DC: Center for Economic and Policy Research, 2016): 81–2, https://deanbaker.net/images/stories/documents/Rigged.pdf.
38 Atsuko Kamiike, "The TRIPS Agreement and the Pharmaceutical Industry in India," *Journal of Interdisciplinary Economics* 32, no. 1 (December 5, 2019): 95–113, https://doi.org/10.1177/0260107919875573.
39 An Act to Amend the Federal Food, Drug, and Cosmetic Act to Revise the Procedures for New Drug Applications, to Amend Title 35, United States Code, to Authorize the Extension of the Patents for Certain Regulated Products, and for Other Purposes.," Pub. L. No. 98–417 (1984), https://www.congress.gov/bill/98th-congress/senate-bill/1538; John R. Thomas, "The Hatch-Waxman Act: A Primer," Congressional Research Service, September 28, 2016, https://www.congress.gov/crs-product/R44643.
40 Christina D. Brown-Marshall and Dexter Whitley, "Hatch-Waxman 101," FISH., April 15, 2024, https://www.fr.com/insights/thought-leadership/blogs/hatch-waxman-101-3/.
41 Alfred Engelberg, "Unaffordable Prescription Drugs: The Real Legacy of the Hatch-Waxman Act," *STAT* (blog), December 16, 2020, https://www.statnews.com/2020/12/16/unaffordable-prescription-drugs-real-legacy-hatch-waxman-act/.
42 Thomas, "The Hatch-Waxman Act: A Primer."
43 FDA, "Small Business Assistance: Frequently Asked Questions for New Drug Product Exclusivity," US Food & Drug Administration, February 11, 2016, https://www.fda.gov/drugs/cder-small-business-industry-assistance-sbia/small-business-assistance-frequently-asked-questions-new-drug-product-exclusivity.
44 Thomas, "The Hatch-Waxman Act: A Primer"; Ryan Timmis, "The Biologics Price Competition and Innovation Act: Potential Problems in the Biologic-Drug Regulatory Scheme," *Northwestern Journal of Technology and Intellectual Property*

13, no. 2 (Fall 2015): 215–32, https://scholarlycommons.law.northwestern.edu/njtip/vol13/iss2/6.

45 "Policy Proposal: Reducing the Exclusivity Period for Biological Products," Pew, September 8, 2017, http://pew.org/2eLeXav.

46 "FDA Issues Draft Guidance on Regulatory Exclusivity for Biologics," Nutter, August 13, 2014, https://www.nutter.com/ip-law-bulletin/fda-issues-draft-guidance-on-regulatory-exclusivity-for-biologics; Engelberg, "Unaffordable Prescription Drugs."

47 Baker, *Rigged*, 96; CBO, "Prescription Drugs: Spending, Use, and Prices," Congressional Budget Office, January 2022, https://www.cbo.gov/publication/57772.

48 Raghav Mahobe, "Moderna Considers Pricing COVID Vaccine at $110-$130—WSJ," *Reuters*, January 9, 2023, sec. Healthcare & Pharmaceuticals, https://www.reuters.com/business/healthcare-pharmaceuticals/moderna-considers-pricing-covid-vaccine-110-130-wsj-2023-01-09/.

49 FDA, "Generic Drugs: Questions & Answers," US Food & Drug Administration, March 16, 2021, https://www.fda.gov/drugs/frequently-asked-questions-popular-topics/generic-drugs-questions-answers#:~:text=The%20reduction%20in%20upfront%20research,of%20the%20brand%2Dname%20medicine.

50 Ryan Conrad and Kristin Davis, "Estimating Cost Savings from New Generic Drug Approvals in 2021," US Food and Drug Administration, September 2023, https://www.fda.gov/media/172608/download?attachment.

51 Nathan E. Wineinger, Yunyue Zhang, and Eric J. Topol, "Trends in Prices of Popular Brand-Name Prescription Drugs in the United States," *JAMA Network Open* 2, no. 5 (May 31, 2019): e194791, https://doi.org/10.1001/jamanetworkopen.2019.4791; "Value of $1 from 2012 to 2017," CPI Inflation Calculator, accessed June 14, 2024, https://www.in2013dollars.com/us/inflation/2012?amount=1.

52 Inmaculada Hernandez et al., "Changes in List Prices, Net Prices, and Discounts for Branded Drugs in the US, 2007–2018," *JAMA* 323, no. 9 (March 3, 2020): 854–62, https://doi.org/10.1001/jama.2020.1012; "Value of $1 from 2007 to 2018," CPI Inflation Calculator, accessed June 14, 2024, https://www.officialdata.org/us/inflation/2007?endYear=2018&amount=1.

53 CBO, "Research and Development in the Pharmaceutical Industry."

54 Richard G. Frank and Kathleen Hannick, "Five Things to Understand about Pharmaceutical R&D," Brookings, June 2, 2022, https://www.brookings.edu/articles/five-things-to-understand-about-pharmaceutical-rd/.

55 Aris Angelis et al., "High Drug Prices Are Not Justified by Industry's Spending on Research and Development," *BMJ* 380, no. 8371 (February 15, 2023): e071710, https://doi.org/10.1136/bmj-2022-071710.

56 Committee on Oversight and Reform, "Drug Pricing Investigation: Majority Staff Report," US House of Representatives, December 2021, https://oversightdemocrats.house.gov/sites/evo-subsites/democrats-oversight.house.gov/files/DRUG%20PRICING%20REPORT%20WITH%20APPENDIX%20v3.pdf.

57 William Lazonick et al., "US Pharma's Financialized Business Model," *Institute for New Economic Thinking Working Paper Series No. 60*, July 13, 2017, https://doi.org/10.2139/ssrn.3035529.

58 Öner Tulum and William Lazonick, "Setting Pharmaceutical Drug Prices: What the Medicare Negotiators Need to Know About Innovation and Financialization," *Institute for New Economic Thinking Working Paper Series No. 60*, September 9, 2024, https://doi.org/10.36687/inetwp226.

59 "Inflation Reduction Act of 2022," Pub. L. No. 117–69 (2022), https://www.congress.gov/bill/117th-congress/house-bill/5376.
60 Jishian Ravinthiran, "Profits Over Patients," Public Citizen, January 18, 2024, https://www.citizen.org/article/profits-over-patients/.
61 Fred D. Ledley et al., "Profitability of Large Pharmaceutical Companies Compared with Other Large Public Companies," *JAMA* 323, no. 9 (March 3, 2020): 834–43, https://doi.org/10.1001/jama.2020.0442.
62 Government Accountability Office, "Drug Industry: Profits, Research and Development Spending, and Merger and Acquisition Deals," November 2017, https://www.gao.gov/assets/gao-18-40.pdf.
63 Ibid; Mulcahy, Schwam, and Lovejoy, "International Prescription Drug Price Comparisons"; Michael Christel, "2023 Pharm Exec Top 50 Companies," Pharmaceutical Executive, June 10, 2023, https://www.pharmexec.com/view/2023-pharm-exec-top-50-companies; EFPIA, "The Pharmaceutical Industry in Figures: Key Data 2024," European Federation of Pharmaceutical Industries and Associations, November 28, 2023, https://efpia.eu/media/2rxdkn43/the-pharmaceutical-industry-in-figures-2024.pdf; Michael Christel, "2024 Pharm Exec Top 50 Companies," Pharmaceutical Executive, June 14, 2024, https://www.pharmexec.com/view/2024-pharm-exec-top-50-companies; EFPIA, "The Pharmaceutical Industry in Figures: Key Data 2025," European Federation of Pharmaceutical Industries and Associations, November 28, 2024, https://www.efpia.eu/media/uj0popel/the-pharmaceutical-industry-in-figures-2025.pdf; "Pharma 50: The Top Pharma Companies in the World for 2025," Drug Discovery & Development, accessed July 8, 2025, https://www.drugdiscoverytrends.com/pharma-50-the-50-largest-pharmaceutical-companies-in-the-world-for-2025/.
64 Olivier J. Wouters et al., "Association of Research and Development Investments with Treatment Costs for New Drugs Approved from 2009 to 2018," *JAMA Network Open* 5, no. 9 (September 26, 2022): e2218623, https://doi.org/10.1001/jamanetworkopen.2022.18623.
65 Office of the Assistant Secretary for Planning and Evaluation, "Comparing Prescription Drugs in the U.S. and Other Countries: Prices and Availability," US Department of Health & Human Services, January 31, 2024, https://aspe.hhs.gov/reports/comparing-prescription-drugs.
66 Kerstin N. Vokinger and Huseyin Naci, "Negotiating Drug Prices in the US—Lessons from Europe," *JAMA Health Forum* 3, no. 12 (December 22, 2022): e224801, https://doi.org/10.1001/jamahealthforum.2022.4801.
67 Common Cause, "The Medicare/Prescription Drug Bill: A Study in How Government Shouldn't Work," June 3, 2004, https://www.govinfo.gov/content/pkg/CREC-2004-06-04/html/CREC-2004-06-04-pt1-PgE1038-4.htm.
68 Sarnak et al., "Paying for Prescription Drugs around the World."
69 Committee on Oversight and Reform, "Drug Pricing Investigation: Majority Staff Report," xvii.
70 Ibid., xvii, 90.
71 "Overpatented, Overpriced Special Edition: Humira," I-MAK, September 2021, https://www.i-mak.org/wp-content/uploads/2021/09/i-mak.humira.report.3.final-REVISED-2021-09-22.pdf.
72 Committee on Oversight and Reform, "Drug Pricing Investigation: Majority Staff Report," 173.

73 Rebecca Robbins, "How a Drug Company Made $114 Billion by Gaming the U.S. Patent System," *The New York Times*, January 28, 2023, sec. Business, https://www.nytimes.com/2023/01/28/business/humira-abbvie-monopoly.html.
74 "The Truth about America's Top Selling Drugs in 2021," I-MAK, June 2022, https://www.i-mak.org/2021-top-selling/.
75 Feldman, "May Your Drug Price Be Evergreen."
76 William B. Feldman et al., "Patents and Regulatory Exclusivities on Inhalers for Asthma and COPD, 1986–2020," *Health Affairs* 41, no. 6 (May 17, 2022): 787–96, https://doi.org/10.1377/hlthaff.2021.01874.
77 Frank and Hannick, "Five Things to Understand about Pharmaceutical R&D."
78 Osipenko et al., "Provenance and Clinical Benefit of Medicines Introduced to the French Market, 2008 to 2018"; Wieseler, McGauran, and Kaiser, "New Drugs."
79 Alexander C. Egilman, Benjamin N. Rome, and Aaron S. Kesselheim, "Added Therapeutic Benefit of Top-Selling Brand-Name Drugs in Medicare," *JAMA* 329, no. 15 (April 18, 2023): 1283–9, https://doi.org/10.1001/jama.2023.4034.
80 Baker, *Rigged*, 101.
81 David Dranove, Craig Garthwaite, and Manuel Hermosilla, "Pharmaceutical Profits and the Social Value of Innovation" (Cambridge, MA: National Bureau of Economic Research, 2014), https://doi.org/10.3386/w20212.
82 Gupta, Meenu, and Mohan, "The Tamiflu Fiasco and Lessons Learnt."
83 Baker, *Rigged*, 101.
84 Heidi L. Williams, "Intellectual Property Rights and Innovation: Evidence from the Human Genome," *Journal of Political Economy* 121, no. 1 (2013): 1–27, https://doi.org/10.1086/669706.
85 DiStefano et al., "Association between Drug Characteristics and Manufacturer Spending on Direct-to-Consumer Advertising."
86 Sanne Magnan, "Social Determinants of Health 101 for Health Care: Five Plus Five," National Academy of Medicine, October 9, 2017, https://nam.edu/social-determinants-of-health-101-for-health-care-five-plus-five/#:~:text=Medical%20care%20is%20estimated%20to,socioeconomic%20factors%2C%20and%20environmental%20factors.
87 Moses et al., "The Anatomy of Medical Research."
88 Sepideh Soltani et al., "Adherence to the Mediterranean Diet in Relation to All-Cause Mortality: A Systematic Review and Dose-Response Meta-Analysis of Prospective Cohort Studies," *Advances in Nutrition* 10, no. 6 (2019): 1029–39, https://doi.org/10.1093/advances/nmz041.
89 Shafqat Ahmad et al., "Mediterranean Diet Adherence and Risk of All-Cause Mortality in Women," *JAMA Network Open* 7, no. 5 (May 31, 2024): e2414322, https://doi.org/10.1001/jamanetworkopen.2024.14322; "2015–2020 Dietary Guidelines for Americans," US Department of Health and Human Services and US Department of Agriculture, accessed June 14, 2024, https://health.gov/our-work/food-nutrition/previous-dietary-guidelines/2015; Alice H. Lichtenstein et al., "2021 Dietary Guidance to Improve Cardiovascular Health: A Scientific Statement from the American Heart Association," *Circulation* 144, no. 23 (November 2, 2021): e472–87, https://doi.org/https://doi.org/10.1161/CIR.0000000000001031; Francesco Cosentino et al., "2019 ESC Guidelines on Diabetes, Pre-Diabetes, and Cardiovascular Diseases Developed in Collaboration with the EASD," *European Heart Journal* 41, no. 2 (2020): 255–323, https://doi.org/10.1093/eurheartj/ehz486.

90 Diabetes Prevention Program Research Group, "Reduction in the Incidence of Type 2 Diabetes with Lifestyle Intervention or Metformin."
91 Abramson, *Sickening*, 76–7.
92 Charlie Katebi, "Patent Abuses Keep Prescription Drugs Unaffordable," AFPI, February 14, 2024, https://americafirstpolicy.com/issues/patent-abuses-keep-prescription-drugs-unaffordable.
93 HSGAC Minority Staff, "Manufactured Crisis: How Devastating Drug Price Increases Are Harming America's Seniors," US House of Representatives, December 2021, https://strategichealthcare.net/wp-content/uploads/2018/03/McCaskill-Drug-Report.pdf.
94 Lunna Lopes et al., "Americans' Challenges with Health Care Costs," *KFF* (blog), March 1, 2024, https://www.kff.org/health-costs/issue-brief/americans-challenges-with-health-care-costs/.
95 "The U.S. Generic Biosimilar Medicines Report," Association for Accessible Medicines, September 2022, https://accessiblemeds.org/sites/default/files/2022-09/AAM-2022-Generic-Biosimilar-Medicines-Savings-Report.pdf.
96 Baker, *Rigged*, 103–11.
97 Ibid., 104.
98 Ibid., 105.
99 Moses et al., "The Anatomy of Medical Research"; Magnan, "Social Determinants of Health 101 for Health Care: Five Plus Five."
100 Dennis J. Kucinich, "Free Market Drug Act," H.R. 5155 (2004), https://www.congress.gov/bill/108th-congress/house-bill/5155/text.
101 Susan Jaffe, "Kucinich Wants Government to Oversee Drug Research," *PNHP* (blog), September 29, 2004, https://pnhp.org/news/kucinich-wants-government-to-oversee-drug-research/.
102 Kucinich, Free Market Drug Act.
103 Emily Connelly and Stacie Propst, "2004 Investment in U.S. Health Research: About 6¢ of Every Health Dollar Is Spent on Research," Research!America, May 2005, https://www.researchamerica.org/wp-content/uploads/2022/09/healthdollar2004.pdf.
104 Kucinich, Free Market Drug Act.
105 Jocelyn Kaiser, "Final NIH Budget for 2024 Is Essentially Flat," *Science*, March 21, 2024, https://www.science.org/content/article/final-nih-budget-2024-essentially-flat#:~:text=Congress%20has%20given%20the%20National,partial%20government%20shutdown%20this%20weekend; Laurie Harris et al., "Federal Research and Development (R&D) Funding: FY2024," Congressional Research Service, May 19, 2023, https://crsreports.congress.gov/product/pdf/R/R47564; "Budget," National Institutes of Health, October 24, 2023, https://www.nih.gov/about-nih/what-we-do/budget.
106 Galkina Cleary et al., "Comparison of Research Spending on New Drug Approvals by the National Institutes of Health vs the Pharmaceutical Industry, 2010–2019."
107 "U.S. Investments in Medical and Health Research and Development: 2016–2020."
108 US Bureau of Economic Analysis, "National Data: National Income and Product Accounts (2020)," BEA, May 30, 2024, https://apps.bea.gov/iTable/?reqid=19&step=2&isuri=1&categories=survey&_gl=1*1jdfet1*_ga*MTk0OTc2Mjc0NC4xNzE3MjU5NzA5*_ga_J4698JNNFT*MTcxNzI1OTcwOS4xLjEuMTcxNzI1OTc2Mi43LjAuMA..#eyJhcHBpZCI6MTksInN0ZXBzI

jpbMSwyLDMsM10sImRhdGEiOltbImNhdGVnb3JpZXMiLCJTdXJ2ZXkiXSxbIk5JUEFfVGFibGVfTGlzdCIsIjUiXSxbIkZpcnN0X1llYXIiLCIyMDIwIl0sWyJMYXN0X1llYXIiLCIyMDIwIl0sWyJTY2FsZSIsIi05Il0sWyJTZXJpZXMiLCJBIl1dfQ==; CBO, "The Federal Budget in Fiscal Year 2020: An Infographic," Congressional Budget Office, April 30, 2021, https://www.cbo.gov/publication/57170.

109 Baker, *Rigged*, 105–6.

110 "Defense Lobbying," OpenSecrets, accessed June 1, 2025, https://www.opensecrets.org/industries/lobbying?ind=D.

111 USASpending.gov, "Advanced Search," accessed June 1, 2025, https://www.usaspending.gov/search?hash=1b5fceaae0c7bdce691869b131697cc8.

112 Blanes I Vidal, Draca, and Fons-Rosen, "Revolving Door Lobbyists"; Ridge, Ingram, and Hill, "Beyond Lobbying Expenditures."

113 Bernie Sanders, "Defense Contractors Are Bilking the American People," Bernie Sanders: US Senator for Vermont, February 27, 2024, https://www.sanders.senate.gov/op-eds/defense-contractors-are-bilking-the-american-people/; "Value of $1 from 1991 to 2024," CPI Inflation Calculator, accessed June 14, 2024, https://www.in2013dollars.com/us/inflation/1991?amount=1.

114 Peter C. Gøtzsche, "Patients Not Patents: Drug Research and Development as a Public Enterprise," *European Journal of Clinical Investigation* 48, no. 2 (December 15, 2017): e12875, https://doi.org/10.1111/eci.12875.

115 Jeff Maskell, "Lobbying Regulations on Non-Profit Organizations," Congressional Research Service, May 7, 2008, https://www.everycrsreport.com/files/20080507_96-809_51cff1bb115b22678b6a4d27ed5e2474a7d5b674.pdf.

116 J. P. Finet, "Do Nonprofits Pay Taxes?," FindLaw, May 23, 2024, https://www.findlaw.com/smallbusiness/business-taxes/do-nonprofits-pay-taxes-.html.

117 "Lobbying," IRS, June 4, 2024, https://www.irs.gov/charities-non-profits/lobbying; "O. SCIENTIFIC RESEARCH UNDER IRC 501(c)(3)," Internal Revenue Service, 1986, https://www.irs.gov/pub/irs-tege/eotopico86.pdf; "Measuring Lobbying Activity: Expenditure Test," IRS, October 18, 2024, https://www.irs.gov/charities-non-profits/measuring-lobbying-activity-expenditure-test.

118 Abramson, *Sickening*, 109–13.

119 "Medical Innovation Prize Fund (MIPF)," iMed, Art / Earth / Tech, accessed June 22, 2024, https://imedproject.org/proposals-database/mipf/.

120 Bernard Sanders, "Medical Innovation Prize Fund Act," S.495 (2017), https://www.congress.gov/bill/115th-congress/senate-bill/495.

121 Chris Micheli, "The Use of notwithstanding Clauses in California Legislation," *Capitol Weekly*, March 29, 2024, https://capitolweekly.net/the-use-of-notwithstanding-clauses-in-california-legislation/.

122 Cisneros v. Alpine Ridge Group, 508 U.S. 10 (US Supreme Court 1993).

123 Sanders, Medical Innovation Prize Fund Act.

124 US Bureau of Economic Analysis, "National Data: National Income and Product Accounts (2023)," BEA, May 30, 2024, https://apps.bea.gov/iTable/?reqid=19&step=2&isuri=1&categories=survey&_gl=1*1volvk*_ga*MTk0OTc2Mjc0NC4xNzE3MjU5NzA5*_ga_J4698JNNFT*MTcxNzI4MjIwOS4yLjEuMTcxNzI4MjIzMC4zOS4wLjA.#eyJhcHBpZCI6MTksInN0ZXBzIjpbMSwyLDMsM10sImRhdGEiOltbImNhdGVnb3JpZXMiLCJTdXJ2ZXkiXSxbIk5JUEFfVGFibGVfTGlzdCIsIjUiXS

xbIkZpcnN0X1llYXIiLCIyMDIzIl0sWyJMYXN0X1llYXIiLCIyMDIzIl0sWyJTY2FsZSIsIi05Il0sWyJTZXJpZXMiLCJBIl1dfQ==.

125 "U.S. Investments in Medical and Health Research and Development: 2016–2020."

126 US Bureau of Economic Analysis, "National Data: National Income and Product Accounts (2019)," BEA, May 30, 2024, https://apps.bea.gov/iTable/?reqid=19&step=2&isuri=1&categories=survey&_gl=1*1volvk*_ga*MTk0OTc2Mjc0NC4xNzE3MjU5NzA5*_ga_J4698JNNFT*MTcxNzI4MjIwOS4yLjEuMTcxNzI4MjIzMC4zOS4wLjA.#eyJhcHBpZCI6MTksInN0ZXBzIjpbMSwyLDMsM10sImRhdGEiOltbImNhdGVnb3JpZXMiLCJTdXJ2ZXkiXSxbIk5JUEFfVGFibGVfTGlzdCIsIjUiXSxbIkZpcnN0X1llYXIiLCIyMDE5Il0sWyJMYXN0X1llYXIiLCIyMDE5Il0sWyJTY2FsZSIsIi05Il0sWyJTZXJpZXMiLCJBIl1dfQ==.

127 Sanders, Medical Innovation Prize Fund Act.

128 "The Medical Innovation Prize Fund," Knowledge Ecology International, May 26, 2011, https://keionline.org/sites/default/files/big_prize_fund_overview_26may2011_a4.pdf.

129 Sanders, Medical Innovation Prize Fund Act.

130 "Cost-Effectiveness, the QALY, and the EvLYG," ICER, accessed June 14, 2024, https://icer.org/our-approach/methods-process/cost-effectiveness-the-qaly-and-the-evlyg/.

131 Pettitt Da et al., "The Limitations of QALY: A Literature Review," *Journal of Stem Cell Research & Therapy* 6, no. 4 (2016): 1000334, https://doi.org/10.4172/2157-7633.1000334.

132 Sanders, Medical Innovation Prize Fund Act.

133 US Bureau of Economic Analysis, "National Data: National Income and Product Accounts (2023)."

134 "The Medical Innovation Prize Fund."

135 "Declaration on the TRIPS Agreement and Public Health," World Trade Organization, November 20, 2001, https://www.wto.org/english/thewto_e/minist_e/min01_e/mindecl_trips_e.htm.

136 "Part II—Standards Concerning the Availability, Scope and Use of Intellectual Property Rights," World Trade Organization, accessed June 14, 2024, https://www.wto.org/english/docs_e/legal_e/27-trips_04c_e.htm.

137 Aaron O'Neill, "Countries with the Largest Gross Domestic Product (GDP) 2025," Statista, May 28, 2025, https://www.statista.com/statistics/268173/countries-with-the-largest-gross-domestic-product-gdp/; "Chart Pack: Defense Spending," Peter G. Peterson Foundation, February 3, 2025, https://www.pgpf.org/article/chart-pack-defense-spending/.

138 Lisa Forman, "The Intergovernmental Working Group on Public Health, Innovation and Intellectual Property," in *Realizing the Right to Development* (Office of the United Nations High Commissioner for Human Rights, 2013), https://www.ohchr.org/sites/default/files/Documents/Issues/Development/RTDBook/PartIIIChapter22.pdf.

139 James Love and Tim Hubbard, "The Big Idea: Prizes to Stimulate R&D for New Medicines," *Chicago-Kent Law Review* 82, no. 3 (June 2007): 1547, https://scholarship.kentlaw.iit.edu/cklawreview/vol82/iss3/16.

## 10 The COVID-19 Case Study

1 Elizabeth Cohen, Dakin Andone, and Ben Tinker, "US Government Declares the Novel Coronavirus a Public Health Emergency," CNN, January 31, 2020, https://www.cnn.com/2020/01/31/health/us-coronavirus-friday/index.html; WHO Declares Coronavirus a Pandemic, Urges Aggressive Action," AP, March 12, 2020, https://apnews.com/article/united-nations-michael-pence-religion-travel-virus-outbreak-52e12ca90c55b6e0c398d134a2cc286e.

2 Government Accountability Office, "Operation Warp Speed: Accelerated COVID-19 Vaccine Development Status and Efforts to Address Manufacturing Challenges," February 2021, https://www.gao.gov/assets/gao-21-319.pdf; Simi V. Siddalingaiah, "Operation Warp Speed Contracts for COVID-19 Vaccines and Ancillary Materials," Congressional Research Service, December 9, 2022, https://crsreports.congress.gov/product/pdf/IN/IN11560; Jamey Keaten, Maria Cheng, and John Leicester.

3 "Timeline," Congressman Tom Cole, accessed June 14, 2024, http://cole.house.gov/coronavirus/timeline.

4 Siddalingaiah, "Operation Warp Speed Contracts for COVID-19 Vaccines and Ancillary Materials."

5 Government Accountability Office, "Operation Warp Speed: Accelerated COVID-19 Vaccine Development Status and Efforts to Address Manufacturing Challenges."

6 "Vaccine Research & Development," Johns Hopkins Coronavirus Resource Center, accessed June 14, 2024, https://coronavirus.jhu.edu/vaccines/timeline.

7 Catherine Clifford, "How the Moderna Covid-19 MRNA Vaccine Was Made So Quickly," CNBC, July 3, 2021, https://www.cnbc.com/2021/07/03/how-moderna-made-its-mrna-covid-vaccine-so-quickly-noubar-afeyan.html.

8 David J. Sencer and CDC Museum, "CDC Museum COVID-19 Timeline," Centers for Disease Control and Prevention, accessed June 14, 2024, https://www.cdc.gov/museum/timeline/covid19.html.

9 Hussain S. Lalani et al., "US Public Investment in Development of MRNA Covid-19 Vaccines: Retrospective Cohort Study," *BMJ* 380, no. 8373 (March 1, 2023): e073747, https://doi.org/10.1136/bmj-2022-073747.

10 "Analysis: Pfizer Vaccine Relies on U.S. Government-Developed Spike Protein Technology," Public Citizen, November 10, 2020, https://www.citizen.org/news/analysis-pfizer-vaccine-relies-on-u-s-government-developed-spike-protein-technology/.

11 Zain Rizvi, "The NIH Vaccine," Public Citizen, June 25, 2020, https://www.citizen.org/article/the-nih-vaccine/.

12 Sheryl Gay Stolberg and Rebecca Robbins, "Moderna and U.S. at Odds over Vaccine Patent Rights," *The New York Times*, November 11, 2021, sec. U.S., https://www.nytimes.com/2021/11/09/us/moderna-vaccine-patent.html.

13 Moderna, "Moderna Reports Fourth Quarter and Fiscal Year 2022 Financial Results and Provides Business Updates," Access Newswire, February 23, 2023, https://www.accesswire.com/740439/Moderna-Reports-Fourth-Quarter-and-Fiscal-Year-2022-Financial-Results-and-Provides-Business-Updates; Eric Sagonowsky, "Moderna Pays US Government $400M 'Catch-Up Payment' under New COVID-19 Vaccine License," Fierce Pharma, February 24, 2023, https://www.fiercepharma.com/pharma/moderna-pays-us-government-400m-catch-payment-under-new-covid-19-vaccine-license.

14 Benjamin Mueller, "After Long Delay, Moderna Pays N.I.H. for Covid Vaccine Technique," *The New York Times*, February 23, 2023, sec. Science, https://www.nytimes.com/2023/02/23/science/moderna-covid-vaccine-patent-nih.html.
15 Office of Infectious Disease and HIV/AIDS Policy, "Vaccine Types," US Department of Health and Human Services, December 22, 2022, https://www.hhs.gov/immunization/basics/types/index.html; Mary West, "MRNA Vaccine vs. Traditional Vaccines," Medical News Today, March 28, 2023, https://www.medicalnewstoday.com/articles/mrna-vaccine-vs-traditional-vaccine.
16 "Messenger RNA (MRNA) Vaccines for COVID-19: How Do They Work?," Memorial Sloan Kettering Cancer Center, December 6, 2021, https://www.mskcc.org/coronavirus/messenger-rna-vaccines-covid-19.
17 Selam Gebrekidan and Matt Apuzzo, "Rich Countries Signed Away a Chance to Vaccinate the World," *The New York Times*, March 21, 2021, sec. World, https://www.nytimes.com/2021/03/21/world/vaccine-patents-us-eu.html.
18 Siddalingaiah, "Operation Warp Speed Contracts for COVID-19 Vaccines and Ancillary Materials."
19 Matej Mikulic, "Number of COVID-19 Vaccine Doses Administered in the United States as of April 26, 2023, by Vaccine Manufacturer," Statista, May 2, 2023, https://www.statista.com/statistics/1198516/covid-19-vaccinations-administered-us-by-company/.
20 Administration for Strategic Preparedness and Response, "COVID-19 Portfolio," MedicalCountermeasures.gov, accessed June 14, 2024, https://www.medicalcountermeasures.gov/app/barda/coronavirus/COVID19.aspx.
21 Jennifer Kates, Cynthia Cox, and Josh Michaud, "How Much Could COVID-19 Vaccines Cost the U.S. after Commercialization?," KFF, March 10, 2023, https://www.kff.org/coronavirus-covid-19/issue-brief/how-much-could-covid-19-vaccines-cost-the-u-s-after-commercialization/.
22 Administration for Strategic Preparedness and Response, "COVID-19 Portfolio"; Jennifer Kates, Cynthia Cox, and Josh Michaud, "How Much Could COVID-19 Vaccines Cost the U.S. after Commercialization?," KFF, March 10, 2023, https://www.kff.org/coronavirus-covid-19/issue-brief/how-much-could-covid-19-vaccines-cost-the-u-s-after-commercialization/.
23 Kevin Dunleavy, "While Moderna Moves off COVID, Spikevax Posts Market-Share Gains on Pfizer Rival," Fierce Pharma, February 22, 2024, https://www.fiercepharma.com/pharma/while-moderna-moving-covid-its-vaccine-gaining-share-pfizers-comirnaty#:~:text=During%20their%20heyday%20in%202021,versus%20%2436%20billion%20for%20Spikevax.
24 Gebrekidan and Apuzzo, "Rich Countries Signed Away a Chance to Vaccinate the World."
25 "Pfizer Inc. Covid-19 Vaccine Contract," US. Department of Health and Human Services, July 21, 2020, https://www.hhs.gov/sites/default/files/pfizer-inc-covid-19-vaccine-contract.pdf.
26 Jon Miltimore, "Understanding the 500% Price Increase of Pfizer's Covid Vaccine," Foundation for Economic Education, October 22, 2023, https://fee.org/articles/understanding-the-500-price-increase-of-pfizers-covid-vaccine/; Patrick Wingrove, "Moderna Expects to Price Its COVID Vaccine at about $130 in the US," *Reuters*, March 21, 2023, sec. Healthcare & Pharmaceuticals, https://www.reuters.com/business/healthcare-pharmaceuticals/moderna-expects-price-its-covid-vaccine-about-130-us-2023-03-20/.

27 Guillermo Aquino-Jarquin, "The Patent Dispute over the Breakthrough MRNA Technology," *Frontiers in Bioengineering and Biotechnology* 10 (November 3, 2022): 1049873, https://doi.org/10.3389/fbioe.2022.1049873.
28 Blake Brittain, ""Pfizer, BioNTech Countersue Moderna over COVID-19 Vaccine Patents," *Reuters*, December 6, 2022, sec. Legal, https://www.reut ers.com/legal/pfi zerbiontech-cou nter sue-mode rna-over-covid-19-vacc ine-pate nts-2022-12-05/.
29 Blake Brittain, "Pfizer Convinces US Patent Office to Cancel Two Moderna COVID-19 Vaccine Patents," *Reuters*, March 5, 2025, https://www.reuters.com/legal/pfizer-biontech-countersue-moderna-over-covid-19-vaccine-pate nts-2022-12-05/; Oliver Barnes and Ian Johnston, "Moderna Wins Covid Jab Patent Dispute over Pfizer and BioNTech," *Financial Times*, May 17, 2024, https://www.ft.com/content/50c5078c-c9f0-4b35-b916-3475b641c773.
30 Shayerah I. Akhtar, "World Trade Organization: 'TRIPS Waiver' for COVID-19 Vaccines," Congressional Research Service, August 31, 2022, https://crsreports.congr ess.gov/product/pdf/R/R47231/2.
31 Elizabeth Cohen Nedelman Michael, "The Secretive Group at the Center of the Nation's Largest Vaccine Trials," CNN, October 3, 2020, https://www.cnn.com/2020/10/03/health/dsmb-role-coronavirus-vaccine-trial/index.html; Steven Joffe et al., "Data and Safety Monitoring of COVID-19 Vaccine Clinical Trials," *The Journal of Infectious Diseases* 224, no. 12 (May 19, 2021): 1995–2000, https://doi.org/10.1093/infdis/jiab263.
32 Michael Nedelman Gumbrecht Jamie, "Trial Review Board Raises Concerns about AstraZeneca Vaccine Data," CNN, March 23, 2021, https://www.cnn.com/2021/03/23/health/astrazeneca-vaccine-dsmb-statement/index.html; Lauren Neergaard and Zeke Miller, "AstraZeneca Accused of Cherry-Picking Vaccine Study Data," AP, March 23, 2021, https://apnews.com/article/astrazeneca-may-have-used-outdated-info-vacc ine-trial-a98ef616f4e861a4b7568891d06b7da8.
33 Niamh Kennedy, "AstraZeneca Vaccine Is 79% Effective against Symptomatic Covid-19, Company Says," CNN, March 22, 2021, https://www.cnn.com/2021/03/22/health/astrazeneca-vaccine-efficacy-us-based-clinical-trial/index.html.
34 Rebecca Robbins et al., "Blunders Eroded U.S. Confidence in Early Vaccine Front-Runner," *The New York Times*, October 5, 2021, sec. Business, https://www.nytimes.com/2020/12/08/business/covid-vaccine-oxford-astrazeneca.html.
35 Sarah Tanveer et al., "Transparency of COVID-19 Vaccine Trials: Decisions without Data," *BMJ Evidence-Based Medicine* 27, no. 4 (August 9, 2021): 199–205, https://doi.org/10.1136/bmjebm-2021-111735.
36 Steven J. Ellison, "Can I Sue a Vaccine Manufacturer for Side Effects?," FindLaw, January 3, 2024, https://www.findlaw.com/litigation/filing-a-lawsuit/can-i-sue-a-vacc ine-manufacturer-.html; "Public Readiness and Emergency Preparedness (PREP) Act," ASPR, accessed June 14, 2024, https://aspr.hhs.gov/legal/PREPact/Pages/default.aspx#:~:text=Public%20Readiness%20and%20Emergency%20Preparedn ess%20(PREP)%20Act&text=The%20declaration%20provides%20immunity%20f rom,to%20diseases%2C%20threats%20and%20conditions.
37 MacKenzie Sigalos, "You Can't Sue Pfizer or Moderna If You Have Severe Covid Vaccine Side Effects. The Government Likely Won't Compensate You for Damages Either," CNBC, December 17, 2020, https://www.cnbc.com/2020/12/16/covid-vacc ine-side-effects-compensation-lawsuit.html.

38 US Department of Health & Human Services, "12th Amendment to Declaration Under the Public Readiness and Emergency Preparedness Act for Medical Countermeasures Against COVID-19," Federal Register, December 11, 2024, https://www.federalregister.gov/documents/2024/12/11/2024-29108/12th-amendment-to-declaration-under-the-public-readiness-and-emergency-preparedness-act-for-medical.
39 Cheri Falvey, "PREP Act Protections for COVID-19 Vaccine Liability," PharmExec, January 11, 2021, https://www.pharmexec.com/view/prep-act-protections-for-covid-19-vaccine-liability; "National Childhood Vaccine Injury Act of 1986," Pub. L. No. 99–660 (1986), https://www.congress.gov/99/statute/STATUTE-100/STATUTE-100-Pg3743.pdf.
40 Tanveer et al., "Transparency of COVID-19 Vaccine Trials."
41 "US Coronavirus Vaccine Tracker," USAFacts, May 10, 2024, https://usafacts.org/visualizations/covid-vaccine-tracker-states/.
42 Peter Doshi and Linda Wastila to BMJ Editor, "Rapid Response: Key Pfizer Covid-19 Vaccine Trial Dataset Still Not Released," Comment on "Covid-19: Researchers Face Wait for Patient Level Data from Pfizer and Moderna Vaccine Trials," October 7, 2022, https://www.bmj.com/content/378/bmj.o1731/rr-1.
43 Greene, "Paramount Importance."
44 Pittman, "Public Health and Medical Professionals for Transparency v. Food and Drug Administration, No. 4:21-Cv-1058-P: Document 35."
45 "US Coronavirus Vaccine Tracker."
46 Daniel A. Cox et al., "America's Crisis of Confidence: Rising Mistrust, Conspiracies, and Vaccine Hesitancy after COVID-19," American Enterprise Institute, accessed June 14, 2022, https://www.aei.org/research-products/report/americas-crisis-of-confidence-rising-mistrust-conspiracies-and-vaccine-hesitancy-after-covid-19/.
47 "2024 Edelman Trust Barometer—Special Report: Trust and Health," Edelman Trust Institute, 2024, https://www.edelman.com/trust/2024/trust-barometer/special-report-health.
48 Kearney et al., "KFF Tracking Poll on Health Information and Trust."
49 Grace Sparks et al., "KFF COVID-19 Vaccine Monitor: April 2022," KFF, May 4, 2022, https://www.kff.org/coronavirus-covid-19/poll-finding/kff-covid-19-vaccine-monitor-april-2022/.
50 Cox et al., "America's Crisis of Confidence: Rising Mistrust, Conspiracies, and Vaccine Hesitancy after COVID-19."
51 Tej D. Azad et al., "Assessment of Public Opinion on Transparency at the US Food and Drug Administration," *JAMA Network Open* 5, no. 2 (February 18, 2022): e220026, https://doi.org/10.1001/jamanetworkopen.2022.0026.
52 Pittman, "Public Health and Medical Professionals for Transparency v. Food and Drug Administration, No. 4:21-Cv-1058-P: Document 35," 2.
53 Bill Chappell, "1st Known U.S. COVID-19 Death Was Weeks Earlier than Previously Thought," *NPR*, April 22, 2020, sec. The Coronavirus Crisis, https://www.npr.org/sections/coronavirus-live-updates/2020/04/22/840836618/1st-known-u-s-covid-19-death-was-on-feb-6-a-post-mortem-test-reveals; CDC, "Surveillance and Data Analytics: COVID-19 Surveillance Data in the United States," July 9, 2025, https://www.npr.org/sections/coronavirus-live-updates/2020/04/22/840836618/1st-known-u-s-covid-19-death-was-on-feb-6-a-post-mortem-test-reveals; CDC, "Surveillance and Data Analytics: COVID-19 Surveillance Data in the United States," July 9, 2025, https://www.cdc.gov/nchs/nvss/vsrr/covid19/index.htm.

54 Patrick Boyle, "How Are COVID-19 Deaths Counted? It's Complicated," AAMC, February 18, 2021, https://www.aamc.org/news/how-are-covid-19-deaths-counted-it-s-complicated.

55 Katharine Lang, "Are We Overcounting COVID-19 Deaths?," Medical News Today, March 11, 2022, https://www.medicalnewstoday.com/articles/how-are-covid-19-deaths-counted-and-what-does-this-mean; Eugenio Paglino et al., "Excess Natural-Cause Mortality in US Counties and Its Association with Reported COVID-19 Deaths," *Proceedings of the National Academy of Sciences* 121, no. 6 (February 1, 2024): e2313661121, https://doi.org/10.1073/pnas.2313661121.

56 FDA, "Emergency Use Authorization for Vaccines Explained," US Food & Drug Administration, November 20, 2020, https://www.fda.gov/vaccines-blood-biologics/vaccines/emergency-use-authorization-vaccines-explained.

57 "Vaccine Research & Development."

58 Fernando P. Polack et al., "Safety and Efficacy of the BNT162b2 MRNA Covid-19 Vaccine," *New England Journal of Medicine* 383, no. 27 (December 10, 2020): 2603–15, https://doi.org/10.1056/NEJMoa2034577; Lindsey R. Baden et al., "Efficacy and Safety of the MRNA-1273 SARS-CoV-2 Vaccine," *New England Journal of Medicine* 384, no. 5 (December 30, 2020): 403–16, https://doi.org/10.1056/NEJMoa2035389.

59 Polack et al., "Safety and Efficacy of the BNT162b2 MRNA Covid-19 Vaccine."

60 Baden et al., "Efficacy and Safety of the MRNA-1273 SARS-CoV-2 Vaccine"; Claudio Marabotti, "Efficacy and Effectiveness of Covid-19 Vaccine—Absolute vs. Relative Risk Reduction," *Expert Review of Vaccines* 21, no. 7 (April 19, 2022): 873–5, https://doi.org/10.1080/14760584.2022.2067531.

61 "Paul A. Offit, MD," Children's Hospital of Philadelphia, accessed June 14, 2024, https://www.chop.edu/doctors/offit-paul-a.

62 Paul A. Offit, *Tell Me When It's Over: An Insider's Guide to Deciphering Covid Myths and Navigating Our Post-Pandemic World* (Washington, DC: National Geographic Partners, 2024), 70.

63 Ibid., 137–41.

64 "Symptoms of COVID-19," CDC, March 15, 2024, https://web.archive.org/web/20240331012544/https://www.cdc.gov/coronavirus/2019-ncov/symptoms-testing/symptoms.html.

65 Offit, *Tell Me When It's Over*, 137–41.

66 Polack et al., "Safety and Efficacy of the BNT162b2 mRNA Covid-19 Vaccine"; Baden et al., "Efficacy and Safety of the mRNA-1273 SARS-CoV-2 Vaccine."

67 Anderson E. Ikeokwu et al., "Unveiling the Impact of COVID-19 Vaccines: A Meta-Analysis of Survival Rates among Patients in the United States Based on Vaccination Status," *Cureus* 15, no. 8 (August 10, 2023): e43282, https://doi.org/10.7759/cureus.43282.

68 Fiona P. Havers et al., "COVID-19-Associated Hospitalizations among Vaccinated and Unvaccinated Adults 18 Years or Older in 13 US States, January 2021 to April 2022," *JAMA Internal Medicine* 182, no. 10 (September 8, 2022): 1071–81, https://doi.org/10.1001/jamainternmed.2022.4299.

69 "People with Certain Medical Conditions and COVID-19 Risk Factors," CDC, January 6, 2025, https://www.cdc.gov/covid/risk-factors/?CDC_AAref_Val=https://www.cdc.gov/coronavirus/2019-ncov/need-extra-precautions/people-with-medical-conditions.html.

70 "United States: COVID-19 Weekly Death Rate by Vaccination Status," Our World in Data, accessed June 14, 2024, https://ourworldindata.org/grapher/united-states-rates-of-covid-19-deaths-by-vaccination-status?facet=metric&country=~65-79.

71 Betzaida Tejada-Vera and Ellen A. Kramarow, "COVID-19 Mortality in Adults Aged 65 and Over: United States, 2020," National Center for Health Statistics, October 2022, https://www.cdc.gov/nchs/data/databriefs/db446.pdf.

72 Havers et al., "COVID-19-Associated Hospitalizations among Vaccinated and Unvaccinated Adults 18 Years or Older in 13 US States, January 2021 to April 2022."

73 Jason Robert C. Singson et al., "Factors Associated with Severe Outcomes among Immunocompromised Adults Hospitalized for COVID-19—COVID-NET, 10 States, March 2020–February 2022," *MMWR Morbidity and Mortality Weekly Report* 71, no. 27 (2022): 878–84, https://doi.org/10.15585/mmwr.mm7127a3; Andrea Antinori and Mary Bausch-Jurken, "The Burden of COVID-19 in the Immunocompromised Patient: Implications for Vaccination and Needs for the Future," *The Journal of Infectious Diseases* 228, no. Supplement 1 (August 4, 2023): S4–12, https://doi.org/10.1093/infdis/jiad181.

74 Rachael A. Evans et al., "Impact of COVID-19 on Immunocompromised Populations during the Omicron Era: Insights from the Observational Population-Based INFORM Study," *The Lancet Regional Health—Europe* 35 (October 12, 2023): 100747, https://doi.org/10.1016/j.lanepe.2023.100747.

75 Lyudmyla Kompaniyets et al., "Body Mass Index and Risk for COVID-19–Related Hospitalization, Intensive Care Unit Admission, Invasive Mechanical Ventilation, and Death—United States, March–December 2020," *MMWR Morbidity and Mortality Weekly Report* 70, no. 10 (2021): 355–61, https://doi.org/10.15585/mmwr.mm7010e4.

76 Satoshi Yoshiji et al., "Causal Associations between Body Fat Accumulation and COVID-19 Severity: A Mendelian Randomization Study," *Frontiers in Endocrinology* 13 (August 2, 2023): 899625, https://doi.org/10.3389/fendo.2022.899625.

77 "Obesity, Race/Ethnicity, and COVID-19," CDC, accessed July 13, 2025, https://web.archive.org/web/20250714012211/https://www.cdc.gov/obesity/data/obesity-and-covid-19.html.

78 Bryan Stierman et al., "National Health and Nutrition Examination Survey 2017–March 2020 Prepandemic Data Files—Development of Files and Prevalence Estimates for Selected Health Outcomes," National Center for Health Statistics, June 14, 2021, https://www.cdc.gov/nchs/data/nhsr/nhsr158-508.pdf.

79 Fryar et al., "Prevalence of Overweight, Obesity, and Severe Obesity among Adults Aged 20 and Over: United States, 1960–1962 through 2017–2018."

80 "People with Certain Medical Conditions."

81 Robert Sallis et al., "Physical Inactivity Is Associated with a Higher Risk for Severe COVID-19 Outcomes: A Study in 48 440 Adult Patients," *British Journal of Sports Medicine* 55, no. 19 (April 13, 2021): 1099–105, https://doi.org/10.1136/bjsports-2021-104080.

82 Offit, *Tell Me When It's Over*, 141–2.

83 Catherine M. Brown et al., "Outbreak of SARS-CoV-2 Infections, Including COVID-19 Vaccine Breakthrough Infections, Associated with Large Public Gatherings—Barnstable County, Massachusetts, July 2021," *MMWR Morbidity and Mortality Weekly Report* 70, no. 31 (2021): 1059–62, https://doi.org/10.15585/mmwr.mm7031e2.

84 Molly K. Steele et al., "Estimated Number of COVID-19 Infections, Hospitalizations, and Deaths Prevented Among Vaccinated Persons in the US, December 2020 to September 2021," JAMA Network Open 5, no. 7 (2022): e2220385, https://doi.org/10.1001/jamanetworkopen.2022.20385; Virat Agrawal, Neeraj Sood, and Christopher Whaley, "The Impact of the Global COVID-19 Vaccination Campaign on All-Cause Mortality" (Cambridge, MA: National Bureau of Economic Research, 2023), https://doi.org/10.3386/w31812.

85 Our World in Data, "United States: COVID-19 Weekly Death Rate."

86 Antinori and Bausch-Jurken, "The Burden of COVID-19 in the Immunocompromised Patient."

87 Offit, *Tell Me When It's Over*, 210–15.

88 Tomás M. León et al., "COVID-19 Cases and Hospitalizations by COVID-19 Vaccination Status and Previous COVID-19 Diagnosis—California and New York, May–November 2021," *MMWR Morbidity and Mortality Weekly Report* 71, no. 4 (January 28, 2022): 125–31, https://doi.org/10.15585/mmwr.mm7104e1.

89 Caroline Stein et al., "Past SARS-CoV-2 Infection Protection against Re-infection: A Systematic Review and Meta-Analysis," *The Lancet* 401, no. 10379 (February 16, 2023): 833–42, https://doi.org/10.1016/S0140-6736(22)02465-5.

90 Meredith Wadman, "Having SARS-CoV-2 Once Confers Much Greater Immunity than a Vaccine—but Vaccination Remains Vital," Science, August 25, 2021, https://www.science.org/content/article/having-sars-cov-2-once-confers-much-greater-immunity-vaccine-vaccination-remains-vital.

91 "The Lancet: Most Comprehensive Study to Date Provides Evidence on Natural Immunity Protection by COVID-19 Variant and How Protection Fades over Time," Institute for Health Metrics and Evaluation, February 16, 2023, https://www.healthdata.org/news-events/newsroom/news-releases/lancet-most-comprehens ive-study-date-provides-evidence-natural.

92 FDA, "FDA Approves First COVID-19 Vaccine," US Food & Drug Administration, August 23, 2021, https://www.fda.gov/news-events/press-announcements/fda-approves-first-covid-19-vaccine#:~:text=Today%2C%20the%20U.S.%20Food%20and,years%20of%20age%20and%20older.

93 Philip R. Krause, "Follow the Science?: Oversight of the Biden Covid-19 Administrative State Response," Congressional Hearing Testimony, June 26, 2024, https://judiciary.house.gov/sites/evo-subsites/republicans-judiciary.house.gov/files/evo-media-document/Krause%20Testimony.pdf.

94 Marion Gruber to Peter Marks and Celia Witten, "Pfizer COVID-19 Vaccine BLA Review Timeline," July 15, 2021, https://www.fda.gov/media/168263/download.

95 Krause, "Follow the Science?: Oversight of the Biden Covid-19 Administrative State Response," June 26, 2024.

96 Alexander Gaffney, "FDA Today | Peter Marks' Defense of CBER's Vaccine Approach," LinkedIn, September 14, 2021, https://www.linkedin.com/pulse/fda-today-peter-marks-defense-cbers-vaccine-approach-alexander.

97 Lloyd Austin, "Mandatory Coronavirus Disease 2019 Vaccination of Department of Defense Service Members," Memorandum, August 24, 2021, https://media.defense.gov/2021/Aug/25/2002838826/-1/-1/0/Memorandum-for-mandatory-coronavirus-disease-2019-vaccination-of-department-of-defense-service-members.pdf; U.S. Department of Defense, "2021 Demographics: Profile of the Military Community"

(2022), https://download.militaryonesource.mil/12038/MOS/Reports/2021-demog raphics-report.pdf.

98 Joseph R. Biden Jr., "Executive Order 14043: Requiring Coronavirus Disease 2019 Vaccination for Federal Employees," Federal Register, September 9, 2021, https:// www.federalregister.gov/documents/2021/09/14/2021-19927/requiring-coronavi rus-disease-2019-vaccination-for-federal-employees; Sheryl Gay Stolberg and Katie Rogers, "New Vaccine Requirements Apply to a Broad Range of the National Work Force.," *The New York Times*, September 9, 2021, sec. U.S., https://www.nytimes. com/2021/09/09/us/politics/federal-employee-vaccine-mandate.html; Heidi M. Peters and L. Elaine Halchin, "Executive Order 14042 Requirements for COVID-19 Vaccination of Federal Contractors," Congressional Research Service, November 19, 2021, https://www.congress.gov/crs_external_products/IN/PDF/IN11803/IN11 803.1.pdf; State of Texas, "State of Texas v. Biden et al., No. 3:21-Cv-00309 Document 1" (United States District Court for the Southern District of Texas Galveston Division, October 29, 2021), https://www.texasattorneygeneral.gov/sites/default/ files/global/images/20211029_TX%20v%20Biden%20et%20al%20%28file%20mar ked%29.pdf.

99 Roy Maurer, "Biden Orders Vaccination Mandates for Larger Employers, Federal Workforce," SHRM, September 9, 2021, https://www.shrm.org/topics-tools/news/tal ent-acquisition/biden-orders-vaccination-mandates-larger-employers-federalworkforce.

100 CMS, "Biden-Harris Administration Issues Emergency Regulation Requiring COVID-19 Vaccination for Health Care Workers," CMS.Gov, November 4, 2021, https://www.cms.gov/newsroom/press-releases/biden-harris-administration-issues-emergency-regulation-requiring-covid-19-vaccination-health-care.

101 Katie Rogers and Sheryl Gay Stolberg, "Biden Mandates Vaccines for Workers, Saying, 'Our Patience Is Wearing Thin,'" *The New York Times*, November 12, 2021, sec. U.S., https://www.nytimes.com/2021/09/09/us/politics/biden-mandates-vacci nes.html.

102 Joseph R. Biden Jr., "Remarks by President Biden on Fighting the COVID- 19 Pandemic," The White House Briefing Room, September 9, 2021, https://bidenwhi tehouse.archives.gov/briefing-room/speeches-remarks/2021/09/09/remarks-by-president-biden-on-fighting-the-covid-19-pandemic-3/.

103 CDC, "COVID-19 Vaccinations in the United States,Jurisdiction."

104 "Coronavirus (COVID-19) Vaccinations," Our World in Data, accessed June 14, 2024, https://ourworldindata.org/covid-vaccinations.

105 ZDoggMD, "Boosters, Masking Kids, Vaccine Mandates & More (w/Dr. Vinay Prasad)," YouTube, September 15, 2021, at 14:28–17:46, https://www.youtube.com/ watch?v=Fe9boK1jKCM; "New Vintage 2021 Population Estimates Available for the Nation, States and Puerto Rico," United States Census Bureau, December 21, 2021, https://www.census.gov/newsroom/press-releases/2021/2021-population-estima tes.html.

106 FDA, "Antibody (Serology) Testing for COVID-19: Information for Patients and Consumers," US Food & Drug Administration, April 25, 2024, https://www.fda.gov/ medical-devices/coronavirus-covid-19-and-medical-devices/antibody-serology-test ing-covid-19-information-patients-and-consumers.

107 Andrea Hsu, "Thousands of Workers Are Opting to Get Fired, Rather than Take the Vaccine," *NPR*, October 24, 2021, sec. Business, https://www.npr.org/2021/10/24/104 7947268/covid-vaccine-workers-quitting-getting-fired-mandates; Andrea Hsu,

"Thousands of Workers Were Fired over Vaccine Mandates. For Some, the Fight Goes On," WUSF, December 27, 2022, https://www.wusf.org/health-news-florida/2022-12-27/thousands-of-workers-were-fired-over-vaccine-mandates-for-some-the-fight-goes-on.
108 David Henry et al., "No Jab, No Job: Citigroup to Fire Unvaccinated Staff This Month - Memo," *Reuters*, January 8, 2022, https://www.reuters.com/business/finance/citi-terminate-employees-unvaccinated-jan-14-source-2022-01-07/.
109 Andy Thomason and Brian O'Leary, "Here's a List of Colleges That Require Students or Employees to Be Vaccinated Against Covid-19," The Chronicle of Higher Education, January 26, 2022, https://archive.is/6Kxd5#selection-1663.9-1670.0.
110 Oren Liebermann, "Only 43 of More than 8,000 Discharged from US Military for Refusing Covid Vaccine Have Rejoined," CNN Politics, October 2, 2023, https://www.cnn.com/2023/10/02/politics/us-military-covid-vaccine.
111 National Federation of Independent Business v. Department of Labor, Occupational Safety and Health Administration, 595 U.S. (US Supreme Court 2022).
112 Patricia Anderson Pryor and Laura A. Mitchell, "Nationwide Injunction Against Federal Contractor COVID-19 Vaccine Mandate Overturned," Jackson Lewis, August 29, 2022, https://www.jacksonlewis.com/insights/nationwide-injunction-against-federal-contractor-covid-19-vaccine-mandate-overturned.
113 David Shepardson et al., "U.S. Judge Blocks Biden Federal Employee COVID Vaccine Mandate," *Reuters*, January 21, 2022, https://www.reuters.com/legal/government/us-judge-blocks-biden-federal-employee-covid-19-vaccine-mandate-2022-01-21/; Dan Diamond, "Most Federal Covid Vaccine Mandates to End May 11," *The Washington Post*, May 1, 2023, https://www.washingtonpost.com/health/2023/05/01/covid-vaccine-requirements-end-international-travelers/.
114 "The Biden-Harris Administration Will End COVID-19 Vaccination Requirements for Federal Employees, Contractors, International Travelers, Head Start Educators, and CMS-Certified Facilities," The American Presidency Project, May 1, 2023, https://www.presidency.ucsb.edu/documents/white-house-press-release-the-biden-harris-administration-will-end-covid-19-vaccination.
115 "Influenza Vaccine," C-SPAN, October 11, 2004, 30:07–30:34, https://www.c-span.org/video/?183885-2/influenza-vaccine#!
116 Madeline Holcombe, Maggie Fox, and Holly Yan, "Covid-19 Vaccine Mandates Work, Dr. Anthony Fauci Says," CNN, October 11, 2021, https://www.cnn.com/2021/10/11/health/us-coronavirus-monday/index.html.
117 Offit, *Tell Me When It's Over*, 214–15.
118 Emily Kopp, "EXCLUSIVE: 'People Were Angry': Inside One Biden Admin COVID Decree That Upended Countless Careers," Daily Caller, March 19, 2025, https://dailycaller.com/2025/03/19/exclusive-inside-one-biden-admin-covid-decree-upeneded-careers/.
119 Offit, *Tell Me When It's Over*, 214–15.
120 FDA, "Coronavirus (COVID-19) Update: FDA Authorizes Pfizer-BioNTech COVID-19 Vaccine for Emergency Use in Adolescents in Another Important Action in Fight against Pandemic," US Food & Drug Administration, May 10, 2021, https://archive.is/eaDAK#selection-679.0-679.78.
121 FDA, "FDA Authorizes Pfizer-BioNTech COVID-19 Vaccine for Emergency Use in Children 5 through 11 Years of Age," US Food & Drug Administration, October 29, 2021, https://web.archive.org/web/20211223221752/https://www.fda.gov/news-eve

ucsb.edu/documents/remarks-the-covid-19-response-and-national-vaccination-efforts-0.
170 Offit, *Tell Me When It's Over*, 142–3.
171 Yinon M. Bar-On et al., "Protection of BNT162b2 Vaccine Booster against Covid-19 in Israel," New England Journal of Medicine 385, no. 15 (September 15, 2021): 1393–400, https://doi.org/10.1056/NEJMoa2114255.
172 Offit, *Tell Me When It's Over*, 143.
173 Sara G. Miller, Reynolds Lewis, and Erika Edwards, "FDA Advisory Group Rejects Covid Boosters for Most, Limits to High-Risk Groups," NBC News, September 17, 2021, https://www.nbcnews.com/health/health-news/fda-advisory-group-rejects-covid-boosters-limits-high-risk-groups-rcna2074.
174 Offit, *Tell Me When It's Over*, 143.
175 "Marion F. Gruber, Ph.D., MS," LinkedIn, accessed July 6, 2025, https://www.linkedin.com/in/marion-gruber/details/experience/; Ashley Collman, "2 Top FDA Officials Resigned over the Biden Administration's Booster-Shot Plan, Saying It Insisted on the Policy before the Agency Approved It, Reports Say," Business Insider, September 1, 2021, https://www.businessinsider.com/2-top-fda-officials-resigned-biden-booster-plan-reports-2021-9.
176 Philip R. Krause et al., "Considerations in Boosting COVID-19 Vaccine Immune Responses," *The Lancet* 398, no. 10308 (September 13, 2021): 1377–80, https://doi.org/10.1016/S0140-6736(21)02046-8.
177 "167th Vaccines and Related Biological Products Advisory Committee (VRBPAC) Meeting," Web-Conference, U.S. Food & Drug Administration, October 26, 2021, https://www.fda.gov/media/154871/download.
178 FDA, "FDA Authorizes Booster Dose of Pfizer-BioNTech COVID-19 Vaccine for Certain Populations," US Food & Drug Administration, September 22, 2021, https://www.fda.gov/news-events/press-announcements/fda-authorizes-booster-dose-pfizer-biontech-covid-19-vaccine-certain-populations.
179 Maggie Fox, "CDC Advisers Recommend Booster Doses of Covid-19 Vaccine for Certain Adults Only," CNN, September 23, 2021, https://www.cnn.com/2021/09/23/health/pfizer-acip-booster-recommendation/index.html; Sarah Mbaeyi et al., "The Advisory Committee on Immunization Practices' Interim Recommendations for Additional Primary and Booster Doses of COVID-19 Vaccines—United States, 2021," *MMWR Morbidity and Mortality Weekly Report* 70, no. 44 (November 5, 2021): 1545–52, https://doi.org/10.15585/mmwr.mm7044e2.
180 Apoorva Mandavilli and Benjamin Mueller, "C.D.C. Chief Overrules Agency Panel and Recommends Pfizer-BioNTech Boosters for Workers at Risk," *The New York Times*, November 21, 2021, sec. World, https://www.nytimes.com/2021/09/24/world/covid-boosters-vaccine-cdc-director.html.
181 CDC, "CDC Statement on ACIP Booster Recommendations," CDC Archive, September 24, 2021, https://archive.cdc.gov/www_cdc_gov/media/releases/2021/p0924-booster-recommendations-.html.
182 Mandavilli and Mueller, "C.D.C. Chief Overrules Agency Panel and Recommends Pfizer-BioNTech Boosters for Workers at Risk."
183 FDA, "Coronavirus (COVID-19) Update: FDA Expands Eligibility for COVID-19 Vaccine Boosters," US Food & Drug Administration, November 19, 2021, https://web.archive.org/web/20211120122706/https://www.fda.gov/news-eve

nts/press-announcements/coronavirus-covid-19-update-fda-expands-eligibil ity-covid-19-vaccine-boosters.

184 Philip Krause, Marion F. Gruber, and Paul A. Offit, "We Don't Need Universal Booster Shots. We Need to Reach the Unvaccinated.," *The Washington Post*, November 29, 2021, https://www.washingtonpost.com/outlook/2021/11/29/boos ter-shots-universal-opinion/.

185 CDC, "CDC Expands COVID-19 Booster Recommendations," CDC Archive, November 29, 2021, https://archive.cdc.gov/#/details?url=https://www.cdc.gov/media/releases/2021/s1129-booster-recommendations.html.

186 FDA, "Coronavirus (COVID-19) Update: FDA Expands Eligibility for Pfizer-BioNTech COVID-19 Booster Dose to 16- and 17-Year-Olds," US Food & Drug Administration, December 9, 2021, https://www.fda.gov/news-events/press-announcements/coronavirus-covid-19-update-fda-expands-eligibility-pfizer-biont ech-covid-19-booster-dose-16-and-17#:~:text=The%20FDA%20has%20determi ned%20that,serious%20consequences%20that%20can%20occur.

187 Philip Krause and Luciana Borio, "The Biden Administration Has Been Sidelining Vaccine Experts," *The Washington Post*, December 16, 2021, https://www.washingtonpost.com/outlook/2021/12/16/vaccines-fda-cdc-boosters-exp ert-panel/.

188 FDA, "Coronavirus (COVID-19) Update: FDA Takes Multiple Actions to Expand Use of Pfizer-BioNTech COVID-19 Vaccine," U.S. Food & Drug Administration, January 3, 2022, https://web.archive.org/web/20220107183841/https://www.fda.gov/news-events/press-announcements/coronavirus-covid-19-update-fda-takes-multi ple-actions-expand-use-pfizer-biontech-covid-19-vaccine.

189 FDA, "Coronavirus (COVID-19) Update: FDA Takes Key Action by Approving Second COVID-19 Vaccine," US Food & Drug Administration, January 31, 2022, https://web.archive.org/web/20220207175703/https://www.fda.gov/news-events/press-announcements/coronavirus-covid-19-update-fda-takes-key-action-approv ing-second-covid-19-vaccine.

190 FDA, "Coronavirus (COVID-19) Update: FDA Expands Eligibility for Pfizer-BioNTech COVID-19 Vaccine Booster Dose to Children 5 through 11 Years," U.S. Food & Drug Administration, May 17, 2022, https://web.archive.org/web/202 20524072628/https://www.fda.gov/news-events/press-announcements/coronavi rus-covid-19-update-fda-expands-eligibility-pfizer-biontech-covid-19-vaccine-boos ter-dose.

191 CDC, "CDC Expands COVID-19 Booster Recommendations," CDC Archive, November 29, 2021, https://archive.cdc.gov/#/details?q=CDC%20Recommends%20 vaccine%20booster%20COVID&start=0&rows=10&url=https://www.cdc.gov/media/releases/2021/s1129-booster-recommendations.html; CDC, "CDC Expands COVID-19 Booster Recommendations to 16-and-17-Year-Olds," CDC Archive, December 9, 2021, https://archive.cdc.gov/#/details?q=CDC%20Recommends%20 vaccine%20booster%20COVID&start=0&rows=10&url=https://www.cdc.gov/media/releases/2021/s1208-16-17-booster.html; CDC, "CDC Expands Booster Shot Eligibility and Strengthens Recommendations for 12-17 Year Olds," CDC Archive, January 5, 2022, https://archive.cdc.gov/#/details?q=CDC%20Recommends%20 &start=0&rows=10&url=https://www.cdc.gov/media/releases/2022/s0105-Boos ter-Shot.html; CDC, "CDC Recommends Pediatric COVID-19 Vaccine for Children 5 to 11 Years," CDC Archive, November 2, 2021, https://archive.cdc.gov/#/deta

ils?url=https://www.cdc.gov/media/releases/2021/s1102-PediatricCOVID-19Vaccine.html.

192 "United States: Coronavirus Pandemic Country Profile," Our World in Data, accessed June 14, 2024, https://ourworldindata.org/coronavirus/country/united-states.

193 "Coronavirus (COVID-19) Hospitalizations," Our World in Data, accessed June 14, 2024, https://ourworldindata.org/covid-hospitalizations.

194 "Coronavirus (COVID-19) Deaths," Our World in Data, accessed June 14, 2024, https://ourworldindata.org/covid-deaths.

195 Benjamin Mueller and Eleanor Lutz, "During the Omicron Wave, Death Rates Soared for Older People," *The New York Times*, May 31, 2022, sec. Health, https://www.nytimes.com/2022/05/31/health/omicron-deaths-age-65-elderly.html.

196 "Deaths by Select Demographic and Geographic Characteristics," CDC, September 27, 2023, https://www.cdc.gov/nchs/nvss/vsrr/covid_weekly/index.htm#SexAndAge.

197 Mueller and Lutz, "During the Omicron Wave, Death Rates Soared for Older People."

198 Prasad and Haslam, "COVID-19 Vaccines."

199 Alex Sigal et al., "Estimating Disease Severity of Omicron and Delta SARS-CoV-2 Infections," *Nature Reviews Immunology* 22 (April 2022): 267–9, https://doi.org/10.1038/s41577-022-00720-5.

200 Maya Pottiger, "Three DC Universities Will Require Covid Booster Shots by Early 2022," *Washingtonian*, December 16, 2021, https://www.washingtonian.com/2021/12/16/three-dc-universities-will-require-covid-booster-shots-by-early-2022/; Michael T. Nietzel, "Expect All Of America's Top 20 Colleges to Require Booster Vaccines for Next Semester," *Forbes*, December 20, 2021, https://www.forbes.com/sites/michaeltnietzel/2021/12/20/expect-every-one-of-americas-top-20-colleges-to-require-booster-vaccines-for-next-semester/.

201 Yinon M. Bar-On et al., "Protection against Covid-19 by BNT162b2 Booster across Age Groups," *New England Journal of Medicine* 385, no. 26 (December 8, 2021): 2421–30, https://doi.org/10.1056/NEJMoa2115926.

202 Prasad and Haslam, "COVID-19 Vaccines"; Marty Makary, "The Dangerous Push to Give Boosters to Teens," The Wall Street Journal, December 21, 2021, https://www.wsj.com/articles/dangerous-push-to-give-boosters-to-teens-vacccine-covid-19-omicron-vaxx-requirement-mandate-11640107759.

203 Kevin Bardosh et al., "COVID-19 Vaccine Boosters for Young Adults: A Risk Benefit Assessment and Ethical Analysis of Mandate Policies at Universities," *Journal of Medical Ethics* 50, no. 2 (December 5, 2022): 126–38, https://doi.org/10.1136/jme-2022-108449.

204 Ibid.

205 FDA, "Coronavirus (COVID-19) Update: FDA Authorizes Moderna and Pfizer-BioNTech COVID-19 Vaccines for Children Down to 6 Months of Age," US Food & Drug Administration, June 17, 2022, https://web.archive.org/web/20220617125738/https://www.fda.gov/news-events/press-announcements/coronavirus-covid-19-update-fda-authorizes-moderna-and-pfizer-biontech-covid-19-vaccines-children.

206 CDC, "CDC Recommends COVID-19 Vaccines for Young Children," CDC Archive, June 18, 2022, https://archive.cdc.gov/#/details?url=https://www.cdc.gov/media/releases/2022/s0618-children-vaccine.html.

207 "FDA Briefing Document: EUA Amendment Request for Use of the Moderna COVID-19 Vaccine in Children 6 Months through 17 Years of Age," Vaccines

and Related Biological Products Advisory Committee Meeting, June 14, 2022, https://www.fda.gov/media/159189/download; Prasad and Haslam, "COVID-19 Vaccines."

208 FDA, "Coronavirus (COVID-19) Update: FDA Authorizes Moderna and Pfizer-BioNTech COVID-19 Vaccines for Children Down to 6 Months of Age."

209 Kristie E. N. Clarke et al., "Seroprevalence of Infection-Induced SARS-CoV-2 Antibodies—United States, September 2021–February 2022," *MMWR Morbidity and Mortality Weekly Report* 71, no. 17 (April 29, 2022): 606–8, https://doi.org/10.15585/mmwr.mm7117e3.

210 Prasad and Haslam, "COVID-19 Vaccines"; "FDA Briefing Document: EUA Amendment Request for Use of the Moderna COVID-19 Vaccine in Children 6 Months through 17 Years of Age"; "FDA Briefing Document: EUA Amendment Request for Pfizer-BioNTech COVID-19 Vaccine for Use in Children 6 Months through 4 Years of Age," Vaccines and Related Biological Products Advisory Committee Meeting, June 15, 2022, https://www.fda.gov/media/159195/download; "FDA Briefing Document: EUA Amendment Request for Pfizer-BioNTech COVID-19 Vaccine for Use in Children 5 through 11 Years of Age," Vaccines and Related Biological Products Advisory Committee Meeting, October 26, 2021, https://www.fda.gov/media/153447/download; Denise M. Hinton "Pfizer-BioNTech COVID-19 Vaccine EUA Letter of Authorization Reissued 05-10-2021," to Elisa Harkins, May 10, 2021, https://www.fda.gov/media/144412/download.

211 Paul A. Offit, "Bivalent Covid-19 Vaccines—A Cautionary Tale," *New England Journal of Medicine* 388, no. 6 (January 11, 2023): 481–3, https://doi.org/10.1056/NEJMp2215780.

212 175th Vaccines and Related Biological Products Advisory Committee (VRBPAC) Meeting," Web-Conference, U.S. Food & Drug Administration, June 28, 2022, https://www.fda.gov/media/160778/download.

213 Elizabeth Cohen and Naomi Thomas, "FDA Vaccine Advisers 'Disappointed' and 'Angry' That Early Data about New Covid-19 Booster Shot Wasn't Presented for Review Last Year," CNN, January 11, 2023, https://www.cnn.com/2023/01/11/health/moderna-bivalent-transparency/index.html.

214 FDA, "Coronavirus (COVID-19) Update: FDA Authorizes Moderna, Pfizer-BioNTech Bivalent COVID-19 Vaccines for Use as a Booster Dose," US Food & Drug Administration, August 31, 2022, https://web.archive.org/web/20220901035343/https://www.fda.gov/news-events/press-announcements/coronavirus-covid-19-update-fda-authorizes-moderna-pfizer-biontech-bivalent-covid-19-vaccines-use?utm_medium=email&utm_source=govdelivery.

215 U.S. Food & Drug Administration, "Pfizer Bivalent Division Memo 08312022," August 31, 2022, https://www.fda.gov/media/161595/download; U.S. Food & Drug Administration, "Moderna EUA Decision Memo 08312022," August 31, 2022, https://www.fda.gov/media/161554/download; Kena A. Swanson, "Pfizer/BioNTech COVID-19 Omicron-Modified Vaccine Options," Presentation, Pfizer-BioNTech, June 28, 2022, https://www.fda.gov/media/159496/download; Jacqueline Miller, "Booster Doses of Moderna COVID-19 Vaccines in Adults, Adolescents & Children," Presentation, Moderna, September 1, 2022, https://web.archive.org/web/20220915022130/https://www.cdc.gov/vaccines/acip/meetings/downloads/slides-2022-09-01/06-COVID-Miller-508.pdf.

216 Robert M. Califf, X (Twitter), September 9, 2022, https://archive.ph/FXIMB.

217 CDC, "CDC Recommends the First Updated COVID-19 Booster," CDC Archive, September 1, 2022, https://archive.cdc.gov/#/details?url=https://www.cdc.gov/media/releases/2022/s0901-covid-19-booster.html.

218 FDA, "Coronavirus (COVID-19) Update: FDA Authorizes Moderna and Pfizer-BioNTech Bivalent COVID-19 Vaccines for Use as a Booster Dose in Younger Age Groups," US Food and Drug Administration, October 12, 2022, https://web.archive.org/web/20221024174258/https://www.fda.gov/news-events/press-announcements/coronavirus-covid-19-update-fda-authorizes-moderna-and-pfizer-biontech-bivalent-covid-19-vaccines; CDC, "CDC Expands Updated COVID-19 Vaccines to Include Children Ages 5 Through 11," CDC Archive, October 12, 2022, https://archive.cdc.gov/www_cdc_gov/media/releases/2022/s1012-COVID-19-Vaccines.html.

219 FDA, "Coronavirus (COVID-19) Update: FDA Authorizes Updated (Bivalent) COVID-19 Vaccines for Children Down to 6 Months of Age," U.S. Food and Drug Administration, December 8, 2022, https://web.archive.org/web/20221216223935/https://www.fda.gov/news-events/press-announcements/coronavirus-covid-19-update-fda-authorizes-updated-bivalent-covid-19-vaccines-children-down-6-months; CDC, "CDC Expands Updated COVID-19 Vaccines to Include Children Ages 6 Months through 5 Years," CDC Archive, December 9, 2022, https://archive.cdc.gov/#/details?q=cdc%20recommend%20booster%206%20months%205%20years&start=0&rows=10&url=https://www.cdc.gov/media/releases/2022/s1209-covid-vaccine.html; Danielle L. Moulia et al., "Interim Recommendations for Use of Bivalent mRNA COVID-19 Vaccines for Persons Aged ≥6 Months — United States, April 2023," *MMWR Morbidity and Mortality Weekly Report* 72, no. 24 (2023): 657–62. http://dx.doi.org/10.15585/mmwr.mm7224a3.

220 Kristina Fiore, "Are Doctors Getting Their COVID Boosters?," MedPage Today, September 12, 2022, https://www.medpagetoday.com/special-reports/exclusives/100665.

221 Jason Laughlin, "Paul Offit, Philly's Most Vocal Vaccine Advocate, on Science, Truth, and Why He's Not a Fan of the Latest COVID Boosters," *The Philadelphia Inquirer*, November 8, 2022, https://www.inquirer.com/health/coronavirus/paul-offit-philadelphia-covid-vaccine-bivalent-booster-20221108.html.

222 Annika Kim Constantino, "BA.5 Boosters Could Be Here in the Next 3 Weeks, Says Dr. Jha: 'These Are Substantial Upgrades in Our Vaccines,'" CNBC, August 18, 2022, https://www.cnbc.com/2022/08/18/dr-ashish-jha-covid-ba-5-booster-shots-could-be-just-weeks-away.html.

223 "Pfizer and BioNTech Announce Positive Early Data From Clinical Trial of Omicron BA.4/BA.5-Adapted Bivalent Booster in Individuals 18 Years and Older," Pfizer, October 13, 2022, https://www.pfizer.com/news/press-release/press-release-detail/pfizer-and-biontech-announce-positive-early-data-clinical.

224 MS NOW, "CDC Director Walensky: 'You Need To Get Your Fall Booster Vaccine,'" YouTube, September 7, 2022, 1:00–2:35, https://www.youtube.com/watch?v=0Q6V67AZEHo.

225 Q. Want et al., "Antibody Responses to Omicron BA.4/BA.5 Bivalent MRNA Vaccine Booster Shot," bioRxiv, October 24, 2022, https://www.biorxiv.org/content/10.1101/2022.10.22.513349v1.

226 Ai-ris Y. Collier et al., "Immunogenicity of the BA.5 Bivalent MRNA Vaccine Boosters," bioRxiv, October 25, 2022, https://doi.org/10.1101/2022.10.24.513619.

227 Paul A. Offit, "Bivalent Covid-19 Vaccines—A Cautionary Tale," *New England Journal of Medicine* 388, no. 6 (January 11, 2023), https://doi.org/10.1056/NEJMp 2215780.
228 Reuben Jones, "CDC Likely to Recommend Annual COVID Shot in the Fall, Director Says," Spectrum News, July 27, 2023, https://ny1.com/nyc/all-boroughs/news/2023/07/27/cdc-director-covid-shot-annual-.
229 FDA, "FDA Takes Action on Updated mRNA COVID-19 Vaccines to Better Protect Against Currently Circulating Variants," US Food and Drug Administration, September 11, 2023, https://web.archive.org/web/20230913014025/https://www.fda.gov/news-events/press-announcements/fda-takes-action-updated-mrna-covid-19-vaccines-better-protect-against-currently-circulating; "CDC Recommends Updated COVID-19 Vaccine for Fall/Winter Virus Season," CDC Newsroom, September 12, 2023, https://www.cdc.gov/media/releases/2023/p0912-COVID-19-Vaccine.html.
230 Offit, *Tell Me When It's Over*, 151.
231 "SAGE Updates COVID-19 Vaccination Guidance," World Health Organization, March 28, 2023, https://www.who.int/news/item/28-03-2023-sage-updates-covid-19-vaccination-guidance; UK Health Security Agency, "JCVI Advises on Eligible Groups for 2023 Autumn Booster," GOV.UK, August 8, 2023, https://www.gov.uk/government/news/jcvi-advises-on-eligible-groups-for-2023-autumn-booster; "Information on Coronavirus Vaccination," Federal Ministry of Health, February 15, 2024, https://www.bundesgesundheitsministerium.de/en/coronavirus/faq-covid-19-vaccination; "Vaccines and Coronavirus," Finnish Institute for Health and Welfare, July 12, 2023, https://thl.fi/en/topics/infectious-diseases-and-vaccinations/what-s-new/coronavirus-covid-19-latest-updates/vaccines-and-coronavirus; "COVID-19 Vaccination in Norway," Helsenorge, April 25, 2023, https://www.helsenorge.no/en/coronavirus/covid19-vaccination/; "Current Rules and Recommendations," https://krisinformation.se/, March 19, 2024, https://www.krisinformation.se/en/hazards-and-risks/disasters-and-incidents/2020/official-information-on-the-new-coronavirus/current-rules-and-recommendations.
232 FDA, "FDA Approves and Authorizes Updated MRNA COVID-19 Vaccines to Better Protect against Currently Circulating Variants," US Food & Drug Administration, August 22, 2024, https://www.fda.gov/news-events/press-announcements/fda-approves-and-authorizes-updated-mrna-covid-19-vaccines-better-protect-against-currently; CDC, "CDC Recommends Updated 2024–2025 COVID-19 and Flu Vaccines for Fall/Winter Virus Season," CDC Newsroom, June 27, 2024, https://www.cdc.gov/media/releases/2024/s-t0627-vaccine-recommendations.html.
233 Ezekiel J. Emanuel and Paul A. Offit, "Could Trump Turn a Vaccine Into a Campaign Stunt?," *The New York Times*, June 8, 2020, sec. Opinion, https://www.nytimes.com/2020/06/08/opinion/trump-coronavirus-vaccine.html.
234 Ibid; Stanley A. Plotkin, "Correlates of Protection Induced by Vaccination," Clinical and Vaccine Immunology 17, no. 7 (July 1, 2010): 1055–65, https://doi.org/10.1128/CVI.00131-10.
235 Ashish K. Jha, X (Twitter), August 30, 2020, https://archive.is/ua0Jc.
236 Ghulam Rehman Mohyuddin and Vinay Prasad, "Detecting Selection Bias in Observational Studies—When Interventions Work Too Fast," *JAMA Internal Medicine* 183, no. 9 (June 12, 2023): 897–8, https://doi.org/10.1001/jamainternmed.2023.2067.

237 Ronen Arbel et al., "BNT162b2 Vaccine Booster and Mortality Due to Covid-19," *New England Journal of Medicine* 385, no. 26 (December 8, 2021): 2413–20, https://doi.org/10.1056/NEJMoa2115624.
238 Tracy B. Høeg, Ram Duriseti, and Vinay Prasad, "Potential 'Healthy Vaccinee Bias' in a Study of BNT162b2 Vaccine against Covid-19," *New England Journal of Medicine* 389, no. 3 (July 19, 2023): 284–6, https://doi.org/10.1056/NEJMc2306683.
239 Ronen Arbel et al., "Effectiveness of a Second BNT162b2 Booster Vaccine against Hospitalization and Death from COVID-19 in Adults Aged over 60 Years," *Nature Medicine* 28 (2022): 1486–90, https://doi.org/10.1038/s41591-022-01832-0.
240 Polack et al., "Safety and Efficacy of the BNT162b2 MRNA Covid-19 Vaccine."
241 Vinay Prasad MD MPH, "Why No One Trusts Scientists Anymore | My Lecture to WASH U | COVID19 Policy," YouTube, December 27, 2023, at 42:44–46:26, https://www.youtube.com/watch?v=EIdMMOUgVq4.
242 Abhishek Kumar et al., "Evaluation of the Use of Cancer Registry Data for Comparative Effectiveness Research," *JAMA Network Open* 3, no. 7 (July 30, 2020): e2011985, https://doi.org/10.1001/jamanetworkopen.2020.11985.
243 Centers for Disease Control and Prevention (CDC), "September 12, 2023 ACIP Meeting—Evidence to Recommendations," YouTube, September 18, 2023, at 16:26–24:14, https://youtu.be/lG5OccysvEg?t=986; Centers for Disease Control and Prevention (CDC), "Advisory Committee on Immunization Practices (ACIP) Day 2," YouTube, June 27, 2024, at 2:24:29–2:25:18, https://youtu.be/DQslT3K9L8Y?t=8610.
244 Centers for Disease Control and Prevention (CDC), "Advisory Committee on Immunization Practices (ACIP) Day 2," YouTube, June 27, 2024, at 2:23:52.
245 Kates et al., "How Much Could COVID-19 Vaccines Cost the U.S. After Commercialization?"; Sheryl Gay Stolberg, "The U.S. Agrees to Buy 200 Million More Doses of Moderna's Vaccine, in Case Boosters Are Needed.," *The New York Times*, June 16, 2021, sec. U.S., https://www.nytimes.com/2021/06/16/us/politis/moderna-covid-vaccine-booster-shots.html; Betsy Klein and Naomi Thomas, "Biden Administration Purchases Extra Pfizer Doses to Prepare for Possibility of Children Vaccine Needs and Booster Shots," CNN, July 23, 2021, https://www.cnn.com/2021/07/23/politics/pfizer-vaccine-doses-children-vaccinations-and-boosters/index.html.
246 Apoorva Mandavilli, "The C.D.C. Isn't Publishing Large Portions of the Covid Data It Collects," *The New York Times*, February 20, 2022, sec. Health, https://www.nytimes.com/2022/02/20/health/covid-cdc-data.html.
247 Apoorva Mandavilli, "Younger Americans Benefited Less from Booster Shots than Older People," *The New York Times*, February 4, 2022, sec. Health, https://www.nytimes.com/2022/02/04/health/covid-boosters-older-younger.html.
248 Mandavilli, "The C.D.C. Isn't Publishing Large Portions of the Covid Data It Collects."
249 TODAY, X (Twitter), September 12, 2023, https://twitter.com/TODAYshow/status/1701575004645638440?s=20.
250 Vinay Prasad, "Ashish Jha Has Gone Too Far with False Statements," *Vinay Prasad's Observations and Thoughts* (blog), September 14, 2023, https://www.drvinayprasad.com/p/ashish-jha-has-gone-too-far-with.
251 Ola Andersson et al., "Anticipation of COVID-19 Vaccines Reduces Willingness to Socially Distance," *Journal of Health Economics* 80 (September 15, 2021): 102530, https://doi.org/10.1016/j.jhealeco.2021.102530.

252 CDC, "Long COVID Basics," U.S. Centers for Disease Control and Prevention, July 24, 2025, https://web.archive.org/web/20250724191910/https://www.cdc.gov/long-covid/about/index.html.
253 Elena Azzolini et al., "Association between BNT162b2 Vaccination and Long COVID after Infections Not Requiring Hospitalization in Health Care Workers," *JAMA* 328, no. 7 (July 1, 2022): 676–8, https://doi.org/10.1001/jama.2022.11691.
254 *September 12, 2023 ACIP Meeting—Evidence to Recommendations.*
255 Centers for Disease Control and Prevention (CDC), "September 12, 2023 ACIP Meeting—Public Comment & Vote," YouTube, September 18, 2023, at 09:26–10:47, https://www.youtube.com/watch?v=9btUOBz3XCs.
256 Katherine J. Wu, "The One Thing Everyone Should Know about Fall COVID Vaccines," *The Atlantic*, September 13, 2023, https://www.theatlantic.com/health/archive/2023/09/fall-covid-vaccine-update-cdc-recommendation/675304/.
257 MedPage Today, "Should Scientists Openly Debate Vaccine Policies?," YouTube, October 24, 2023, at 05:31–06:17, https://www.youtube.com/watch?v=Qe4DVSQdSvY.
258 CDC, "COVID-19 Vaccination Coverage and Intent for Vaccination, Adults 18 Years and Older, United States," COVIDVaxView, May 7, 2025, https://www.cdc.gov/covidvaxview/weekly-dashboard/adult-vaccination-coverage.html; CDC, "COVID-19 Vaccination Coverage and Intent for Vaccination, Children 6 Months through 17 Years, United States," COVIDVaxView, May 7, 2025, https://www.cdc.gov/covidvaxview/weekly-dashboard/child-coverage-vaccination.html.
259 Aria Bendix, "Covid Vaccines Will Likely Become Annual like Flu Shots, White House Officials Say," NBC News, September 6, 2022, https://www.nbcnews.com/health/health-news/covid-vaccines-likely-annual-like-flu-shots-rcna46456.
260 Paul Offit, "Does Everyone Need a Yearly Covid Booster?," *Beyond the Noise* (blog), September 18, 2023, https://pauloffit.substack.com/p/does-everyone-need-a-yearly-covid; Jiří Beran et al., "Prevention of Influenza during Mismatched Seasons in Older Adults with an MF59-Adjuvanted Quadrivalent Influenza Vaccine: A Randomised, Controlled, Multicentre, Phase 3 Efficacy Study," *The Lancet Infectious Diseases* 21, no. 7 (February 9, 2021): 1027–37, https://doi.org/10.1016/S1473-3099(20)30694-0.
261 Petra Zimmermann and Nigel Curtis, "Why Does the Severity of COVID-19 Differ with Age?," *Pediatric Infectious Disease Journal* 41, no. 2 (2022): e36–45, https://doi.org/10.1097/INF.0000000000003413.
262 Meredith Wadman, "Fever, Aches from Pfizer, Moderna Jabs Aren't Dangerous but May Be Intense for Some," Science, November 18, 2020, https://www.science.org/content/article/fever-aches-pfizer-moderna-jabs-aren-t-dangerous-may-be-intense-some.
263 FDA, "FDA Takes Action on Updated MRNA COVID-19 Vaccines to Better Protect against Currently Circulating Variants," US Food & Drug Administration, September 11, 2023, https://www.fda.gov/news-events/press-announcements/fda-takes-action-updated-mrna-covid-19-vaccines-better-protect-against-currently-circulating.
264 FDA, "Prescription Drug Advertising | Questions and Answers," US Food & Drug Administration, June 19, 2015, https://www.fda.gov/drugs/prescription-drug-advertising/prescription-drug-advertising-questions-and-answers#law_violation_how.
265 Constantino, "BA.5 Boosters Could Be Here in the next 3 Weeks, Says Dr. Jha."
266 *Review of the FY2022 Budget Blueprint for the Centers for Disease Control and Prevention: Hearing before the Subcommittee on Labor, Health and Human Services,*

*Education, and Related Agencies,* US Senate (2021), at 46:46–47:22, https://www.appropriations.senate.gov/hearings/review-of-the-fy2022-budget-blueprint-for-the-centers-for-disease_control-and-prevention.

267 Ben Hargreaves, "Pfizer and Moderna COVID-19 Sales Beat Expectations, but for How Long?," BioSpace, February 22, 2024, https://www.biospace.com/article/pfizer-and-moderna-covid-19-sales-beat-expectations-but-for-how-long-/.

268 Kates, Cox, and Michaud, "How Much Could COVID-19 Vaccines Cost the U.S. after Commercialization?"

269 Lydia Saad, "Retail, Pharmaceutical Industries Slip in Public Esteem," Gallup, September 13, 2023, https://news.gallup.com/poll/510641/retail-pharmaceutical-industries-slip-public-esteem.aspx.

270 Lunna Lopes et al., "KFF COVID-19 Vaccine Monitor: December 2022," KFF, December 16, 2022, https://www.kff.org/coronavirus-covid-19/poll-finding/kff-covid-19-vaccine-monitor-december-2022/.; Kirzinger et al., "KFF COVID-19 Vaccine Monitor September 2023."

271 Offit, *Tell Me When It's Over*, 232.

## 11 A Path Forward

1 Abramson, *Sickening*, 230.

2 Kapczynski and Morten, "The Big Data Regulator, Rebooted"; FDA, "Driving Biomedical Innovation: Initiatives to Improve Products for Patients."

3 Kapczynski and Morten, "The Big Data Regulator, Rebooted."

4 "An Act to Enact Title 5, United States Code, 'Government Organization and Employees,'" Pub. L. No. 89–554, US Code (1966), https://www.govinfo.gov/content/pkg/STATUTE-80/pdf/STATUTE-80-Pg378.pdf.

5 Chrysler Corporation v. Brown, 441 U.S. 281 (US Supreme Court 1979).

6 Ibid.

7 "Trade Secrets Act," 18 US Code § 1905, accessed April 23, 2024, https://www.law.cornell.edu/uscode/text/18/1905.

8 Food and Drug Administration Amendments Act of 2007.

9 Ibid.; Kapczynski and Morten, "The Big Data Regulator, Rebooted."

10 Lindsey Cowen et al., "Uniform Trade Secrets Act with 1985 Amendments," National Conference of Commissioners on Uniform State Laws, August 1985: 6, https://www.wipo.int/edocs/lexdocs/laws/en/us/us034en.pdf.

11 Kapczynski and Morten, "The Big Data Regulator, Rebooted."

12 Public Citizen Health Research Group v. Department of Health, Education & Welfare, 477 F. Supp. 595 (US District Court for the District of Columbia 1979).

13 Kapczynski and Morten, "The Big Data Regulator, Rebooted," 534.

14 Egilman et al., "Systematic Overview of Freedom of Information Act Requests to the Department of Health and Human Services from 2008 to 2017."

15 Kapczynski and Morten, "The Big Data Regulator, Rebooted."

16 EMA, "External Guidance on the Implementation of the European Medicines Agency Policy on the Publication of Clinical Data for Medicinal Products for Human Use."

17 Loper Bright Enterprises et al. v. Raimondo, Secretary of Commerce, et al., 603 U.S.

18 Katherine Keisler-Starkey and Lisa N. Bunch, "Health Insurance Coverage in the United States: 2023," United States Census Bureau, September 10, 2024, https://www.census.gov/library/publications/2024/demo/p60-284.html.
19 Sargent Jr., "The Office of Technology Assessment: History, Authorities, Issues, and Options."
20 Center for Drug Evaluation and Research, "Advancing Health through Innovation: New Drug Therapy Approvals 2024"; FDA, "2024 Device Approvals," US Food & Drug Administration, March 6, 2025, https://www.fda.gov/medical-devices/recently-approved-devices/2024-device-approvals.
21 Bethany Withycombe et al., "Timing of Pivotal Clinical Trial Results Reporting for Newly Approved Medications Varied by Reporting Source," *Journal of Clinical Epidemiology* 77 (September 2016): 78–83, https://doi.org/10.1016/j.jclinepi.2016.04.007.
22 "The National Guideline Clearinghouse Extent Adherence to Trustworthy Standards (NEATS) Assessments."
23 Committee on Standards for Developing Trustworthy Clinical Practice Guidelines, Board on Health Care Services, and Institute of Medicine, *Clinical Practice Guidelines We Can Trust.*
24 Kung, Miller, and Mackowiak, "Failure of Clinical Practice Guidelines to Meet Institute of Medicine Standards."
25 Scutti, "Government Shuts down Website for Doctors."
26 "What Epidemiologists Do," US Bureau of Labor Statistics, April 17, 2024, https://www.bls.gov/ooh/life-physical-and-social-science/epidemiologists.htm.
27 FDA, "Good Clinical Practice," US Food & Drug Administration, December 11, 2019, https://www.fda.gov/about-fda/center-drug-evaluation-and-research-cder/good-clinical-practice.
28 Wallach et al., "Associations between Surrogate Markers and Clinical Outcomes for Nononcologic Chronic Disease Treatments."
29 Chen, Haslam, and Prasad, "FDA Acceptance of Surrogate End Points for Cancer Drug Approval."
30 Darrow, Avorn, and Kesselheim, "FDA Regulation and Approval of Medical Devices"; Committee on the Public Health Effectiveness of the FDA 510(k) Clearance Process, Board on Population Health and Public Health Practice, and Institute of Medicine, *Medical Devices and the Public's Health.*
31 Committee on the Public Health Effectiveness of the FDA 510(k) Clearance Process, Board on Population Health and Public Health Practice, and Institute of Medicine, *Medical Devices and the Public's Health*, 9.
32 Horton, "Vioxx, the Implosion of Merck, and Aftershocks at the FDA," 1995.
33 Gøtzsche, *Deadly Medicines and Organised Crime*, 270.
34 FDA, "FDA at a Glance October 2024."
35 Drummond Rennie, "When Evidence Isn't: Trials, Drug Companies and the FDA," *Journal of Law and Policy* 15, no. 3 (2008): 1009, https://brooklynworks.brooklaw.edu/jlp/vol15/iss3/18.
36 FDA, "FDA at a Glance October 2024."
37 "How Much Has the U.S. Government Spent This Year?," FiscalData, accessed June 14, 2024, https://fiscaldata.treasury.gov/americas-finance-guide/federal-spending/; "How Much Revenue Has the U.S. Government Collected This Year?," FiscalData, accessed June 14, 2024, https://fiscaldata.treasury.gov/americas-finance-guide/government-revenue/.

38 "18 USC 207: Restrictions on Former Officers, Employees, and Elected Officials of the Executive and Legislative Branches."
39 "Post-employment Restrictions," House Committee on Ethics, accessed June 14, 2024, https://ethics.house.gov/outside-employment-income/post-employment-restrictions.
40 Wood and Mador, "Uncapping Conflict of Interest?"
41 Feder, "POGO Letter Urges FDA Not to Weaken Conflict of Interest Standards at Center for Drug Evaluation and Research"; Darren E. Zinner et al., "Participation of Academic Scientists in Relationships with Industry"; Mendelson et al., "Conflicts of Interest in Cardiovascular Clinical Practice Guidelines
42 Graham et al., "Risk of Acute Myocardial Infarction"; Graham, "Testimony of David J. Graham, MD, MPH"; The Associated Press, "10 on FDA Vioxx Panel Had Ties to Companies."
43 Morning Consult, "Clean Water Act," Walton Family Foundation, November 2023, https://static.waltonfamilyfoundation.org/5e/2b/780176044698ae7535c6941c9 0b2/2310214-wff-clean-water-act-national-deck-2.pdf.
44 Spielmans and Parry, "From Evidence-Based Medicine to Marketing-Based Medicine."
45 Baker, *Rigged*, 106.
46 "Generic vs. Brand Name and the Cost of Bad News," John Hopkins Carey Business School, March 27, 2023, https://carey.jhu.edu/articles/generic-brand-medication-cost.
47 "Syprine Prices, Coupons, Copay & Patient Assistance Programs," Drugs.com, accessed June 2, 2025, https://www.drugs.com/price-guide/syprine.
48 "Trientine HCl (Generic for Syprine)," Mark Cuban Cost Plus Drug Company, accessed June 2, 2025, https://costplusdrugs.com/medications/trientine-hcl-250mg-capsule/.
49 Mulcahy, Schwam, and Lovejoy, "International Prescription Drug Price Comparisons."
50 "Overpatented, Overpriced Special Edition: Humira"; Committee on Oversight and Reform, "Drug Pricing Investigation: Majority Staff Report."
51 Rebecca Robbins, "How a Drug Company Made $114 Billion by Gaming the U.S. Patent System," *The New York Times*, January 28, 2023, sec. Business, https://www.nytimes.com/2023/01/28/business/humira-abbvie-monopoly.html.
52 Tulum and Lazonick, "Setting Pharmaceutical Drug Prices: What the Medicare Negotiators Need to Know About Innovation and Financialization."
53 Abramson, *Sickening*, chap. 1; Graham et al., "Risk of Acute Myocardial Infarction"; Graham, "Testimony of David J. Graham, MD, MPH."
54 Edward M. Scolnick to Deborah R. Shapiro, Alise S. Reicin, and Alan S. Nies, "Vigor," March 9, 2000, https://www.industrydocuments.ucsf.edu/drug/docs/#id=jsww0217.
55 Denis G. Arnold, Oscar Jerome Stewart, and Tammy Beck, "Financial Penalties Imposed on Large Pharmaceutical Firms for Illegal Activities," *JAMA* 324, no. 19 (November 17, 2020): 1995–7, https://doi.org/10.1001/jama.2020.18740.
56 Common Cause, "The Medicare/Prescription Drug Bill: A Study in How Government Shouldn't Work."
57 Sarnak et al., "Paying for Prescription Drugs Around the World."
58 Stuckey, "Tauzin Aided Drug Firms, Then They Hired Him"; Wayne and Armstrong, "Tauzin's $11.6 Million Made Him Highest-Paid Health-Law Lobbyist."
59 Philip Steven and Stephen Ezell, "Delinkage Debunked: Why Replacing Patents with Prizes for Drug Development Won't Work," Information Technology and Innovation Foundation, February 3, 2020, https://itif.org/publications/2020/02/03/delinkage-debunked-why-replacing-patents-prizes-drug-development-wont-work/.

60 Jill Lepore, These Truths: A History of the United States, First edition (New York: W. W. Norton & Company, 2018), 736.
61 Robbins, "How a Drug Company Made $114 Billion by Gaming the U.S. Patent System"; "Overpatented, Overpriced Special Edition: Humira"; Committee on Oversight and Reform, "Drug Pricing Investigation: Majority Staff Report," 80, 90, 118.
62 Tulum and Lazonick, "Setting Pharmaceutical Drug Prices: What the Medicare Negotiators Need to Know About Innovation and Financialization."
63 Osipenko et al., "Provenance and Clinical Benefit of Medicines Introduced to the French Market, 2008 to 2018"; Wieseler, McGauran, and Kaiser, "New Drugs"; Egilman, Rome, and Kesselheim, "Added Therapeutic Benefit."
64 Committee on the Public Health Effectiveness of the FDA 510(k) Clearance Process, Board on Population Health and Public Health Practice, and Institute of Medicine, *Medical Devices and the Public's Health*.
65 Steele et al., "Estimated Number of COVID-19 Infections, Hospitalizations, and Deaths Prevented Among Vaccinated Persons in the US, December 2020 to September 2021"; Agrawal, Sood, and Whaley, "The Impact of the Global COVID-19 Vaccination Campaign on All-Cause Mortality"; Ioannidis et al., "Global Estimates of Lives and Life-Years Saved by COVID-19 Vaccination During 2020-2024"; Watson et al., "Global Impact of the First Year of COVID-19 Vaccination."
66 Policy Cures Research and Global Health Technologies Coalition, "Doing Well by Doing Good," March 14, 2024, https://www.ghtcoalition.org/documents/pdf/Doing-Well-by-Doing-Good.pdf.
67 "U.S. Investments in Medical and Health Research and Development: 2016–2020."
68 Office of Science & Data Policy, "Trends in Prescription Drug Spending, 2016–2021."
69 FDA, "Generic Drugs: Questions & Answers."
70 Mulcahy, Schwam, and Lovejoy, "International Prescription Drug Price Comparisons."
71 "Pharma's Rx for R&D," McKinsey & Company, February 11, 2025, https://www.mckinsey.com/featured-insights/sustainable-inclusive-growth/charts/pharmas-rx-for-r-and-d.
72 Sam Hughes and Nicole Rapfogel, "Following the Money: Untangling U.S. Prescription Drug Financing," Center for American Progress, October 12, 2023, https://www.americanprogress.org/article/following-the-money-untangling-u-s-prescription-drug-financing/.
73 John Cornyn, "Affordable Prescriptions for Patients Act," S.1041 (2025), https://www.congress.gov/bill/119th-congress/senate-bill/1041; Richard Durbin, "Interagency Patent Coordination and Improvement Act of 2025," S.1097 (2025), https://www.congress.gov/bill/119th-congress/senate-bill/1097; "Limiting Evergreening for Name-Brand Prescription Drugs," Committee for a Responsible Federal Budget, July 26, 2021, https://www.crfb.org/papers/limiting-evergreening-name-brand-prescription-drugs.
74 Brooke Singman, "CDC Director Rochelle Walensky Explains What You Need to Know about COVID Vaccines, Boosters and More," Fox News, November 10, 2021, https://www.foxnews.com/health/cdc-director-rochelle-walensky-what-you-need-to-know-about-covid-vaccines-boosters.
75 "Hearing Wrap Up: Dr. Fauci Held Publicly Accountable by Select Subcommittee," United States House Committee on Oversight and Accountability, June 4, 2024, https://oversight.house.gov/release/hearing-wrap-up-dr-fauci-held-publicly-accountable-by-select-subcommittee/.

76 "42 U.S. Code § 247d—Public Health Emergencies," Legal Information Institute, accessed June 15, 2024, https://www.law.cornell.edu/uscode/text/42/247d.
77 "21 U.S. Code § 360bbb-3—Authorization for Medical Products for Use in Emergencies."
78 Steele et al., "Estimated Number of COVID-19 Infections, Hospitalizations, and Deaths Prevented Among Vaccinated Persons in the US, December 2020 to September 2021"; Agrawal, Sood, and Whaley, "The Impact of the Global COVID-19 Vaccination Campaign on All-Cause Mortality."
79 Stein et al., "Past SARS-CoV-2 Infection Protection against Re-infection."
80 Sharon Batt, Judy Butler, and Adriane Fugh-Berman, "What Needs to Change at the FDA?: Protecting and Advancing Public Health," PharmedOut, March 2024: 51, https://georgetown.app.box.com/s/n87us836fpmdhtcvdaqopyobfwx7bymx.
81 Kaiser, "Final NIH Budget for 2024 Is Essentially Flat"; "Budget."
82 "42 U.S. Code § 247d—Public Health Emergencies."

# Conclusion

1 Anna Fleck, "More than Half of Americans Take Prescribed Meds Daily," Statista, November 6, 2023, https://www.statista.com/chart/31183/us-respondents-who-aretaking-prescribed-medicine; Kirzinger et al., "Public Opinion on Prescription Drugs and Their Prices"; "Prescription Drugs," Health Policy Institute (blog), accessed June 14, 2024, https://web.archive.org/web/20240629012748/https://www.hpi.georgetown.edu/rxdrugs/; "Total Population by Child and Adult Populations," Kids Count Data Center, July 2024, https://datacenter.aecf.org/data/tables/99-total-population-by-child-and-adult-populations.
2 Fleck, "Infographic"; Kirzinger et al., "Public Opinion on Prescription Drugs and Their Prices."
3 "Implantable Material and Device Regulation," *AMA Journal of Ethics* 23, no. 9 (September 2021): E667–756, https://journalofethics.ama-assn.org/issue/implantable-material-and-device-regulation; "New 2024 Population Estimates Show Nation's Population Grew by about 1% to 340.1 Million since 2023," United States Census Bureau, December 19, 2024, https://www.census.gov/library/stories/2024/12/population-estimates.html.
4 "Implantable Material and Device Regulation."
5 Susan Perry, "The Medicalization of America: How It's Making Most of Us 'Sick,'" *MinnPost*, May 23, 2016, http://www.minnpost.com/second-opinion/2016/05/medicalization-america-how-its-making-most-us-sick/; John Fauber and Kristina Fiore, "New and Expanded Medical Definitions Create More Patients—and a Lucrative Market for Drug Firms," *Milwaukee Journal Sentinel*, May 22, 2016, https://web.archive.org/web/20160616073529/https://www.jsonline.com/watchdog/watchdogreports/new-and-expanded-medical-definitions-create-more-patients--and-a-lucrative-market-for-drug-firms--379981751.html/.
6 Lisa Cosgrove and Sheldon Krimsky, "A Comparison of DSM-IV and DSM-5 Panel Members' Financial Associations with Industry: A Pernicious Problem Persists," *PLoS Medicine* 9, no. 3 (March 13, 2012): e1001190, https://doi.org/10.1371/journal.pmed.1001190.

7 Byrne et al., "Evaluating the Association between Low-Density Lipoprotein Cholesterol Reduction and Relative and Absolute Effects of Statin Treatment."
8 Abramson, *Sickening*, 48–9; Unite Here!, "American Heart Association Fails to Disclose $100K in Pharma-Funded Research Led by Vice Chair of Cholesterol Guideline."
9 Rakshit and McGough, "How Does U.S. Life Expectancy Compare to Other Countries?"
10 "Heart Disease Facts," CDC, October 24, 2024, https://www.cdc.gov/heart-disease/data-research/facts-stats/index.html; Imani Telesford et al., "How Has the Burden of Chronic Diseases in the U.S. and Peer Nations Changed over Time?," Peterson-KFF Health System Tracker, April 16, 2025, https://www.healthsystemtracker.org/chart-collection/how-has-the-burden-of-chronic-diseases-in-the-u-s-and-peer-nations-changed-over-time/.
11 "Prescription Drug Prices in the U.S. Are 2.78 Times Those in Other Countries," RAND, February 1, 2024, https://www.rand.org/news/press/2024/02/01.html; Bob Herman, "Medical Devices Cost More in U.S. than in Similar Countries," Axios, October 5, 2018, https://www.axios.com/2018/10/05/medical-devices-cost-more-in-us-than-in-similar-countries; Gerard F. Anderson et al., "It's Still The Prices, Stupid: Why The US Spends So Much On Health Care, And A Tribute To Uwe Reinhardt," *Health Affairs* 38, no. 1 (2019): 87–95, https://doi.org/10.1377/hlthaff.2018.05144.
12 Lundh et al., "Industry Sponsorship and Research Outcome."
13 Gupta, Meenu, and Mohan, "The Tamiflu Fiasco and Lessons Learnt."
14 Jefferson et al., "Neuraminidase Inhibitors for Preventing and Treating Influenza in Adults and Children."
15 Balraj S. Heran et al., "Blood Pressure Lowering Efficacy of Angiotensin Converting Enzyme (ACE) Inhibitors for Primary Hypertension," *Cochrane Database of Systematic Reviews* 2008, no. 4 (October 8, 2008): Article CD003823, https://doi.org/10.1002/14651858.CD003823.pub2.
16 Schwartz et al., "ClinicalTrials.Gov and Drugs@FDA."
17 Greene, "Paramount Importance."
18 Kapczynski and Morten, "The Big Data Regulator, Rebooted."
19 Liu et al., "Payments by US Pharmaceutical and Medical Device Manufacturers to US Medical Journal Editors"; Haque et al., "Conflicts of Interest of Editors of Medical Journals"; Wong, Avalos, and Callaham, "Industry Payments to Physician Journal Editors."
20 Smith, "Medical Journals Are an Extension of the Marketing Arm of Pharmaceutical Companies."
21 Wager et al., "JAMA Published Fewer Industry-Funded Studies after Introducing a Requirement for Independent Statistical Analysis."
22 Schwartz and Woloshin, "Medical Marketing in the United States, 1997–2016."
23 DiStefano et al., "Association between Drug Characteristics and Manufacturer Spending on Direct-to-Consumer Advertising."
24 Committee on Standards for Developing Trustworthy Clinical Practice Guidelines, Board on Health Care Services, and Institute of Medicine, *Clinical Practice Guidelines We Can Trust.*
25 National Cholesterol Education Program (NCEP) Expert Panel on Detection, Evaluation, and Treatment of High Blood Cholesterol in Adults (Adult Treatment Panel III), "Third Report of the National Cholesterol Education Program (NCEP)

Expert Panel on Detection, Evaluation, and Treatment of High Blood Cholesterol in Adults (Adult Treatment Panel III) Final Report."
26 Abramson, *Sickening* 42.
27 PeterQ Eichacker and Charles Natanson, "Medical Guidelines and Performance Measures: The Need to Keep Them Free of Industry Influence," *Mens Sana Monographs* 6, no. 1 (2008): 22–8, https://pmc.ncbi.nlm.nih.gov/articles/PMC 3190551/; "Lilly Announces Withdrawal of Xigris® Following Recent Clinical Trial Results"; Prasad and Cifu, *Ending Medical Reversal*, 141.
28 Mooghali et al., "Financial Conflicts of Interest among US Physician Authors of 2020 Clinical Practice Guidelines."
29 See notes 61–62 in Chapter 5.
30 Darrow, Avorn, and Kesselheim, "FDA Regulation and Approval of Medical Devices."
31 Kadakia et al., "Renewing the Call for Reforms to Medical Device Safety—The Case of Penumbra."
32 Kadakia et al., "Use of Recalled Devices in New Device Authorizations under the US Food and Drug Administration's 510(k) Pathway and Risk of Subsequent Recalls."
33 See Figure 9.
34 Hacker and Hilzenrath, "Ten Doctors on FDA Panel Reviewing Abbott Heart Device Had Financial Ties with Company."
35 FDA, "FDA at a Glance October 2024."
36 von Eschenbach, "Toward a 21st-Century FDA."
37 Kane, "Medscape Physician Compensation Report 2023: 'Your Income vs Your Peers.'"
38 Osipenko et al., "Provenance and Clinical Benefit of Medicines Introduced to the French Market, 2008 to 2018"; Wieseler, McGauran, and Kaiser, "New Drugs"; Darrow, Avorn, and Kesselheim, "FDA Regulation and Approval of Medical Devices"; DiStefano et al., "Association between Drug Characteristics and Manufacturer Spending on Direct-to-Consumer Advertising."
39 "Overpatented, Overpriced Special Edition: Humira."
40 Feldman, "May Your Drug Price Be Evergreen."
41 FDA, "Generic Drugs: Questions & Answers."
42 Lalani et al., "US Public Investment in Development of MRNA COVID-19 Vaccines.
43 Mahobe, "Moderna Considers Pricing COVID Vaccine at $110-$130—WSJ"; Miltimore, "Understanding the 500% Price Increase of Pfizer's Covid Vaccine.
44 Pittman, "Public Health and Medical Professionals for Transparency v. Food and Drug Administration, No. 4:21-Cv-1058-P: Document 35."
45 Offit, *Tell Me When It's Over*, 142–53, 231–3.
46 *CDC Director Walensky: "You Need to Get Your Fall Booster Vaccine."*
47 Prasad and Haslam, "COVID-19 Vaccines."
48 Gutentag, "Drug Companies Test New Booster on Eight Mice and Zero Humans, FDA Approves It Anyway."
49 TODAY, X (Twitter), September 12, 2023, https://twitter.com/TODAYshow/sta tus/1701575004645638440?s=20.
50 Offit, *Tell Me When It's Over*, 137–41.
51 Brown et al., "Outbreak of SARS-CoV-2 Infections, Including COVID-19 Vaccine Breakthrough Infections, Associated with Large Public Gatherings—Barnstable County, Massachusetts, July 2021."
52 Bardosh et al., "COVID-19 Vaccine Boosters for Young Adults."

53 D'Angelo Gore, "Scientist Misleads on COVID-19 Vaccine Effectiveness and Vaccine Safety for Children," FactCheck.org, February 1, 2022, https://www.factcheck.org/2022/02/scicheck-scientist-misleads-on-covid-19-vaccine-effectiveness-and-vaccine-safety-for-children/.
54 House Select Subcommittee on the Coronavirus Pandemic, Investigating the Origins of COVID-19.
55 Moses et al., "The Anatomy of Medical Research."
56 Magnan, "Social Determinants of Health 101 for Health Care: Five Plus Five."
57 "Less Is More," *Archives of Internal Medicine* 170, no. 7 (April 12, 2010): 584, https://doi.org/10.1001/archinternmed.2010.48.

## Afterword: A New Regime

1 US Department of Health and Human Services, "Secretary Kennedy Delivers Welcoming Remarks to HHS Staff," YouTube, February 18, 2025, 10:10–10:39, https://www.youtube.com/watch?v=o-BCMG198Yc.
2 Joseph A. Wulfsohn, "CNN Anchor Calls RFK Jr. Endorsing Trump 'Huge' Based on Swing State Polls: 'It Is Everything,'" Fox News, August 24, 2024, https://www.foxnews.com/media/cnn-anchor-calls-rfk-jr-endorsing-trump-huge-based-swing-state-polls-it-everything.
3 Jonathan J. Cooper, "Robert F. Kennedy Jr. Becomes a Frequent Campaigner for Donald Trump," AP, September 16, 2024, https://apnews.com/article/donald-trump-rfk-jr-tulsi-gabbard-821f0edcb154ebcc023c834aacc249a8.
4 Donald J. Trump, "Statement by President-Elect Donald J. Trump Announcing the Nomination of Robert F. Kennedy Jr. as Secretary of Health and Human Services (HHS)," The American Presidency Project, November 14, 2024, https://www.presidency.ucsb.edu/documents/statement-president-elect-donald-j-trump-announcing-the-nomination-robert-f-kennedy-jr.
5 US Department of Health and Human Services, "Secretary Kennedy Delivers Welcoming Remarks to HHS Staff."
6 Donald J. Trump, "Executive Order 14210: Implementing the President's 'Department of Government Efficiency' Workforce Optimization Initiative," Federal Register, February 11, 2025, https://www.federalregister.gov/documents/2025/02/14/2025-02762/implementing-the-presidents-department-of-government-efficiency-workforce-optimization-initiative.
7 Russell T. Vought and Charles Ezell to Heads of Executive Departments and Agencies, "Guidance on Agency RIF and Reorganization Plans Requested by Implementing The President's 'Department of Government' Workforce Optimization Initiative," February 26, 2025, 2, https://www.opm.gov/policy-data-oversight/latest-memos/guidance-on-agency-rif-and-reorganization-plans-requested-by-implementing-the-president-s-department-of-government-efficiency-workforce-optimization-initiative.pdf.
8 Mike Stobbe and Carla K. Johnson, "HHS Is Losing Thousands of Workers under Trump Administration Probationary Job Cuts," AP, February 14, 2025, https://apnews.com/article/trump-job-cuts-health-cdc-0d002fd6f528a7b91ced79628bf68196; Patrick Wingrove and Dan Levine, "Exclusive: US Health Agency Says Employees Can Apply for Early Retirement," *Reuters*, March 4, 2025, https://www.reuters.com/busin

ess/healthcare-pharmaceuticals/us-health-agency-now-says-employees-must-respond-doge-email-2025-03-03/; Noah Tong, "HHS Employees Offered $25K Voluntary Buyout Offer—but Not All FDA Workers," Fierce Healthcare, March 10, 2025, https://www.fiercehealthcare.com/regulatory/hhs-directed-fire-more-employees-submit-agency-reorganization-plans.

9 HHS, "HHS Announces Transformation to Make America Healthy Again," US Department of Health and Human Services, March 27, 2025, https://www.hhs.gov/press-room/hhs-restructuring-doge.html.

10 Ashleigh Fields, "RFK Jr. Defends HHS Job Cuts: 'We're Not Cutting Front-Line Workers,'" *The Hill*, March 28, 2025, https://thehill.com/policy/healthcare/5219280-robert-f-kennedy-jr-hhs-job-cuts/.

11 Christina Jewett and Benjamin Mueller, "H.H.S. Finalizes Thousands of Layoffs after Supreme Court Decision," *The New York Times*, July 15, 2025, https://www.nytimes.com/2025/07/15/us/politics/hhs-layoffs.html; Melissa R. DuBose, "State of New York v. Kennedy, No. 1:25-Cv-00196: Document 73," United States District Court for the District of Rhode Island, July 1, 2025, https://ag.ny.gov/sites/default/files/court-filings/state-of-new-york-et-al-v-robert-f-kennedy-jr-et-al-complaint-2025.pdf.

12 HHS, "Fiscal Year 2026: Budget in Brief," US Department of Health and Human Services, May 2025, https://www.hhs.gov/sites/default/files/fy-2026-budget-in-brief.pdf.

13 Alexander Tin, "RFK Jr. Says 20% of Health Agency Layoffs Could Be Mistakes," CBS News, April 3, 2025, https://www.cbsnews.com/news/rfk-jr-hhs-job-cuts-doge-mistakes/.

14 Rachel Treisman, "After Mass Layoffs, Some Federal Agencies Are Trying to Bring Employees Back," NPR, February 21, 2025, https://www.npr.org/2025/02/21/nx-s1-5304152/federal-government-layoffs-reversed.

15 Hannah Natanson et al., "Trump Administration Races to Fix a Big Mistake: DOGE Fired Too Many People," *The Washington Post*, June 6, 2025, https://www.washingtonpost.com/business/2025/06/06/doge-staff-cuts-rehiring-federal-workers/.

16 Cheyenne Haslett and Youri Benadjaoud, "CDC Rehires 450 Employees Cut in HHS Restructuring, Internal Documents Show," ABC News, June 11, 2025, https://abcnews.go.com/Politics/cdc-rehires-450-employees-cut-hhs-restructuring-internal/story?id=122751330.

17 Culliton, "The Academic-Industrial Complex"; Institute of Medicine, *Funding Health Sciences Research*; Abramson, Sickening, 109–13.

18 Richard G. Frank and Sherry Glied, "The Trump Administration's NIH and FDA Cuts Will Negatively Impact Patients," Brookings, May 14, 2025, https://www.brookings.edu/articles/the-trump-administrations-nih-and-fda-cuts-will-negatively-impact-patients/.

19 Jocelyn Kaiser and Meredith Wadman, "Kennedy, Trump's Health Chief, Confronts Criticism and Praise from U.S. Lawmakers," Science, May 14, 2025, https://www.science.org/content/article/kennedy-trump-s-health-chief-confronts-criticism-and-praise-u-s-lawmakers.

20 Diabetes Prevention Program Research Group, "Reduction in the Incidence of Type 2 Diabetes with Lifestyle Intervention or Metformin."

21 Kyle Munz, "Trump Administration Cancels Crucial Funding for Diabetes Prevention Program," AJMC, March 18, 2025, https://www.ajmc.com/view/trump-administration-cancels-crucial-funding-for-diabetes-prevention-program.

22 Govexec Staff, "RIF Watch: See Which Agencies Are Laying off Federal Workers," *Government Executive*, May 15, 2025, https://www.govexec.com/workforce/2025/02/rif-watch-see-which-agencies-are-laying-federal-workers/403342/.
23 Ben Johansen, "Kennedy Shutters Several FOIA Offices at HHS," *Politico*, April 3, 2025, https://www.politico.com/news/2025/04/03/kennedy-shutters-several-foia-offices-at-hhs-00268646.
24 Rachana Pradhan, "In Reversal, FDA Rehires Staff Tasked with Releasing Public Records," KFF Health News, May 2, 2025, https://kffhealthnews.org/news/article/fda-rehires-foia-staff-public-records-requests-layoffs-trump-hhs/.
25 LiveNOW from FOX, "FULL EVENT: RFK Jr. Announces Food Dye and Artificial Additive Bans," YouTube, April 22, 2025, at 1:09:15, 1:08:58–1:10:18, https://www.youtube.com/watch?v=qBgW5n5YU14.
26 C-SPAN, "Robert F. Kennedy, Jr. Senate Confirmation Hearing to Be Secretary of Health & Human Services," YouTube, January 29, 2025, at 3:09:26, 3:09:10–3:09:35, https://www.youtube.com/watch?v=NeeC7nGm6cI.
27 Martin A. Makary and Vinay Prasad, "Priorities for a New FDA," *JAMA* 334, no. 7 (June 10, 2025): 565–6, https://doi.org/10.1001/jama.2025.10116.
28 FDA, "FDA News Release: FDA to Issue New Commissioner's National Priority Vouchers to Companies Supporting U.S. National Interests," U.S. Food and Drug Administration, June 17, 2025, https://www.fda.gov/news-events/press-announcements/fda-issue-new-commissioners-national-priority-vouchers-companies-supporting-us-national-interests.
29 US Food and Drug Administration, "FDA Roundtable on Cell and Gene Therapy," YouTube, June 5, 2025, https://www.youtube.com/watch?v=0qDhRtnHXdU&t=288s.
30 FDA, "FDA Announces Completion of First AI-Assisted Scientific Review Pilot and Aggressive Agency-Wide AI Rollout Timeline," US Food & Drug Administration, May 8, 2025, https://www.fda.gov/news-events/press-announcements/fda-announces-completion-first-ai-assisted-scientific-review-pilot-and-aggressive-agency-wide-ai.
31 FDA, "FDA Launches Agency-Wide AI Tool to Optimize Performance for the American People," US Food & Drug Administration, June 2, 2025, https://www.fda.gov/news-events/press-announcements/fda-launches-agency-wide-ai-tool-optimize-performance-american-people.
32 Berkeley Lovelace Jr., "FDA's AI Tool for Medical Devices Struggles with Simple Tasks," NBC News, June 3, 2025, https://www.nbcnews.com/health/health-news/fdas-ai-tool-medical-devices-struggles-simple-tasks-rcna210340.
33 "When AI Gets It Wrong: Addressing AI Hallucinations and Bias," MIT Sloan Teaching & Learning Technologies, accessed June 8, 2025, https://mitsloanedtech.mit.edu/ai/basics/addressing-ai-hallucinations-and-bias/.
34 Sarah Owermohle, "FDA's Artificial Intelligence Is Supposed to Revolutionize Drug Approvals. It's Making up Nonexistent Studies," CNN, July 23, 2025, https://www.cnn.com/2025/07/23/politics/fda-ai-elsa-drug-regulation-makary; Make America Healthy Again Commission, "The MAHA Report," The White House, May 2025, https://www.whitehouse.gov/wp-content/uploads/2025/05/WH-The-MAHA-Report-Assessment.pdf.
35 Caitlin Gilbert et al., "The MAHA Report's AI Fingerprints, Annotated," *The Washington Post*, May 30, 2025, https://www.washingtonpost.com/health/2025/05/30/maha-report-ai-white-house/.

36 Emily Kennard and Margaret Manto, "The MAHA Report Cites Studies That Don't Exist," NOTUS, May 9, 2025, https://www.notus.org/health-science/make-america-healthy-again-report-citation-errors.
37 FDA, "FDA Announces Completion of First AI-Assisted Scientific Review Pilot and Aggressive Agency-Wide AI Rollout Timeline."
38 Vinay Prasad and Martin A. Makary, "An Evidence-Based Approach to Covid-19 Vaccination," *New England Journal of Medicine*, May 20, 2025, https://doi.org/10.1056/NEJMsb2506929.
39 Melissa Mendoza and David C. Kaslow to Kathleen Callahan, "Approval Letter—NUVAXOVID," May 16, 2025, https://www.fda.gov/media/186545/download; David C. Kaslow to Trung Ly, "Approval Letter—MNEXSPIKE," May 30, 2025, https://www.fda.gov/media/186740/download?attachment.
40 Secretary Kennedy, X (Twitter), May 27, 2025, https://x.com/seckennedy/status/1927368440811008138?s=46.
41 "COVID-19 Vaccine Advice and Recommendations," Australian Government: Department of Health, Disability and Ageing, November 20, 2024, https://www.health.gov.au/our-work/covid-19-vaccines/getting-your-vaccination; "COVID-19 Vaccinations," Österbottens Välfärdsområde Pohjanmaan Hyvinvointialue, accessed June 27, 2025, https://en.osterbottensvalfard.fi/our-services/health-centre-and-hospital-services/health-centre-services/vaccinations/covid-19-vaccinations/#recommended-basic-series-of-the-coronavirus-vaccine; Prasad and Makary, "An Evidence-Based Approach to Covid-19 Vaccination."
42 CDC, "Child Immunization Schedule Notes," CDC: Vaccines & Immunizations, May 29, 2025, https://www.cdc.gov/vaccines/hcp/imz-schedules/child-adolescent-notes.html.
43 Face the Nation, "FDA Commissioner Marty Makary Discusses COVID Vaccine Recommendations," YouTube, June 1, 2025, https://www.youtube.com/watch?v=WGH23FhqZxY.
44 Ibid., at 05:00–06:14.
45 HHS, "HHS Takes Bold Step to Restore Public Trust in Vaccines by Reconstituting ACIP," US Department of Health and Human Services, June 9, 2025, https://www.hhs.gov/press-room/hhs-restore-public-trust-vaccines-acip.html#:~:text=Washington%2C%20DC%E2%80%94JUNE%209%2C,and%20clinical%20need%20of%20vaccines.
46 Mike Stobbe, "Kennedy's New CDC Panel Includes Members Who Have Criticized Vaccines and Spread Misinformation," AP News, June 12, 2025, https://apnews.com/article/cdc-acip-vaccine-committee-9f58e1f004075b081718ff078de88d76.
47 US Food and Drug Administration, "FDA Direct Ep. 7: This Week at the FDA!," YouTube, June 6, 2025, at 08:15–09:16, https://www.youtube.com/watch?v=96aXvMKCN9o&list=PLey4Qe-UxcxbGI04rUjdaGyNhNnuP5cBO&index=1.
48 Makary and Prasad, "Priorities for a New FDA."
49 FDA, "CEO Forums: An FDA Listening Tour to Engage Pharmaceutical and Biotech CEOs," U.S. Food & Drug Administration, July 28, 2025, https://web.archive.org/web/20250803111641/https://www.fda.gov/industry/ceo-forums-fda-listening-tour-engage-pharmaceutical-and-biotech-ceos.
50 FDA, "FDA Commissioner Makary Announces New Policy on Individuals Serving on FDA Advisory Committees."
51 FDA, "Advisory Committee Industry Representatives," US Food & Drug Administration, accessed January 17, 2009, https://web.archive.org/web/2009011

7094245/https://www.fda.gov/oc/advisory/industry.html; Colleen Davis, "Red Tape Tightrope: Regulating Financial Conflicts of Interest in FDA Advisory Committees," *Washington University Law Review* 91, no. 6 (2014), 1594, https://openscholarship.wustl.edu/law_lawreview/vol91/iss6/8.

52 Food and Drug Administration Safety and Innovation Act.

53 Phil Taylor, "Makary, Prasad Set out Their Vision for the FDA," Pharmaphorum, June 11, 2025, https://pharmaphorum.com/news/makary-prasad-set-out-their-vision-fda.

54 Makary and Prasad, "Priorities for a New FDA."

55 The Associated Press, "10 on FDA Vioxx Panel Had Ties to Companies"; Graham et al., "Risk of Acute Myocardial Infarction"; Graham, "Testimony of David J. Graham, MD, MPH."

56 "18 USC 207: Restrictions on Former Officers, Employees, and Elected Officials of the Executive and Legislative Branches."

57 Laurenza, Gross, and Paulsen, "Ethics Changes for Trump Administration Appointees."

58 Harrow Health, Inc., "Harrow Health Announces Appointments to Its Board of Directors," Harrow, March 31, 2022, https://harrowinc.gcs-web.com/newsreleases/news-release-details/harrow-health-announces-appointments-its-boarddirectors; Amy Baxter, "With Conflicts of Interest in Focus, Trump's Pick to Run FDA Could Face Scrutiny of His Own Industry Ties," BioPharma Dive, December 6, 2024, https://www.pharmavoice.com/news/makary-fda-commissioner-hearings-conflicts-of-interest/734535/.

59 Christina Jewett, "He Fought Claims of Harm from Infant Formula. Now He Regulates It," *The New York Times*, March 4, 2025, https://www.nytimes.com/2025/03/04/health/fda-infant-formula-kyle-diamantas.html.

60 "Robert Fox Foster," LinkedIn, accessed June 8, 2025, https://www.linkedin.com/in/robert-fox-foster-a0aa2145/?locale=es_ES.

61 Robert F. Kennedy Jr., "Trump Can Make America Healthy Again," *The Wall Street Journal*, September 5, 2024, https://www.wsj.com/opinion/trump-can-make-america-healthy-again-rfk-jr-reforms-chronic-disease-crisis-a9b4b8c0.

62 Fraiser Kansteiner, "RFK Jr.'s FDA Staff Cuts Claimed Key User Fee Negotiators, Threatening Renewal Talks with Pharma: Reuters," Fierce Pharma, April 18, 2025, https://www.fiercepharma.com/pharma/kennedys-fda-staff-cuts-claimed-key-user-fee-negotiators-threatening-reauthorization-talks.

63 HHS, "Fiscal Year 2026: Budget in Brief"; FDA, "FDA at a Glance October 2024."

64 Ultimate Human Podcast with Gary Brecka, "Robert F. Kennedy Jr.: How to Fix America's Health Crisis as HHS Secretary | TUH #169," YouTube, May 27, 2025, at 31:31, https://www.youtube.com/watch?v=sODZSAuxTTw.

65 Ibid., at 32:01–32:36.

66 Committee on Standards for Developing Trustworthy Clinical Practice Guidelines, Board on Health Care Services, and Institute of Medicine, *Clinical Practice Guidelines We Can Trust.*

67 Make America Healthy Again Commission, "The MAHA Report," 18–19.

68 Ibid., 72.

69 Dua Hassan, "RFK Jr.'s Report Actually Nails What's Wrong with American Health," *Slate*, June 5, 2025, https://slate.com/technology/2025/06/rfk-jr-maha-report-kids-health-chronic-illness-medication.html.

70 "Health Provisions in the 2025 Federal Budget Reconciliation Bill," KFF, May 22, 2025, https://www.kff.org/tracking-the-medicaid-provisions-in-the-2025-budget-bill/.

# Index

www.ingramcontent.com/pod-product-compliance
Ingram Content Group UK Ltd.
Pitfield, Milton Keynes, MK11 3LW, UK
UKHW022101241026
476999UK00001B/21

9 798216 373636